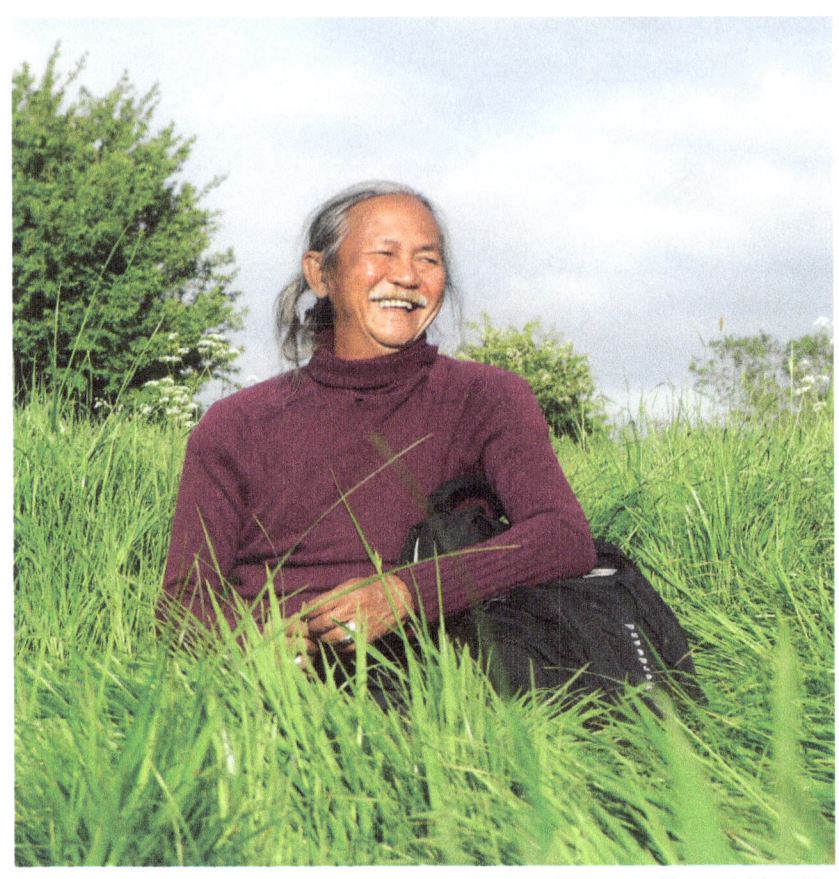

Avebury, UK, 2009. Photo: Keith Miller

"Decades ago, I tried to explore sound becoming voice, becoming words, and becoming sentences. In the beginning, it was just sounds. As time passed, the sounds became an expression. Then, from that expression, I really felt a desire to communicate, to convey something, to create words... Within that process there was an awareness of myself as a word; my presence can create words and arrange words."

EMBODIED LIVES

Reflections on the Influence of
Suprapto Suryodarmo and Amerta Movement

Edited by:
Katya Bloom, Margit Galanter and Sandra Reeve

Published in this first edition in 2014 by:

Triarchy Press
Station Offices
Axminster
Devon
EX13 5PF
England

+44 (0)1297 631456

info@triarchypress.net

www.triarchypress.net

This complete edition copyright © Triarchy Press, 2014

Each chapter, including any images in it, remains copyright © 2014 of the named author of that chapter unless otherwise stated.

The author of each chapter asserts his or her moral right under the Copyright, Designs and Patents Act 1988 to be so identified.

All rights reserved.

No part of this publication may be reproduced, stored in a retrieval system or transmitted in any form or by any means including photocopying, electronic, mechanical, recording or otherwise, without the prior written permission of the publisher.

A catalogue record for this book is available from the British Library.

Cover illustrations by Maxine Yalovitz-Blankenship.

Paperback ISBN: 978-1-909470-32-3

Body-Mind Centering, Feldenkrais Method, HANDLE, Move into Life, Social Dreaming and Somatic Experiencing are registered trade or service marks.

A Balinese Saying

Ilmu Padi (a lesson from the rice plant)

semakin tua semakin berisi, dan semakin merunduk
(the older, the fuller, and the more it bows)

Publisher's Note

Embodied Lives has been set in Bell (the serif font used here and for the bulk of the book) and Corbel (*the sans-serif font used for diary and journal entries, dream sequences and so on*). Bell is well over 200 years old and an early example of so-called Scotch Roman style – exactly the kind of thing that Hadrian's Wall was intended to prevent. Corbel is a relative whippersnapper and not yet ten years old.

In each chapter, we have tried to observe the author's preference for British or American English with respect to grammar, spelling and punctuation. However, to make it easier for readers to move from chapter to chapter, we have standardised some other elements. For example:

- Prapto's words, where they are quoted at length appear in italic font, surrounded by double inverted commas, "*thus*".

- Other people's speech or text, when quoted directly, appear in double inverted commas, "thus".

- Each author's own movement or performance practice (if it is mentioned) appears in single inverted commas, 'thus'.

- Performance titles, like book and workshop titles, as well as many non-English words, terms used by Prapto and terms that the author wants to emphasise, appear in italics, *thus*.

- URLs, for ease of reference, appear in condensed format, thus: http://bit.ly/ELtp02
Most browsers allow you to leave off the http:// prefix when entering a bit.ly URL.

CONTENTS

ACKNOWLEDGEMENTS   xii

INTRODUCTION   1

1. PRESENCE   9
   Beate Stühm (Germany)

2. AMERTA MOVEMENT AND ARCHAEOLOGY   19
   Keith Miller (UK)

3. CULTURAL ASPECTS OF THE MOVEMENT WORK   29
   Christina Stelzer (Germany)

4. AMERTA AND TIBETAN BUDDHISM   37
   Monika Förster (Germany/Holland)

5. THE EYE OF THE HAND   45
   Steve Hopkins (UK)

6. A DOG PRACTICING 'TALKING BODY'   57
   José Mulder van de Graaf (Bolivia)

7. "MAKE LESS THE HOPING"   67
   Sandra Reeve (UK)

8. TOUCHING FORGOTTEN REALITIES   75
   Bettina Mainz (Germany)

9. THE ECHO OF LIFE   87
   Daniela Coronelli (Italy/UK)

10. I ALWAYS DO THREE THINGS   97
    Shantam Zohar (Israel)

11. A PRESENCING DIAL   103
   Margit Galanter (USA)

12. AMERTA MOVEMENT AND SOMATIC COSTUME   113
   Sally E. Dean (USA/UK)

13. CRYSTALLIZATION-PERFORMANCE   127
   Lise Lavelle (Denmark)

14. BEING AND DOING IN THE WILD GARDEN   137
   Susanne Tümpel (Germany)

15. 'MANTRA GERAK'/MOVEMENT MANTRA   147
   Agus Bima Prayitna (Indonesia)

16. THE MUSICAL PORTAL   157
   Tim Jones (UK)

17. NEAR THE UNKNOWN   165
   Franca Fubini (Italy)

18. FAMILY   175
   Una Nicholson (UK)

19. THE INFANT'S LANGUAGE   185
   Katya Bloom (USA/UK)

20. "GOING OUT OF THE SITUATION" AND "STOP, DON'T FOLLOW THAT, WALK!"   195
   Regula Nell (Switzerland)

21. AMERTA MOVEMENT AND AUTISM   201
   Sean Williams (UK)

22. "FIND YOUR POSITION"   211
    Susan Bauer (USA)

23. "BODY BODY"   221
    Helen Poynor (UK)

24. EVER-SPEAKING BEING   231
    Michael Dick (Germany)

25. MOVING IN THE LAW   241
    Simon Slidders (UK)

26. THE BREATHING EYE   249
    Andrea Morein (Germany)

27. JOY   263
    Anita Lüdke (Germany/Bolivia)

28. "RE-MEMBERING" BUTTERFLY BEACH   277
    Melinda Buckwalter (USA)

29. I WILL TRACE THE CONSTELLATION OF MY STARS
    WITH MY FINGERS   285
    Ellin Krinsly (USA/Australia/Mexico/Ethiopia)

30. AWAKENING ART AND DHARMA NATURE TIME   295
    Diane Butler (USA/Indonesia)

AFTERWORD: A PRAPTO COMPANION   306

ACKNOWLEDGEMENTS

The seed of an idea for this book sprouted in late 2011, and has followed an organic process of growing into the garden of shared experience that is *Embodied Lives*. This would not have happened without the involvement of an excellent team, especially the astonishing, dynamic and creative working relationship with my two co-editors, Margit Galanter and Sandra Reeve. Though our meetings all took place in the virtual space of Skype and, to date, they have not met each other face to face, we have flourished by digging together in the same rich soil. I am reminded of the traditional Native-American planting of the 'three sisters', the so-called 'companion plants' of corn, beans and squash that thrive so well in each other's company.

We want to offer heartfelt thanks to all the contributors for their enthusiasm and hard work in offering us their thoughtful writing, and their patience and responsiveness to the editorial process.

Special thanks to Beth Ahlstrand, Harry Blumenthal, Marc Galanter and Hugh Kelly, who gave generously of time, support and feedback, and to Diane Butler for her essential help with translations from Indonesian to English. We also want to thank Maxine Yalovitz-Blankenship for graciously giving us permission to use her artwork on the cover.

Our publisher Andrew Carey, and Michelle Smith and the team at Triarchy Press were wonderfully supportive and skillful, with just the right measure of hands-on guidance, with humility and humor.

And of course our deep gratitude to Prapto, whose work has inspired so many original and unique responses. Finally, as Prapto would surely add, a deep bow of thanks to Life.

KB

INTRODUCTION

The Javanese movement artist and teacher, Suprapto Suryodarmo (Prapto), and his Amerta Movement practice have had widespread influence on people from many cultures and professional backgrounds.

The common denominator for all of us who have had the good fortune to work with Prapto is the exploration of our own movement as a way of deepening our connection to ourselves, to each other and, at the same time, to our world.

The idea for *Embodied Lives* grew out of a wish to bring together reflections from many of us for whom Prapto's work has been transformational in supporting our own lives and work. We were interested in weaving together threads of writing from many practitioners, in the belief that the resulting collection would reveal some of the many different ways in which Amerta Movement has lived, grown and been integrated into their lives. Our intention is to both honour Prapto for his enormously valuable contribution, and to show how Amerta Movement has been, and continues to be, developed and embodied. This collection celebrates some of the fruits of the harvest over many years.

The Practice

Amerta Movement may be seen as cultivating an embodied approach to life through the practice of movement as a skilled art. It seems to reach beyond 'movement meditation' or 'dance' into a movement world that is uniquely sensitizing and integrative.

Amerta Movement differs from most other traditional movement arts, like Tai chi or Yoga, or somatic practices, like the Feldenkrais Method or Alexander Technique, because Amerta has no set form, no pre-existing patterns, or series of movements. There is nothing to follow except one's own experience on all levels, but especially the sensory-motoric – our bodies, on the Earth, and responsive to gravity.

Practitioners interact with both environment and self, while also being in communication with the personalities and cultural heritage of fellow movers. A relationship with the past also comes alive as part of the present. Amerta Movement, thus provides a forum for cultural, artistic, atmospheric, and human interaction. This breadth of the practice affects the quality of experience in the movement itself, as well as perceptions of the world in which we live.

We receive our connection inward and outward simultaneously. From this we follow the moment-by-moment decisions of our beings in time and space, as we follow our intention to deepen our embodied awareness of the ever-changing here and now. Our bodies listen and speak, choose and allow, as we encounter the border between known and unknown. With an attitude of attentive play, we discover meaning.

For most of our lives, after early childhood, our movement settles into and replicates a limited vocabulary of patterns, in which we use our bodies as tools to carry out our wishes and needs. In Amerta Movement, we regain a sense of our bodies as responsive, sensing organisms, and our vocabulary develops from that very different starting place. When we allow our bodies to 'speak' or express from that place, with ordinary, daily life movements and their variations – such as lying, rolling, crawling, sitting, walking, jumping – what arises is an enlivening experience, which Prapto calls *blossoming*. Prapto's image for the common field of practice, when a group moves together, is that of a garden, where each being is a unique expression of life, and where the micro and the macro levels of one's experience can connect.

The nature of the practice is that we slow things down, relaxing both body and mind. With roots in Vipassana (mindfulness) meditation, daily life movement, non-stylized movement and a Javanese meditation form called Sumarah, the practice helps us to open our senses, to receive what is present and, crucially, to recognize that the present is always changing. The Buddhist principle of non-attachment is central to the Amerta practice, though we are more actively involved in witnessing what comes and goes than we would be in traditional meditation. In this way we discover different points of view, different ways of moving, listening and speaking with our bodies.

There are many movement themes which guide practitioners in this process of change in body/time/space, and support our own ability to move with clarity, comfort and a sense of safety. A wide variety of these are brought to life in a range of different contexts by the contributors to this book.

Prapto is skilled at creating an atmosphere of openness and dialogue, so that each participant can be seen and can recognize their own unique qualities. We have always been asked to interpret his work through our own experience, and to learn, not only from Prapto, but also from each other. He has insisted that he studies from each of us, as much as we study with him.

The stated aim is *sharing movement*. This approach has given value to each person, as it instils a sense of responsibility. This originates, in part, from giving value to the changing body in a changing environment. The emphasis on change means that even the practice itself isn't fixed. We are part of a live, embodied, evolving community of practice.

Time to Harvest

The Balinese word *biukukung* is the name for the ritual offering made by farmers when the rice stalks are full of grain and bowing over, ready to be harvested. The expression is also seen as a metaphor for life – as we grow older and fill with wisdom, we share what we have learned from our many years of experience. *Biukukung* is sometimes translated as blossoming.

This book is a response to the feeling that the time was ripe for a harvest of mature reflections blossoming from some of those who have integrated the practice of Amerta Movement into their work/lives over time. We sent a call to all the dialoguers[1] in the worldwide 'circulation' of Amerta Movement. In answer to the call we gathered these thirty responses from people in fourteen countries. Each of the writers has made the work their own, each with different questions to investigate. As well as illustrating the variety of ways Amerta Movement has been applied, their contributions together uncover the common ground we share – the 'unity in diversity' – a defining principle of the practice.

The writing that comprises *Embodied Lives* is as individual as the people writing, as individual as their expression in movement would be. They bring different styles of writing – academic, poetic, descriptive, imaginal, and historical – from different points of view,

---

1 Instead of teachers, Prapto has created over time a list of around 90 'dialoguers' who have his permission to share practice within the tradition of Amerta Movement.

and different cultural, professional, and familial backgrounds. The book is, therefore, as unique and unusual as the practice itself. Each of the chapters shares the potency that comes from writing out of lived experience, rather than writing *about* something with distance and detachment. The common ground in which the chapters are rooted is the search for something of the truth of what has seeped into our lives from the experience of working with Prapto.

The writers, for many of whom English is not their first language, have each found their own way to put their experience into words. While we have aided the translation of complex ideas into English, we have not necessarily 'corrected' all turns of phrase, so that the flavour of individual voices can remain intact.

Reading 'Embodied Lives'

As editors, we were presented with the creative challenge of weaving the disparate threads together and finding organizing themes and categories. As you can see from the image on the next page, it was difficult to define a single category for each chapter. Rather than represent the material in a list, we have sought to express the constellations and gatherings that occurred around themes in the authors' writings. The image attempts to demonstrate the overlapping and interactive nature of the chapters, their movement, expressed as a web.

We have recognized several main areas of application – the art of teaching, the art of art, the art of life, the art of work, the art of healing, the art of the unknown, and movement itself. The various themes and ideas in the book are both epigenetic[2] and mutually informing; thus, all the different fields enrich our understanding altogether. In the web, we were trying to embody the interrelatedness of the material and tones of the chapters. Movement is placed in the center to communicate its primacy within and through all the arts. The connections come both from the authors themselves, as well as from the perspectives of the editors.

We decided to allow our final arrangement of the chapters to remain fluid, in motion, as it were, as long as we could. We chose a presentation for the book order that is not arranged by category.

---

2 In any *epigenetic* process, as seen in embryology or learning, growth and understanding comes through the foundations of one element informing the next. And at the same time, each field of understanding is reciprocally illuminating in relation with the others. This is beautifully described in Maturana Romesin, H. & Verden-Zoller, G., (2008) *The Origins of Humanness in the Biology of Love*. Imprint Academic.

INTRODUCTION

Instead, we opted to draw on some of the interesting links and juxtapositions between disparate fields in arranging the chapters, creating dynamic counterpoints rather than similarities. In this looser way of weaving the threads from chapter to chapter, we hope to allow space for the movement of your own creative thinking, and to highlight the richness of the common field of practice.

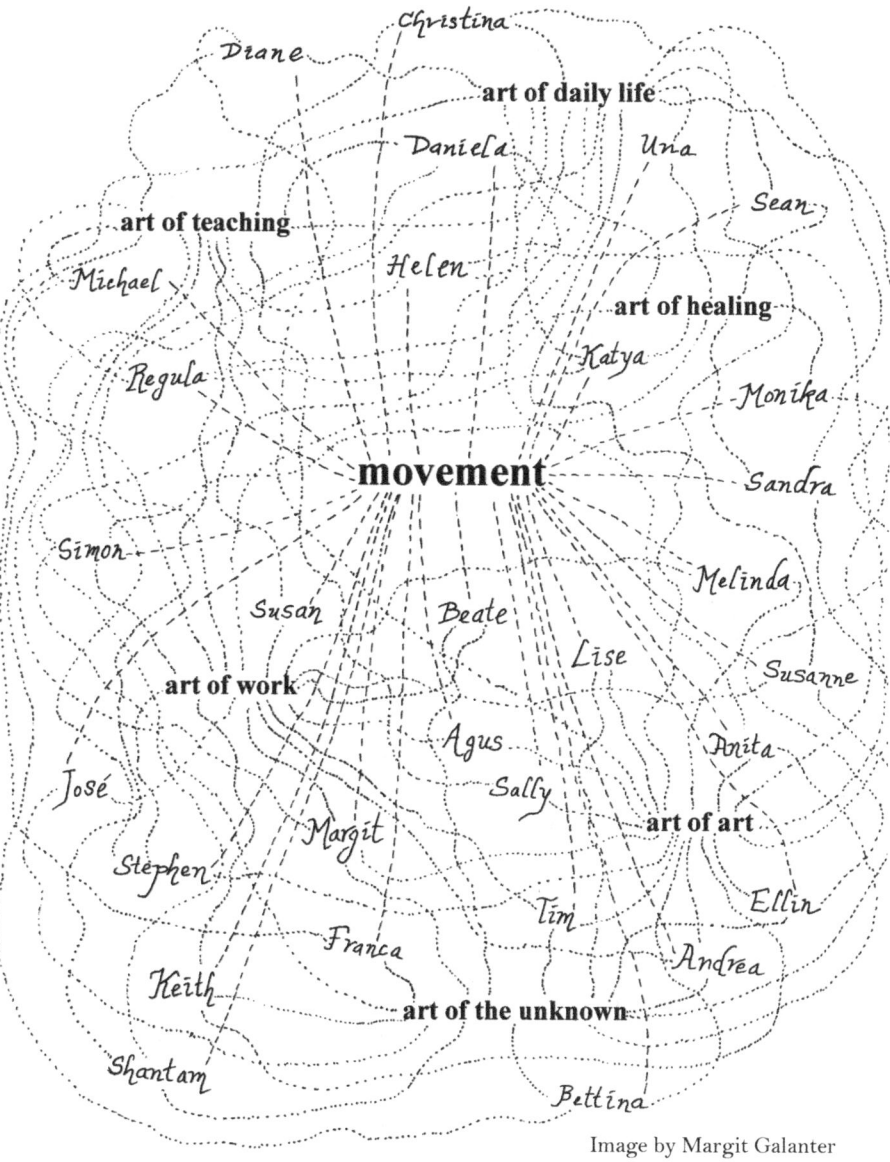

Image by Margit Galanter

Here are some glimpses of these threads: **Beate Stühm** writes from her moment-to-moment experience of moving, allowing us to enter the immediacy of the practice with her. **Keith Miller** takes us on a journey through a weave of movement and archeology. **Christina Stelzer** reflects on how her early studies and longtime experiences in Java gave her a unique perspective on the culture there. **Monika Förster** describes "mind as an ally", and "giving awareness without creating stagnation" amongst other practices as she writes about Tibetan Buddhism and Amerta.

Steve Hopkins describes his embodied film practice, and the experience of a 3m (movement, meditation and movie) group. He situates this approach within a broader reflection on the art of filmmaking. **José Mulder van de Graaf** writes about how his movement practice bridged communication between humans and an animal, and how research in science supports his views. **Sandra Reeve** reveals the four Borobudur mudras in her daily life ritual and speaks about guiding through movement. **Bettina Mainz** writes from the point of view of a child of 1980s' Germany, and how her unconscious cultural attitudes toward life were made conscious through work with Prapto.

Daniela Coronelli chooses the theme of resonance to describe Amerta's influence in her work as a teacher and healing practitioner in traditions of the movement arts. **Shantam Zohar** writes a poignant story about a crucial relationship between artistic flowering, channeling, and *semadi* (meditation). **Margit Galanter** coins a stimulating term, the 'presencing dial', to describe how we modulate qualities of appearance and experience. **Sally Dean** describes her ongoing research, in teaching and performing, into 'somatic costumes'. **Lise Lavelle** writes about a particular performance she made in Java, and how crystallization is an art form in its own right.

Susanne Tümpel describes her fascinating movement therapy work in a psychosomatic hospital in former East Germany, and relates it to Prapto's ideas of *organism* and *organization*. **Agus Bimo** brings us 'Mantra Gerak' (Movement Mantra) from Java, describing the origins of Javanese mantra, how his practice was influenced by Amerta and its current applications. **Tim Jones**'s chapter describes the 'musical portal', the relationship between movement and sound. He describes a workshop exploring that interface, called *Music*

Garden Chatting. **Franca Fubini** describes the process of bringing Amerta Movement into the practice of Social Dreaming in her work with groups; she refers to Prapto's ideas of *Dreamworld* and *Realityworld*.

Una Nicholson writes about the way Amerta has informed her approach to the complexities of family life. **Katya Bloom** describes her experience "conferring with infants" in a Neonatal Intensive Care Unit, as she explores the roots of dialogue before words. **Regula Nell** speaks of how her work with children is informed by two phrases Prapto said to her years ago in Java. **Sean Williams**, a developmental specialist, also works with children, mostly on the autism spectrum. He describes how his intention has changed dramatically through working with Prapto.

Susan Bauer writes about the long-lasting effects of Prapto's idea of *finding your position* and its relation to her practice 'Moving-from-Within'. **Helen Poynor** writes about Prapto's practice of *Body Body*, which has continued to inform her work as a teacher, performer and practitioner of movement. **Michael Dick** describes the qualities he derived from Amerta and which he applies to his work with actors, and offers a practice session as a case study example. **Simon Slidders** takes us into the realm of the law, and describes principles from Amerta that have guided his mindful work at the Royal Courts of Justice in London.

Andrea Morein illustrates how the practice and her experience with mindfulness training have informed her work as a visual artist. **Anita Lüdke** inventively illustrates how Amerta initially influenced her way of teaching students of architecture about the experience of space and now informs her daily life. **Melinda Buckwalter** describes a personal journey through time with Prapto, to find herself everchanging yet always right here. **Ellin Krinsly** describes her engaged performance work in many cultures, and how Prapto helped her locate a sense of home on the road. **Diane Butler** also describes her varied inter-culture work, and points toward its development in the future through the International Foundation for Dharma Nature Time.

Collectively these pieces may be seen as a constellation of happenings at particular places and moments. Though writing about movement fixes it in time, for all the writers, the ongoing influence of Amerta Movement inevitably means discovery, change, and growth.

Touched by Amerta

As editors, we have brought multiple perspectives, inspired both by our studies in Amerta Movement and by sources and approaches in our respective practices; these kinds of resources affected how the editing and shaping of the book unfolded. For example, Sandra brings an understanding of systems and constellations through her research with the ecological body; Margit is influenced by fascinations with feltedness and the embodiment of language; and Katya brings a longstanding interest in free association.

As readers you will inevitably approach the book with your own questions, arising from your own personal or professional background. You may find particular chapters closer to your own starting points, but we encourage you to look for inspiration and insight from all the chapters. Like walking around a garden, we recommend that you allow yourself to be surprised by the unexpected, perhaps finding your own route through the book.

We hope *Embodied Lives* will be of interest not only to those who are already familiar with Prapto's work, but to all who are interested in the value of an embodied approach to life and work. Current thinking about the brain and body point to the crucial importance of nonverbal, embodied perception and communication, and Amerta Movement offers an important path toward growth in this broad terrain.

To state the obvious, movement is a nonverbal and a three-dimensional experience, and any translation from that lived experience to the written word does not altogether represent this fullness. A book is limited by the parameters of its form, and yet, these limitations offer their own kind of liveness, so the process of writing and the composition of these elements onto the page have created a new evolution of Amerta Movement. We hope that the material itself can provide readers with a multi-dimensional, whole-bodied reading experience, and that it provides a new forum for translating and sharing the richness of the practice.

Visit **www.triarchypress.net/embodiedlives** *for further resources related to the book, including information about each author, additional images and information on how you can contribute your thoughts and experiences in an ongoing dialogue.*

1. PRESENCE

Beate Stühm (Germany)

I am in a tropical paradise – unfortunately the mosquitoes are here too.

I feel a bit imprisoned. My choices are: being covered with 'off' repellent, covering up with clothes, being bitten or staying inside. "How to be happy in prison?" I hear Prapto speaking in my mind. Or, I think he said, "being confident in hell", but it is not really that bad.

I go inside – my head is busy, keep it simple, just walking is always a good start, walking and variations, running.

My intention: to get into my body and out of my head – this is my other prison.

This piece wants to be written and of course it should be the best, should be written with space and humour, profound, rich, light, poetic and with a sense of three-dimensional embodiment; all of this, and maybe more.

I walk, I run, head in front – yes – I enjoy this stupid run.

Head in front... it reminds me of my Self Portrait Dance *30 years ago at the San Francisco Dancers' Workshop. My head separate from my body, being in a box full of judgements. It was a great self-caricature, funny and sad. My head was making me feel crazy.*

Stopping now in my movement, I see a bamboo stick, it looks friendly, I ...take it and move with it. Sounds come and – no – I do not follow this known melody, I am curious what evolves when I relax into listening while moving.

I come to sit on the cool grey floor, the bamboo in my hands, deep sounds arise from a deep place and an image from a movie comes –
The Long Walk Home *– the bamboo is brown, has segments and is warm in my hands. I look at my feet, the bamboo, my hands; I see my clothes and my position in the space and think "this would make a*

great photo". I hear the birds, lean into my back and 'wait' for a new movement to come.

I 'wait', open, receiving the presence of life.

I hold the bamboo and the bamboo holds me; looking through the window, I remember the first feedback I got from Prapto, on my first visit to Java in 1987: "look near".

It was like zooming with my eyes from far to near, to myself. While zooming I became aware of the space and sensing the space made me breathe. I touched the way to be connected with space and, through the space, with the far and near.

I am here now, in my body, in the space with the bamboo and enjoy the colours, the movements of the leaves and the play of light and shadow, the birds singing.

Summertime and the living is easy.....I sing the few words I know.

Reflecting

The movement described above is a snapshot, an awareness practice, an 'improvisation' in Bolivia in December 2012.

It is filled with the atmosphere of this particular environment. However the essence of my movement practice and the witnessing of myself could happen anywhere.

I moved alone, but that is only true if I count only human beings. There were different sounds from insects and all kinds of animals, there was the atmosphere of my friend, who created this space, the hot air and who knows who else was also taking part, hiding in corners and holes. I was happy to share and be part of this living environment.

Entering the flow of a movement process is deeply satisfying, but it does not always happen.

Working in and with the 'here and now' is exciting for me.

I am curious about what the body offers, which movements come, which images or feelings arise, what will unfold. I am interested in what the body receives and in how it responds, in what it has to say, what knowledge it holds and when it gives it freely.

When I went inside (into the movement space) I had my intention: to get into my body. I was guided by my awareness and mindfulness.

I started from what I have, as Prapto used to say, which means with all my resources gathered in my life, including my familiar judge. I do not have to think any more what to do or how to start.

No preparation any more: every movement counts on the stage of life. Movement is not seen as a symbol nor is it seen as functional; it is not for getting better, it simply is.

Starting with walking felt good; it is so basic, my feet on the ground, taking a step, stamping in different directions, playing with balancing, falling on the feet, jumping, being creative, silly, all variations; it helps not to get stuck, not to become too serious or go too deep into a search for meaning. Being simple, just muscles, body and having fun and enjoying it.

Now I wonder how to bring the directness and aliveness of it *into writing*. How to write or speak not *about* the experience, but *from* it. Speaking 'about' often feels like drawing a veil over the experience, so we can control it; it creates distance, which sometimes is needed too. Finding the words, speaking from the experience, from being engaged and present with all the senses and feelings is so exciting, almost scary at times; it is real, alive and vibrant. Sometimes there are no words... maybe a poem, a sound, maybe only stillness.

Learning to trust my intuition and allowing for magical moments.

One needs the *Dreieinige Gehirn*, the Triune Brain, the interplay of all our brain areas, no hierarchy, a great field to be in; unfortunately the judge thinks he is the boss.

He comes in when my prefrontal cortex is stressed.

But the sanest and most subtle task of this prefrontal part of the brain is to give space for our listening to (sensing) the body and our feelings – and to be aware of it, reflect on it, understand its meaning.

An Experiment

Some time ago I was asked to offer a short walking experiment in a dance research group.

I had chosen an awareness experiment.

I asked the group members to lift one foot – noticing how they did it and whether they still had a sense of the ground – then to put that foot down – how did it arrive on the ground? I asked them to notice if they followed the foot with the whole body. Did they bring their whole being to the new place... maybe facing a different direction? Being in a new place means being closer or further away from, for example, walls, windows, the others. Did their eyes follow the movement? Or the movement follow their eyes? What did they see, and how did it feel? What did they sense?

Later I read my instructions as written down by a group member as she had heard them; she said: "...lifting the foot for the next step and putting it in a new place... how do the eyes react?"

"Interesting", I thought, "that task sounds and feels quite different". I sensed the speed in it, the forward orientation. The "for the next step" indicates for me the functional, the next and the new, the future. As if all is there, outside, in front. The action described is the same, but the attitude and process of awareness is very different.

Culturally, we in the West are very much forward oriented: the front is interesting and the future too. This became very clear to me after I had lived for some time in Java. I had noticed many times how much I was in front, in the future; I was already there. Food was already prepared, in my mind, while I was still ordering it; I was impatient.

In my movement practice as well as in Sumarah – a Javanese meditation, a path of awareness and acceptance (translated literally: giving up the fight, surrender) – the back is important, the physical back, becoming aware of one's own back, one's own background, the support one can get from having someone behind. There is space and time behind too.

Having a back, feeling it and leaning into it, can be like resting in a *Lehnstuhl,* an easy chair. It gives us space and breathing, then our body has volume, is three-dimensional and becomes our container.

Fields of Awareness

The experience of the participants in this research group was calmness, expanse and a space of awareness. I sensed the aliveness of the space and the more the space was filled with awareness, the more we began to be connected, a sharing of one field for which we all were responsible.

How to stay alive in interdependency and not shrink into dependency? This could be the next task.

We have an effect on each other and on our environment, through our being and our doing, and the environment has an effect on us too.

We resonate: this gives us a sense of what is present in ourselves and in the space.

It can be written down quickly – 'being in resonance' – but not quickly achieved.

It is a never-ending process, a refinement of awareness, of

consciousness, of sensing and feeling, also of understanding and distinguishing.

In a group, if we are in tune and one person changes their place or position or shifts their awareness, then we all need to change too; we respond, adapt, improvise; it is an ongoing process. Someone releases some stress, a tightness, lets go of a burden, and often the whole group will take a deep breath: the release is in the air. Everyone contributes, everyone's creation, expression and release, everyone's change makes a difference to the whole.

At my first encounter with Prapto's work I was amazed (I was just back from California and had learnt to be amazed) by the differences in participants' movement qualities and style; everyone moved in their own unique way, and at the same time there was something special in the air, a connecting atmosphere.

Something in common was in the space and between people moving, like a soft energy. I got interested, even though nothing very exciting seemed to happen.

Seeing them being supported in their own ways and still being connected, sharing the space, was just the opposite of what I had experienced in my family, but I did not think of it then.

Gerald Hüther, a German neurobiologist, says: we human beings have two longings: one is to be free and the other is to be *verbunden*. The dictionary offers me for *verbunden*: connected, related, etc. I add 'being a part of'.

Moving in a group can be like being part of one organism, with a heightened awareness. Sometimes it feels like being under a microscope.

Form and structure evolves from the contact and being in resonance with the living and organised organism.

Following the body and being connected with the living environment we enter the unpredictable nature of life, at times not understanding why we need to move like this, or in that direction, and at the same time being clear that this is what needs to happen, what needs to be done.

Having an intention or a task helps to start the movement practice, it gives a guideline for moving (and living): for being aware, witnessing oneself, growing the ability to respond, to be present and connected to the energy of life. It requires trust in the wisdom of the body and its knowledge. It is surprising, touching, cleansing, authentic, easy, somehow limitless, free and connected. We compose, we create, *wir gestalten* while we move/dance.

Our physical presence, being rooted and grounded in the body, is our base, our home. The body is our instrument, this is where it happens, here we speak – nonverbally – here we receive the nonverbal. It is important to get to know and be present in the body otherwise there is no : body, and we are lost, in the world of fine energy, vibrations and resonances.

I was in Parangtritis, a village in Java on the Indian Ocean. I watched a group practising movement in the endless white dunes. Why did their range of movement and use of space get smaller and smaller and they themselves too? Was it the width of the environment and its constant change due to the wind and the currents in the sea?

Prapto shared his perception, predicting what movement activities would happen next. My mouth probably dropped open: how could he know? My memory is that he said something like: *"by their pattern of communication in action and reaction in movement they affect each other"*. They got stuck, almost completely motionless... He asked me to join the group without entering their communication system, without being absorbed and without using them, but helping to open the space again. I did not believe that this would be possible, but I did go in and worked on opening the space in movement; Prapto witnessed and prayed, and it was possible.

How did I do it? I do not remember. I have the image of a sticky spider's web now and I think I did a cleaning job then, by being clear in my body and my movement.

I saw the documentary film *The Artist is Present* about performance artist Marina Abramovic. She is sitting in MOMA in New York, and is 'just' looking into the eyes of every person who comes to sit in front of her. Some are smiling; from some people's eyes tears are flowing. The 'audience' around is with them. Being seen, being in contact, sitting with someone, present, just this, is so powerful. I left the cinema refreshed after a long day. I felt cleansed.

Just staying with what is.

"When I look, I am seen, so I exist," says British psychoanalyst D.W. Winnicott (1967).

Presence makes the difference, in the art of movement/dance, of performance and the art of healing. Presence deepens the experience, it speaks, verbally sometimes, nonverbally always. Being seen, with an inner attitude of compassion, is an experience beyond any method or technique.

Further Development

At some point I realised that I needed something that I could not get in movement practice, or in meditation. I missed the transformation I was longing for.

I was searching for a method of therapy, for a person who would embody and be connected to at least some essentials I cherish in this movement work.

I ran away from many therapists in the first hour. Until one day when I knew already on the phone that this was it. I felt seen, taken seriously, acknowledged.

Somatic Experiencing (SE) is a resources-oriented and body-centred method of resolving trauma and stress. It is a practice of working with what is present, bringing past and future into the now, and helping to release the effects left in the body from traumatic experiences. It also provided theory, explanations and references that I needed personally and professionally.

In the Amerta practice I had become aware of my reactions; sometimes I went beyond them and moved free, free.

In SE I stayed with my 'reactions' and 'patterns', I felt them, got to know and understand my emotions, my helplessness and my pain, which I released bit by bit.

An SE session is usually a one-to-one situation and I needed someone who would stay with me for a whole hour and more. I needed someone holding the space, creating a safe container, taking my hand, literally. I needed words, and my own language for understanding my story in the context of German history.

Slowing down in movement often happens naturally, by practising refinement, and it often happens in nature. In trauma release work, we are invited to slow down the spontaneous movements and gestures that we often make while speaking, so we can feel every inch of the movement and the inherent feelings and emotions. It makes us aware of all the information our bodies hold. A little movement moment can reveal so much richness, excitement, weakness or important images. The slowing down helps us to find these moments which we tend to skip and jump over. And we are helped by someone who gently reminds us to stay present by asking: "If that is allowed: how does it feel in your body?" Allowing opens the space for us to land in the body.

When we get behind/beyond the judgements, explanations, reasonings, smart thoughts (of the prefrontal brain) and have the courage to feel (the limbic brain), acknowledge the instincts (brain stem), and allow this experience to just be and give time for release to happen, we come into the present and closer to ourselves.

The release seems to drop into every cell, we breathe, cry sometimes or laugh; we have space; a profound relaxation happens as well as a deep transformative process.

SE has deepened my practice in many ways. It gives me a clearer and deeper understanding of what is happening in the body, in movement and in resonance. It deepened my practice of acknowledging the truth and of acceptance.

Acceptance

Acceptance sounds great, but how do we do it? Often the word acceptance is in the realm of judgement itself, because accepting is good and rejecting is bad. What does it require to be able to accept? There are conditions when we cannot accept, not yet or not alone; we need help and sometimes we need a lot of time. "If you have all the time in the world: how does it feel in your body?"

There are ways that can help us find acceptance in movement practice, for instance working on adaptation to a new situation or to a changed physical ability – or working on measurements: how big is my step? how open are my arms? how bright is the light I can be in? – or giving space by relaxing, being thankful and lessening the fear, not letting the fear go, but moving step by step into more confidence; to name but a few. It is a process. Humour and creativity are wonderful ways too.

Accepting is happening; one cannot do it, but one can prepare for it.

Having spent many months in Java, where Prapto and this movement practice originate, I experienced a sensing and feeling culture, a flow of time, of music and traffic, smile and laughter, a grounded physical presence, an attitude of relaxing into what is and the presence of prayer and meditation which taught me a lot.

I am thankful for the free spirit of art of Anna Halprin, the deep and free spiritual connectedness and wisdom of Prapto and the free research mind of Peter Levine.

Blossoming

I have a garden. I find rest there; I stop, listen and see.

It reminds me that there is more than human activity. It is refreshing. I discover wonderful things, learn to understand the needs of plants and my own need to put my hands into the earth, see the sky and create beautiful breathing compositions.

I love to dance connecting to my wild side, to stillness and to the energy of life.

I enjoy teaching, guiding and witnessing growth and creation, development and the unfolding of potential – stimulating more aliveness in what we do, what we have and who we are.

I feel at home with going beyond rules and tools, with inner attitudes of space, compassion, passion and curiosity.

I call my work 'Blossoming'.

~ ~ ~

References

Winnicott D.W. (1967) 'The location of cultural experience', *International Journal of Psychoanalysis*, 48:368–372

Beate Stühm works as a freelance Movement/Dance teacher and artist and, since 2009, as a Somatic Experiencing Practitioner. She trained in Aikido; then graduated from Anna Halprin's San Francisco Dancers' Workshop (SFDW)/Tamalpa Institute. Beate practised intensively in Java at Padepokan Lemah Putih and in Europe with Prapto, 1987-1997; she is a Messenger Art teacher. In Java she also practised Sumarah Meditation and did Meditation Guidance Training with Laura Romano. She edited *Impressions*, a Sharing Movement Magazine (1995-2005), made video documentations 'moving movies' of movement works. She sings in a polyphonic choir and is training in Neuro-Affective Psychotherapy.

BeateStuehm@web.de

www.BeateStuehm.de

2. AMERTA MOVEMENT AND ARCHAEOLOGY

Excavation Without Digging

Keith Miller (UK)

I dream that I'm with my university archaeology lecturer and a fellow archaeology student, walking along an abandoned railway line in the Highlands where we'd been excavating a prehistoric site. They're ahead of me as we go through a cutting and into a tunnel. Halfway along in the darkness I see something glint in the wall. I retrace my steps and see a relief carving, shiny black like coal, of a face in a frame. Looking closer I see that it's the bearded face of a figure sitting behind an opening like a window. Then I see the eyes are shining, alive. With a start, I realise that it is Jesus. He says yes, he is alive. Amazed, I wonder what to do – whether to stay and continue this extraordinary dialogue or go and tell my companions who by now are out of the tunnel. But how can I describe what I'm seeing? It occurs to me that I have no measuring tape or drawing materials to make an archaeological record and, even if I had, how can I convey that the face is alive, let alone that it's Jesus and he's black? Nevertheless, I decide to go and tell my fellow archaeologists at least something about what I had seen...

Archaeology

Archaeology is the study of material culture, the physical evidence of past human behaviour. The timespan stretches from the earliest hominids, over a million years ago, to just a moment ago. The most intensive and immersive archaeological practice is excavation, carefully digging a site to uncover and record the buried remains and residues of human activity. The remains themselves – 'finds' of pottery, bone, insects, seeds and so on – are then 'processed': cleaned, sorted and studied in a kind of micro-excavation. But archaeology is much wider than this; it embraces the study of landscapes and buildings, earthworks and marks in the soil or in growing crops produced by buried features, and the microscopic signatures and changes in the environment brought by human activity.

Archaeological remains are fragments of people's movements and activities, intentions and experiences. Most remains relate to the ordinary daily lives of our anonymous forebears. Even in palaces and temples, it is often the incidental marks and traces of everyday life that are the most telling. All human behaviour, all human artefacts, 'speak'. Archaeologists reveal and interpret these messages, these material memories, bringing them into consciousness, re-presenting and expressing them as part of an ongoing cultural story. With its focus on the study of human behaviour and the material world we have created, archaeology holds a mirror up to our culture and to our own lives and daily experiences of moving through a world layered in history and memory, making marks as we go. Archaeology tells stories about people and places, and at its best it enriches the texture of places and communities and offers insights into personal and cultural identity.

Sometimes we feel a close connection with people from the past, for instance through their personal possessions, or their burial sites (think of those dark slumbering bodies from the European peat bogs). At other times we have a more generalised feeling of the presence of the past, seeing things as they are now as the outcome of past processes and sensing through them the passage of time.

The Embodied Archaeological Experience

There is a particular feeling to archaeological excavation – the elemental experience of digging the earth, exposed to the weather; of repetitive and often demanding physical activity, working through the ground, uncovering the buried shapes of archaeological features, scraping and sifting the crumbling soils and separating out the fragments of broken pottery or bone. Likewise in landscape work; walking to and fro looking for traces, combing the ground for clues, tuning into the texture and shape of the landform and teasing out the human patterns. At the same time we are working with the imagination, sifting through our 'mind objects' – our perceptions, feelings and hunches, our memories and academic facts – reading the human story in the environment.

Whether we dig physically or with our imagination, the process is a kind of ritual undoing of what had been created before; deconstructing and deciphering the remains, whilst at the same time reconstructing them into imagined versions of the past until one particular story seems to fit. Here we touch the essence, the bones, of storytelling: interpreting phenomena in alternative ways, seeing different paths, other worlds.

Time and Place

We usually see time in spatial terms: the past and future as other places, near or distant, behind or in front of us. Academic archaeology follows a conventional version of this, with its emphasis on objective chronological timelines where we locate different ages and cultures and measure progress.

In the embodied archaeological experience, however, the conventional arrangement of time becomes dislocated. As 13th-century Zen master Dōgen observed, there is no time apart from things; and I now find myself among things of different ages, all simultaneously present. I am not on a neat timeline stretching behind and before me, but 'among' time. In the layered strata of an archaeological section, all the times are co-present, and when I scrape across the section with my trowel I am encountering centuries or millennia with each stroke. In the landscape too, features of different ages are simultaneously present underfoot and around me. Past, present and future are not located elsewhere, in separate places, but co-exist and intermingle. There is a feeling of being suspended in time, moving to and fro between the past represented by the archaeological remains, the process of uncovering them in the present, and the story that I am creating out of this material, unfolding into the future.

Our sense of place, too, is changed by the archaeological experience. History and archaeology are site-specific; all events take place *in* place. As we delve, we experience place-making at first hand: how the landscape has rhythms, textures and densities, degrees of 'whereness' composed into sites and places; how places are living relationships, temporary constellations of events and features of different ages, the outcome of many processes through time. Each place is in movement too and has no fixed identity but is many places, with many 'layers' and possible stories.

Archaeological experience is a kind of non-ordinary state of consciousness, but one we are all familiar with. At root, it is simply awareness of a historic dimension – a 'before' – manifest in the environment. When we dig the garden and pick out a piece of broken crockery, or walk down the street wondering why it bends in a particular way, or unwrap an old ticket from the depths of our pocket, we are doing archaeology: investigating layers of memory and meaning, reconstructing past human activity.

But whilst archaeologists are good at describing the minutiae of sites and finds, we tend to forget ourselves. My student dream encounter expressed the conundrum of formal academic archaeology: the lived archaeological experience, the very thing that emotionally engages us with these remains from the past, cannot be easily mapped and measured and is largely absent from academic accounts[1]. Personal subjective experience is not seen as relevant to the scientific archaeological enquiry; the wider environment, including ourselves as active participants, is not part of the story.

Amerta Movement

For me, Amerta practice offers a way to explore and bridge these gaps and to integrate the academic with the experiential; non-stylised environmental movement and archaeology can inform and complement each other.

Amerta movement practice, like archaeology, is rooted in, and inspired by, place. Working, individually and with others, in different places, in all weathers and conditions, returning time and again to places chosen for their natural, historical and cultural importance, has always been at the heart of Prapto's practice. In such places, the environment and their significance for previous generations combine to support our own movement work. Of the many historic sites in the UK that have been used for Amerta work, the prehistoric stone circle at Avebury has seen the most activity and has much in common with places in Java where Prapto works. This has been my main study area. Movement sessions at Avebury up to two weeks long have been held regularly over several years, a pattern not unlike archaeological fieldwork with its seasons of survey and excavation.

Working with Layers

Recognition of layers is fundamental to human understanding. As well as being familiar in daily life (think for instance of clothing, cooking, gardening), the theme of layers, levels and sequences is

---

1 Exceptions include the work of Chris Tilley, Julian Thomas and others taking a phenomenological approach. Others, such as historic re-enactors and neo-pagans, pursue forms of archaeological experience but mostly outside the mainstream.

common in the humanities, arts and sciences, whilst for archaeology and geology, the investigation of successive historic layers and deposits is the very foundation of the disciplines.

Amerta also works with layers. A key practice is the investigation of sensations, perceptions, feelings and memories; starting from daily life movement and then *"excavating, skin by skin, layer by layer, to discover what is the story, the motive, the source"*.[2] The process whereby memory and past experience arises, or is retrieved, to meet the present, is a form of somatic survey, excavation and processing of 'finds', where bodymind itself is an archaeological site.

On a historic site like Avebury, through movement-based research I can explore different layers of myself and the environment: the material and functional (my body, the earth and sky around me), the perceptual and sensual, emotional and attitudinal, cultural and historical, social and religious.

Whatever the focus of my attention, the aim is to maintain an awareness of both subject and object. Through a process of continuous self-reflexive investigation, a dialogue develops between 'subject' – myself as mover-in-the-environment, and the object of my research in the environment – an 'environment-with-mover' that includes me as an active participant. I am reading both myself and my context; surveying 'inner' and 'outer' landscapes – but as different views on a continuum rather than as separate places.

By moving and changing my position and attitude, my pace and focus of attention, I can investigate various perspectives and points of view. I become familiar with different aspects of the object I am investigating and I also acknowledge my own responses throughout the process: the feelings, memories and associations that arise. Attending to subtle sensations and perceptions, I notice phenomena that I may have previously overlooked or ignored because of habitual patterns of posture, movement or attitude. As I pass to and fro among the layers, I am as imaginative and exploratory as I can be without losing my reference point, my home 'anchor', or losing the line I am following. This line, a path of enquiry and expression, is a creative dialogue between myself and the environment, a co-creation through mutual influence and interaction.

Living Measurement

For exploring layers we need measurement. Archaeology, using tools ranging from hand-tapes to lasers, has refined the practice of

---

2 Prapto speaking at Lemah Putih, 23 July, 2013.

objective measurement. But inevitably, these tools narrow attention to particular viewpoints and perspectives. Above all, they reflect our visually-dominated cultural perspective which privileges sight, 'the sense of science', and visual information. With this comes a sense of distance and separateness from an environment which, 'flattened' and objectified, lends itself to sub-division and two-dimensional representation. The measurements tend to replace the things they measure.

Embodied archaeological experience, engaging all the senses, challenges the primacy of sight and its view of a static objectified world, and points to a wider reality, to something more alive. Amerta movement too, through its multi-sensory exploration, loosens the hold of the hungry eye and broadens perceptions.

Amerta recognises that, consciously or not, we are in constant communication and adaptation with our environment, measuring our relationships with our surroundings and each other. To help me recognise this process, and maintain awareness of position and proportion in my movement and my relationships with the surrounding environment, I use the Amerta practice of *living measurement*. This is a dynamic, subjective measuring of body, mind and relationship which takes the basic movements of daily life – walking, sitting, standing, crawling and lying down – as a reference. Through this I check my 'form' – my shape and position, sensations and feelings; the focus and extent of my awareness, and how I am receiving and digesting information and experience.

Combining this personal measured approach with a creative exploration of varied points of view, I perceive differently and sense more connections than I would from conventional body positions or through narrowly-focused instruments. Various techniques help with this: *stopping* (pausing in my movement and becoming aware of my own form and condition and that of my surroundings); *window* (changing my viewpoint, my frame and perspective, opening fresh choices in direction and awareness); and *naming* (simple recognition and naming of the object of attention, sensation or activity at any moment). The techniques are similar to the Bare Attention technique used in Theravada Buddhist mindfulness meditation. As with meditation, there is both distance and involvement at the same time. By maintaining my connection with ordinary everyday movement and experience, and by expanding my awareness, giving value to the gaps and spaces between and not jumping through the layers or across distances, I develop a fuller appreciation and understanding of relationships between myself and the environment.

Position and Perspective

The Amerta technique *point, spot, place and space* enables me to work with different positions and perspectives, from close focus on a point to the whole of a place and its wider context. For close work at Avebury, I might focus on one stone in the circle, or just a small part of it. Using all my senses, I explore its materiality and the 'functional' realm of angle, line, volume, shape, texture, density, temperature – not just as objective data, but as psychophysical experiences – receiving, responding, translating and expressing the information and experience through my movement. At the same time I am aware of my wider context and surroundings: the grass and trees on the earthworks, other people, the weather and wider landscape.

Having established my home position, I extend my exploration into feelings and attitudes, imagination and ideas; the realm of personal and cultural stories. What am I, and the objects of my attention, 'saying'? What stories are unfolding? I try to observe my choices and to notice habitual patterns in my movement, in my thoughts and feelings, and in my cultural preferences and attitudes – all of which might limit perception and awareness. In these ways, embodied movement-based research can assist academic interpretations, for instance by 'ground-truthing' ideas about the form and function of ancient sites and their relationships with the landscape.

Through these movement practices, I become more aware of the process of widening my perspective and view, and learn to recognise occasions when I hold my position too tightly or when I get pulled into the distance, lose my home position and 'fly away' into disembodied thought and speculation. Maintaining my sense of measurement and proceeding step-by-step, giving value to the 'space' between myself and the object I am investigating, I notice my tendencies to become absorbed or lost, or to unthinkingly assume a 'stand-point' or 'leap' to conclusions, in pursuit of particular sensations and outcomes.

There are direct equivalents in archaeology: becoming so absorbed in looking for coins that you miss the pottery; 'chasing features' but missing their context; digging too deep or too quickly through the layers in pursuit of desired results, or simply ignoring the evidence that doesn't fit. A *living measurement* approach is required, with the right pace, right attention and intensity of looking, attending both to objects and their context; and also with a watchful eye on personal and collective habits and motivations.

Using Objects or Tools

Archaeology still retains a strong element of physical human interaction through digging in excavations or working in the landscape. Alongside the latest scientific instruments, the simplest tools – spades, trowels, buckets and barrows – are still the basic equipment for excavation. The physical work, and the textures, smells and sounds, help to balance our habitual emphasis on sight and open other pathways of knowing.

In movement-based work, simple items like a stick, a leaf, a stone or a cloth can be used as 'tools' to excavate the layers of personal and cultural memory and experience. Prapto introduced this to me whilst working on an Indonesian temple site. To my surprise, moving with a leaf and a stone opened the site to me, providing me with a 'handle', a way of orientating myself and of measuring my investigation of the many layers of the place; giving me a link to the people around me both past and present, and a way of understanding their own interactions with the many manifestations of leaf and stone.

The more time spent in a place, the more attuned and receptive we can become. It is unusual to spend longer than a few hours on a heritage site unless you are working there, and in both Amerta work and archaeological investigations, a site can become a 'home' – its latest phase of human activity. Whilst there, our activities and experiences may resonate with those of the earlier builders or users, providing a bridge between past and present. Movement-based research, extending beyond the reach of spoken or written language, expands these possibilities for correspondence with our forebears. When I trudge up the hillside or haul a bucket of excavated soil, when I bow or sing, or sweep the ground with a handful of grass, or walk along an old pilgrims' path, I may well be following earlier footsteps, echoing previous activities and stirring similar areas of the autonomic nervous system with its deep layers of memory and experience. I cannot objectively verify such 'correspondences', but if I heed my own intentions and the environment around me, maintaining my connection with everyday life in steering between sentimental wishful thinking and cynical detachment, then I can deepen my experience and understanding of my relationship with a place and with its communities both past and present.

Circle, Oval, Square

Academic archaeology, like anthropology, employs categories like religion, ritual, economy, social networks and so on. In Amerta work, for exploring different aspects of personal and cultural activity and belief, Prapto uses various open experiential forms or themes, such as *Human, Nature, God*; *Home, Road, Temple, Stage*; *Circle, Oval, Square*. These last three have been particularly useful in Amerta work at Avebury. Circle relates to the world of devotion and the attitude of "*bowing and praying*"; Oval relates to nature and the process of "*purification in circulation*"; Square relates to the marketplace and human dialogue, with the theme of "*unity in diversity*". Working with other people in groups on these different themes offers insights into the functions and qualities of places and how they shift and change; and insights into our attitudes, behaviour and beliefs and how these colour how we see and relate to places and to each other. These themes also provide a language and shared ground for inter-cultural dialogue, both with contemporary cultures and those of the past.

Ritual, myth and personal belief are not usually recognised by archaeologists as being actively present in their own work. The relationship with 'ancestor' similarly goes unacknowledged except, perhaps, in a genealogical sense; ancestor is not seen as an active environmental presence. But archaeological practice inevitably expresses the practitioner's attitudes and beliefs. It takes only a small shift of perspective to see the archaeological excavation of a site and its dutiful recording as a ritual of respect and devotion, of cleansing and purification, of translation and expression; and the archaeological approach itself, with its recognition and respect for the traces of the past and the people who left them, as a commitment honouring a shared history, a process of remembrance and an offering to the ancestors and to ourselves and our successors.

The Art Approach

The more I work with historic sites, the more I am aware of their multiple layers and multiple stories. They do not have a single story or fixed identity – any more than we do. There is no single Avebury: there are, and always were, many Aveburys. This diversity provides many openings and opportunities for understanding and many seeds for creative expression and art; many bridges to heal the sense of fragmentation and separation from a 'lost' past and an objectified environment. This creative diversity is central to Prapto's *Gardening* approach, based on mutual respect and co-creative partnership.

Amerta movement work on historic sites usually culminates in crystallisations: individual and collaborative presentations, installations and site-specific performances. Art, rather than academic reports, is the medium of expression. The world of archaeology and heritage is rich ground for artistic expression, and although academic archaeology is dominated by the paradigm of scientific objectivity, fieldwork is still essentially a craft, and art is never far away. Art is essential for interpretation: only through archaeological experience and imagination can archaeological facts be transformed into stories for understanding. And archaeology itself can be art: excavation and survey as sculpture, performance, storytelling.

Heritage sites are also frequently used for art events. Often, though, the site is simply used as a background setting, rather than as a partner in a creative dialogue between present and past. The most successful 'archaeological' art[3] is embodied and participatory, responsive to place, recognises the role of ritual, and has breathing space for the unseen and unknown. Through such work archaeology and subjective personal experience can be integrated and expressed together. For me, Amerta Movement and its 'art approach' offers a way of individually and collectively exploring and creatively expressing the many layers, stories and manifestations of time and place, whilst still remaining embodied and connected; not using or exploiting places as background or simply 'material', but offering a collaborative expression, where environment and human, past and present, are in dialogue, speaking together.

~ ~ ~

Keith Miller has worked for many years as an archaeologist and landscape and buildings historian, and now works for English Heritage, managing the conservation of sites and buildings in southern England ranging from the Stone Age to last century. He first encountered movement work in the 1980s as part of his Satipatthāna mindfulness meditation practice with teacher John Garrie Rōshi, and has been practising Amerta Movement with Prapto and with fellow Amerta practitioners since the 1990s. A keen artist and musician, for several years Keith and his wife Kristina Bourdillon, with Simon Slidders, have been running movement workshops at Avebury in the UK.

kayarmiller@gmail.com

---

3 I am thinking of site-specific performances like those of Prapto himself, Sandra Reeve, Helen Poynor and Brighton-based Red Earth; writing by Kathleen Jamie and Robert Macfarlane; Seamus Heaney's bog burial poems; Andy Goldsworthy's work; and music and song, for me a basic constituent of place.

3. CULTURAL ASPECTS OF THE MOVEMENT WORK

Christina Stelzer (Germany)

Living on the island of Java for three years from 1985 to 1988 and experimenting together with Prapto in a culture and environment quite different in many ways to my European background, marked a turning point in my life. Although I came back to the West, I never came back to seeing the world the way I had seen it before. That is why it seems to me essential to shed some light on the cultural context in which the movement practice that Prapto named Joged Amerta – and that others have brought into the world with their own names – is rooted. Rather than writing about applying the principles of this movement approach to my practice and teaching, I would like to take you into the atmosphere of an island whose people by their very nature had a fundamental impact on my future life and work.

Java is an island with a tropical climate, where the warmth in the air has a soothing quality at night, and where the daytime heat can immobilize you for most of the afternoon. Living in Java meant not only living in weather conditions quite unlike those I had grown up with but, moreover, it meant living with people who have another relationship altogether to time and space. The ways of relating to each other that I encountered are determined by an awareness rooted in qualities of "right timing" rather than following the clock, and by a very refined sense of atmospheres.

The daily exposure to this very different way of life for such a length of time had a tremendous influence on me, but one that is hard to describe. It all took place in the context of a movement practice that was in the process of emerging, where concepts and structures to work within were minimal. Looking back to this time, there are three cultural aspects I would like to highlight. These aspects are: **waiting, hearing the world** and **respect**.

Waiting

This is a state of being that I call 'waiting' for lack of a more appropriate term.

To me it felt like a quarter of my time in Java was spent waiting. Waiting was part of daily life and living: waiting for transport, waiting impatiently in the immigration office, waiting for Prapto to come, waiting for the monsoon rain to stop, waiting in long lines at the post office, waiting for a dance performance to begin, waiting for the heat to pass to be able to leave the house... And it did not mean just a few minutes; no, often it meant hours. It was so fundamental and had gone so deep under my skin, becoming a state of being rather than a waiting for something, that in the end it was not seen as waiting any more; it became an attitude of relaxing deeply into the situation and giving in.

Things will just not work for you in Javanese culture if you cannot arrive at this inner place of surrender. It is difficult in the beginning for the Western attitude of wanting things our way, and not only our way but right away! We are confronted by our restlessness, our impatience and our concepts of efficiency. Yet when we can give in to the moment and let go, we experience the world from a different point of view. Doors open towards sensing the way in which Javanese people are receiving their environment and each other.

In the West we are commonly very forward-oriented. The planning and following of set schedules dominates our lives. Living in the Javanese culture and moving with Prapto, I began to experience a rhythm that was of a quite different melody.

We often went with Prapto to a place near Wonogiri, a hilly area where Prapto had built a small temple. We practiced there in this beautiful natural environment, surrounded by rice fields and a mountain range and with a view to a lake. There was always this 'arriving', which meant a settling into the place. Prapto would speak a few words with the caretakers of the place, we would look for the mats and spread them, and later the caretakers brought tea. Prapto would come and sit with us, smoking a cigarette. Time to watch butterflies dancing, to listen to the insects and the soft rattling of bamboo. Nothing much happening, it seemed. When do we begin?

Actually, it had already begun. What was happening was already part of the movement process, its opening moment. Opening to more than oneself.

It was a moment of connecting; connecting to one's own state of being as well as to that of others and the surrounding environment.

Most Javanese people would never think of those moments as waiting. Even before a performance or another event begins, the attitude is one of just being there and knowing that what is about to happen will begin when all that is needed is ready. Needed does not mean the functional side only, but the overall atmosphere in which events take place.

'Waiting' as described here means slowing down. In slowing down, there is time to see, to feel, and to tune into your environment. You leave your tunnel view and open. In 'waiting', you let go of your expectations, your holding on to how things should be. And things may as well get done without your doing.

There is a moment that stays with me clearly to this day. It was at the end of my time in Java. A friend and I were in Jakarta and wanted to go to Yogyakarta by bus. Upon entering the bus station we realized it was *Idul Fitri* (the end of Ramadan with its special festivities). Oh my God, we had not thought about it! The bus station was crowded with people, and at first sight it did not look like we would get a ticket for our planned ride that day. We would be uncomfortably stuck in Jakarta. We stood at the side, watching the buses coming into the station, the people running and squeezing in. Bus after bus was packed. We stood there just waiting, standing still next to each other, completely relaxed. There was not much thought at all. Just this presence of being there, watching, receiving the scene, connecting. After quite a while a man approached us asking where we wanted to go. We told him our destination and he said, "come with me!" As we did not have anything to lose, we followed him, leaving the terminal and walking in the direction of the empty buses which were coming in. He finally approached one of the buses and stopped it, spoke with the driver and then shuffled us in with a friendly gesture, refusing the money we wanted to offer. A few minutes later we drove into the terminal, smiles on our faces, where more people climbed into the bus. Was it luck or was it the result of patience, receptivity and just being present?

The process of 'waiting' not only slows you down but also loosens the impulse towards grasping. There is always something we long for, aim at, grasp for, expect. When you live in a culture where buses do not run on schedule (if there are any at all), where things you would like to get repaired are just getting done in a timing that stays mysterious to you, where your teacher arrives according to what he feels is the right moment rather than a set hour, where a gathering begins only after people change their seats as often as necessary so everybody feels the arrangement is *cocok* (fitting), you slowly but surely change. Your mind gets put to rest.

You are in your environment in a different, more subtle way. You open more to your senses; you see, listen, smell, touch and feel. This leads you to sense atmospheres while your awareness has a chance to expand.

You enter into *rasa*, a quality of feeling. *Rasa* is a state of being, highly valued in the Javanese culture. It basically means sensing what is around you, relating to others from your feeling nature rather than your mind. From an inner place that, when cleaned and refined, can be a place of feeling, unclouded by emotions.[1]

Hearing the World

The door bell to our house in Baluwarti, Solo, Central Java had been ringing. Suparmi, our housekeeper, was already at the door before the bell rang, ready to open it for the guest. It was not by chance. She always approached the door before someone rang the bell. How magical! She must have a sixth sense!

Java is a mystical place full of mysterious events, yet what in the beginning might be a mystery to you is often just a different way to live. Javanese people listen to the world. What I came to understand is that they perceive the world mainly through hearing rather than through looking.

It took quite a while to find out that Suparmi had been hearing a bird that was announcing the visitor. Birds do that. They inform the environment about changes in the atmosphere, especially about people entering their sphere. Suparmi was just attentive to sounds. It was natural to her.

It could be quite irritating to be in the presence of a Javanese group who were talking together. We would not have direct eye contact as I had been previously used to when talking. In Europe, it is common to look directly at the person with whom we are speaking, whereas in Java communication takes place through hearing one other. Looking at one other is considered very direct and somehow excluding. In staying connected to hearing, awareness can open 360 degrees. The eyes soften and adopt a receptive quality.

---

[1] On the concept of *rasa* and the Javanese world view, see Laura Romano (2013).

This sensing and indirectness is a characteristic of Javanese culture, approaching life from an angle that I was not used to. Try and listen to the world instead of looking at it. See the effect it has on your body and the way you perceive the world and meet people. For example, you might become more sensitive to the feeling quality in speech. The eyes can close, the ears never do. They can just select incoming information by focusing on near or far, but they always stay open.

It was quite a challenge for us during our first stay in Gadjahan[2] in 1984 when we practiced in the *pendopo* (a space that serves to connect the private part of a house and the public and is often open on three sides), while a man who had come to sell coffee beans was grinding them close to us in a very noisy machine. There were also people passing by; Hendra, the owner of the house, repairing his car in a corner of the garden and talking loudly to other people; *pembantus* (housekeepers) chatting with each other.

In Java there is never complete silence. For example, there may be sound at night from a radio in your neighbor's house, where they are listening to a shadow puppet play until the early morning. The sound is a continuously shifting carpet that just changes its patterns, and everybody is comfortable and relaxed on it... except most of the Westerners, who feel easily disturbed. One reason is the Western cultural tendency to focus on oneself whereas the Javanese usually stay open to collective moods and movements.

Focusing in general is not the principal attitude in Java. With focusing you exclude. You create a central point, pushing aside all else that seems unrelated. You decide what is right and necessary for your chosen focus and what is not. Javanese culture does not function this way, nor does the individual living in it.

Focusing creates boundaries, but in the Javanese attitude it is not by exclusion that boundaries get established. Looking at the language, for example, one can see that Javanese people try to avoid the word *tidak* which means no, because it is considered to be too strong. It is preferred to leave more openness, using words like *belum* (not yet) or *kurang* (less). Instead of saying *tidak baik* (not good), one would say *kurang baik* (less than good, not really good) to make it softer. This way, everything is seen to be in motion, still able to manifest. Also, there are various ways of saying 'yes.' The tone of the 'yes' indicates how close it is to a real 'yes' or if it means 'no.'

---

2 Gadjahan is an area of Solo where Laura Romano with her former husband Hendra used to run a homestay, which became well known Prapto's students.

In my experience the ears are connected to feelings. Perceiving the world predominantly through the ears rather than the eyes means that feelings become refined. It was not only the outer world that I learned to perceive in a different way, but also it was a shift into perceiving inner worlds. Receiving the condition of my physical and emotional presence let information come into my awareness from deep layers of my being. With growing sensitivity this process became more and more subtle.

'Hearing the world' affects the awareness of spatial relationship and timing – timing in the sense of connectedness. We are individual beings, yet connected in various ways, and the qualities of what I call here 'waiting' and 'hearing the world' brought me closer to this experience.

Respect

There exists in Javanese culture a special sense for placing and positioning yourself in relation to others.

This cultural sense of appropriate positioning becomes visible in the home, particularly if you are not a member of the family, in which case you are received in the *pendopo*, between the public and the private area. It can also be seen in people's ways of lowering themselves when passing in front of others already sitting. You become aware of this attitude in relating to each other – it can sometimes be very subtle.

This takes place in all kinds of situations and events, like with the *pembantu* who takes care of a house, as Suparmi did for us. Relating to her challenged me to accept that she would always make sure to place herself lower than me, which meant that if I talked to her while I was sitting on a chair, she would go and sit on the ground. Coming from the West with the idea that everybody is equal and the anti-authoritarian attitude of my generation, this was not so easy to take. Yet she taught me that lowering oneself in space did not mean one has to lose grace and dignity. I learned to respond and to own my position comfortably. Our relationship grew in mutual respect.

Before coming to Java, respect and respectfulness had connotations that belonged to the old days of my parents and a society we had opposed in the sixties. Now, living in a culture that was clearly hierarchically structured, with its visible formalities and expressions of respect, I had to review my opinions. Not only was I touched by the respectfulness in behavior that I met, but also I could see that respectfulness protects one's own and the other person's dignity. And dignity is a human right and value in itself that so often gets stepped on without one even knowing.

It is necessary to give space in relating to each other to keep your own and the other's dignity. The attitude of 'respectfulness' does exactly that: it creates such a space.

The three cultural aspects described have one thing in common: they open awareness to all sides. The attitude of 'waiting' leads to a relaxed state of connectedness to the overall atmosphere one is in, 'hearing the world' shifts one into the center of a circular awareness, and 'respectfulness' creates the space for relating in a way that gives a chance to see the whole rather than only oneself.

Yet only after I had returned to the West and taken on my new task to be a guide and teacher in this movement practice could I begin to see the values I have talked about. I then experienced how they had already become a part of my being, providing a source from which my work evolved.

~ ~ ~

References

Romano, L. (2013) *Sumarah – Spiritual Wisdom from Java*, Lulu Press

Christina Stelzer, Diplom Psychologist, studied Tai chi with Gia-fu Feng (Colorado) and dance therapy with Anna Halprin (California) and was part of the pioneer period 1982-1988 when a small group of people from the West, together with Prapto in Java, created the ground from which Amerta Movement rose. Since then she has continued to develop this movement approach within her work, calling it 'GangArt' (meaning the specific style and attitude of one's walk/approach to life). She teaches in Germany and Austria and takes students regularly for retreats to the Greek island of Paros.

ch.stelzer@gmx.net

www.schule-der-bewegung.net

4. AMERTA AND TIBETAN BUDDHISM

Beyond the Cushion

Monika Förster (Germany/Holland)

It had been a particularly foggy day up on Mount Lawu, where we had gone to practice in Candi Sukuh. With its ornate reliefs and giant stone turtles surrounded by enormous trees, this fertility temple from the 15th or 16th century – its origins remain obscure – is often said to resemble a Mayan structure, plunked down near Solo, Indonesia. There were about a dozen of us students, and the day had brought exertion, exposure... revelation and joy.

That night, during our after-dinner reflection session, I asked Prapto a direct question, but he replied with an observation that has remained with me ever since:

"Very good, you didn't hit yourself with your own mind. That's very hard work. Good luck with it..."

At that moment I realized how – and to what degree – I was constantly judging, evaluating and criticizing myself. It was a realization that brought many tears, and, ultimately, gratefully, a dawning capacity for compassion for myself.

I soon realized that the evening had not freed me from my demons. But through continuing practice I experienced wonderful moments where my mind was at ease, and the beauty of the world spoke to me... The absence of inner struggle was a vast relief.

This is a typical snapshot/example of working with Prapto. Beyond his actual practices and methods, and perhaps more important than them, Prapto establishes a kind of general ambiance for teaching Amerta Movement. I liken it to his rolling out a 'mind carpet' upon which we can all move, learn and interact. The atmosphere is filled with the strength, calmness and quality of his mind – a precious state of pure awareness that accepts (without judging and without attaching) all that comes to consciousness: sense perceptions, thoughts, memories, emotions, all you see, all you hear, all you... everything. Dwelling in this atmosphere, his attitude is contagious; after some time my own mind also became less agitated.

When working with Prapto, the atmosphere allowed me to play, to rest, to explore, to grow, to touch, to be touched, to cry, to listen, to stop, to relax... Memories and emotions often appeared from the well of consciousness; the monsters from the cupboard showed their faces. But supported by Prapto's non-judgmental atmosphere, I was able to let this happen and stay present in the moment, savoring the breezes touching my skin, admiring the colors of the wild Indonesian flowers, relishing the sweet, thick, tropical air. It turned memories that normally overwhelmed me into memories that are just memories. It was deeply healing.

Back Home

When I returned to Amsterdam four months later I, perhaps inevitably, longed for the feelings of being at peace with myself that I had known while working with Prapto. But this was accompanied by the painful insight that it would be nearly impossible for me to return to this way of being at ease without Prapto's support.

I started to search, and eventually found a path – Tibetan Buddhism. In particular, the books of Trungpa Rinpoche and of the great American Buddhist Pema Chödron helped me to understand the processes that Prapto had been guiding me through. Thereafter, through a deep engagement with meditation, my mind started to become more spacious and less judgmental – just what I was looking for. It was both a continuation and development of what I had started to experience with Prapto at Candi Sukuh.

Mind as an Ally?

For me, meditation is a means of "turning my mind into an ally" (as Sakyong Mipham Rinpoche puts it.). In my early meditation practice, I discovered that I couldn't just tell my mind: "Quieten down!" But through recognizing my thinking as thinking, and by simply returning to my own breath, meditation gave me a wonderful opportunity to understand my mind's processes – how emotions and thoughts constantly arise and tickle each other. When approached non-judgmentally, with lots of compassion for oneself, one sees that all of this – the returning thoughts, the repeating patterns of response, the disruptive emotions – is just the dance of the mind. Returning to the simple rhythms of the breath lets us dis-identify with the mind's automatic activity and understand that we are not solely our emotions.

Much the same evolution occurs in Amerta Movement. When we move while remaining in tune with the wisdom of our body, we practice staying present with every sense: with all we hear, all we smell, all we touch and see. At the same time, we also listen to our inner weather report, all those thoughts, emotions, and memories that arise from consciousness.

One part of our movement practice is what Prapto calls *finding proportion*: using the entirety of the body to receive and embody whatever arises in consciousness. This includes all the thoughts, fears, emotions, and perceptions of both the outer and the inner worlds, really everything that we experience. We stay present in our bodies, sometimes expressing, sometimes just listening; and through this, we develop the priceless ability to engage with, in productive ways, whatever presents itself. We're less overwhelmed by all the inputs, promptings, emotions, and demons that dwell in our storebox. And this, in turn, helps reduce the sense – and feeling – that we are victims of our own mind.

Vividly I remember working individually with Prapto one evening after practicing all day at Borobudur, the wonderful huge Buddhist temple. I had been feeling pretty stuck in emotional turmoil for some days, and I had tried everything to get back into my comfort zone, but nothing seemed to work…

…until quite surprisingly I found myself running through the *pendopo* like a bull, using my hands as my horns and with Prapto as my matador.

As funny as it was in its theatrical appearance – the group witnessing burst into laughter – it gave me a strong insight into my way of dealing with difficult emotions: push, push, push!

After some more rounds of crying and laughing while chasing after Prapto, I went out into the garden, moving and singing – letting my tears be washed off by the warm tropical rain.

Letting my 'bull-ness' be seen fully, by myself and the others, was as painful as it was sweet. It helped me enormously to find more gentleness towards myself.

Bowing Towards Daily Life

Amerta Movement starts from the attitude of bowing towards our daily life.

Many spiritual paths start from the idea of retreating from the world to achieve enlightenment.

In Amerta Movement all aspects of our life/experience are welcome.

Many of us have developed habits of forgetting about ourselves in order to adapt and function in our families and in the social situations of our upbringing. Often we apply more or less fixed strategies, patterns of thoughts, and behavior to our life situation. Although these strategies were often functional and even necessary then, now they limit our possibilities of relating to the world as well as relating to our own experience. In practicing Amerta, we not only start to see our patterns, but also have an opportunity to relate in new ways. Moving with each other we can experiment with attitudes/patterns of movement different to those well known to us from our youth.

Staying present, or, if we get lost, just coming back to ourselves, reconnecting with our inner world, we practice perceiving all the different layers of the inner or outer world while being involved in it.

At Candi Sukuh, because the temple has a strong mystical atmosphere, we can easily be absorbed by its energy. In our movement practice up there we were *"building our own place"* by putting down four stones and creating a square on the ground. Again and again we would study the composition, letting our body be informed by it, finding our physical proportion…

After some time of doing the exercise in a physical way I had to face my inability to rest in my own atmosphere, to feel at home on that square meter. Puh! that was so confronting – my 'home' felt deserted and shallow. Jealously I looked at the other students who seemed to be so happy, decorating their 'homes' with leaves and flowers, singing and celebrating their at-homeness. I still remember exactly the first moment of feeling at peace there between my four stones.

My gradually growing capacity to 'stand on my own ground' changed my ability to relate to the other students, to the temple and to the situations of my life in general. Back in Amsterdam I renovated my flat and transformed it into a real home, from where I could move into the world with a sense of having an anchor…

These days I still practice grounding myself through receiving the composition when I feel I have become absorbed by the situations of my daily life. For example: sitting in a team meeting or even in a café, I change the composition by moving the tea cup, lining up the spoon with the table corner, organizing pen and paper. Creating more context allows me to stay embodied throughout situations which would otherwise mentally or emotionally absorb me.

The Blessing of Being Seen

One important aspect of Amerta Movement is the function of the witnesses. Not always, but very often, we practice in smaller groups with the others and Prapto witnessing the practice. This adds another level of awareness to our practice. In being witnessed with kindness we feel seen and heard, we can feel touched and understood.

It also adds a level of understanding to our practice, as we become more aware of our patterns and potentials; for example, sometimes we might be lost in thought… we might be sad or happy or bored… we might do anything to jump out of our experience in order to avoid ourselves. We might be in contact with ourselves, the others, the elements… sometimes we might 'just be' (that is to say we might just be simply present with what is).

Allowing ourselves to be seen helps us to become aware of this whole dance of states, activities, thoughts, and emotions. In time we develop our own friendly witness, which stays with us through the trials and tribulations, the joys and difficulties of our daily lives. Our friendly witness helps us to just perceive what is going on, instead of constantly trying to manipulate our experience. At times this might include having to see that we don't like our experience. Slowly we engage less with acting out or ignoring what's going on.

This attitude helps our process towards crystallization: we learn to bear the knowledge that we are who we are, accepting our shadow and our beauty. At times when strong emotions come up, we witness ourselves in fully feeling them – without having to change anything or find a solution, and without being overwhelmed – we just continue moving and receiving our emotions. Instead of repeating catharsis we can find the door that leads towards a new way of being.

In essence, Amerta Movement is a practice of realization and creativity in daily life.

How to Give Awareness Without Creating Stagnation

For me, and I guess for many others, it is not easy to stay embodied on the meditation cushion. If we don't want to experience our emotions fully, we tend to 'shut down' the connection with our body. Our breathing becomes shallow, our body tenses and our experience becomes less immediate.

In actively integrating my body in Amerta Movement, I experience much less physical stagnation; sometimes inviting expression helps me to get moving again.

In my movement practice I noticed that there was a stream of cultivating awareness through many wonderful techniques: line and point, zooming, naming, three dimensions, body has volume, finding proportion… After being involved in these practices for some time, they often started to feel stale; as if my soul, my emotions had no being; a sort of stagnation of consciousness itself which can happen if we try to hold ourselves too tightly in being aware. Answering my question about this Prapto said:

> *"It is very difficult to teach awareness without giving stagnation."*

My impression is that Prapto invites expression when he feels somebody or the general atmosphere is starting to stagnate. He might say *"find your mouth of movement"* or *"all your body has face."* Often the music he is making supports us in staying out of stagnation within the flow of embodied consciousness.

In my daily practice of meditation – and elsewhere – I often feel and respond to this sense of stagnation and a lack of being witnessed from the outside. In response, I have started to work more and more with my voice. It seems to bridge the gap.

The practice of sounding

In my meditation practice, sometimes I feel less connected with my body or my mind becomes over-active. Often, unseen and unfelt emotions churn beneath this restless mind. At these times, I make vocal sounds to allow me to connect with my inner atmosphere. They can be any sounds at all – gurgling, whining, whispering, humming – or it can just be an out-breath and a well-placed sigh. There's no need to sing a song or construct a melody; each out-breath brings its own music, and I simply let these songs come into being. This free issuing of sound prevents my mind from describing or categorizing my state; I don't fix myself as being sad, angry, happy, or anything else, and so stay open to the further free expression of my soul. Each breath is a new experience and a new allowing, each capable of opening new windows. The 'autopilot' button has not been pressed.

One technique that supports me in this process is to count my out-breaths; usually I go to 108. Regardless of the number, I am frequently – and delightfully – surprised by the range and variety of moods that I make. Furthermore, I am now witnessing myself in the process of making them, providing another and deeper access route towards all the many things I want, and need, to be aware of.

In practicing and teaching Amerta Movement I often work with sound and movement. I invite myself or my students to move and, at the same time, to find sound.

> "…if I move, my body still has sound
>
> …if I make sound, my sound still has body."

It is not that we have to be full-on singing and full-on moving – although that might happen at times. It is particularly the shifting of the focus that helps me to stay present. When we sound, our emotions might take over and we might get lost in them; reminding ourselves to invite our physical bodies in and becoming aware of our senses can bring us back to the present moment. Having our focus on moving and on our perception of sensations, we might lose the connection to our inner world; reminding ourselves that our body has sound reconnects us with our inner 'weather report.'

In Amerta Movement we practice being out in the world and at the same time staying connected with the inner world of perceptions, thoughts and emotions. We learn how to stay more embodied.

In allowing ourselves to be seen, our capacity for witnessing ourselves in a friendly way grows. Speaking with the words of the Sufi tradition, Amerta Movement is a path to learn how "to be in the world but not 'of' it."

Epilogue

Now, in 2013, back at Candi Sukuh again after more than 20 years I can clearly see how Amerta and meditation helped me to find more friendliness and generosity towards myself. Meditation helped me to settle my mind, Amerta kept me from mis-using meditation to suppress emotions; both deeply changed the way I am able to relate to the world and myself. This makes it easier to look further into my patterns and understand them. Instead of judging myself for having those patterns, I am able to experiment with finding new ways of relating – be it towards myself or towards the outside world.

Staying more embodied, my mind is less hyperactive and my emotions have more ground. Though not less intense, I don't experience them as frightening or overwhelming any more. Being more at ease with myself and the world allows my body to relax and my senses to wake up. The dance of life, with all its beauties and difficulties, becomes more spacious, light, and joyous.

~ ~ ~

Monika Förster graduated with a Performance Art degree in New Dance from the Amsterdam Hogeschool van de Kunsten. She has taught movement at the Amsterdam and Utrecht Theater Schools and teaches at the Schule der Bewegung in Germany. Since 1991, Monika has studied regularly with Prapto in Europe and Java. She has hosted his workshops in Amsterdam for 11 years, including the 11th International Movement Arts Meeting in Amsterdam in 2015. Monika is a practicing Buddhist, studies with the Ridhwan School and is a Shiatsu therapist and teacher. Monika's life's work encourages physical awareness, creative expression and body-mind integration.

monikaforster@dds.nl

www.shiatsudansamsterdam.nl

5. THE EYE OF THE HAND

Embodied Filmmaking as Movement Practice

Steve Hopkins (UK)

"Me, it's not movement first." (Prapto)[1]

Although not as troublingly early as the first sit of the day at a Zen sesshin, it's still cold enough for the morning chill to need blunting by a fire. I pile kindling and logs in the fireplace, enough to warm the cavernous shell of the huge old hall. Soon, Prapto and sleepy workshop participants arrive in ones and twos. We sit in two rows, facing one another, on rugs, cushions and chairs, settling into the quiet, still morning. Breath and blood, bone and mind, muscle and flesh; from the smallest cells of the body: "resting/inter-resting", as Prapto puts it. It all starts here.

Over the next five days or so the 3m group – Prapto's name for the meditation, movement and movie groups that have been a part of some of his workshops for the past ten years or so – will explore, express and re-view movement practice on film.[2] At the close of the workshop, we will show their film. But the aim of the 3m group is not to produce a beautiful film – though that may happen – because embodied film is a practice, rather than a product. And although I can draw upon a lifetime's professional engagement with documentary, no prior experience of filmmaking is necessary:

---

[1] All quotations from Prapto, unless otherwise indicated, are from unpublished transcripts of a series of interviews Prapto gave me for *Human Nature Spirit*, a film shot at a workshop held at La Bartra, Spain, in September 2011.

[2] For ease of use, here and throughout I generally use the word 'film' when talking about moving pictures, regardless of the medium on which they were recorded.

embodied film is a matter of attention, attitude and engagement – where you are coming from – rather than technology or technique. It begins with sitting. As Vivian Sobchack (1992) observes, "Embodied perception, whether cinematic or human, is not lived theoretically".

Accordingly, this account's point of departure is, as film critic and screenwriter Yvette Biro puts it, "the function of the film as it has proved itself in practice, and not in the wishes and aspirations of theoreticians" (1992). Like Prapto, it seeks to stay rooted and to journey out, acknowledging "the primacy of the body, not the primacy of perception" (Gendlin 1992), and along the way to provide some answer to Laura Marks's question, "if there is a return to the precious knowledge of the body and the senses, what is that knowledge to be used for?" (2004).

Opening Sequence: The Empty Axis

> *"How can we still listen of nature? How I can also be seen, or the nature see, or speak to me, or touch me, smell me, taste me? Not only I sensing of them, but the nature sensing of me, and my body sensory, or sensing, touch me, not only I touch the sensory or sensing of nature?"* (Prapto)

Touching and being touched; seeing and being seen; hearing and being heard; in an image- and information-soaked culture, the questions Prapto asks himself about openness, receptivity and communication are as important for the 3m groups as they are for him.

Whether experienced movie makers or not, in a digital age we all come with a sophisticated understanding of the image; but the image is only the skin of embodied film. The body of practice lies beneath. To open to it, and to be opened by it, one needs to let go of preconceptions about film, image and story, and sink beneath the surface, in much the same way that meditation enables one to sink beneath other surfaces.

This isn't about the truth claims of photography, its power to shock, or whether film or video or digital images more closely reflect reality, though all of those debates can be had; it's about what avant-garde filmmaker Stan Brakhage put this way:

> "Imagine an eye unruled by man-made laws of perspective, an eye unprejudiced by compositional logic, an eye which does not respond to the name of every-thing but which must know each object encountered in

life through an adventure of perception... Imagine a world alive with incomprehensible objects and shimmering with an endless variety of movement and innumerable gradations of color. Imagine a world before the 'beginning was the word'" (1963).

It's an invitation to a radical openness beyond concerns with narrative, documentary accuracy or realism, in and through which movement practice can be explored and expressed. Today, cheap digital cameras and iPhones have liberated the eye in ways Brakhage could scarcely have imagined, but the new possibilities they raise come with new dangers. Movement practice grounds embodied film, shifting its focus from the eye and head to the body and limbs, toward what David Abram calls a "thinking with the body", the distributed sentience he identifies in a bird in flight (2010). It requires the kind of embodied connectedness that Helen Poynor, writing about Prapto's work in 1986, describes:

> "The body is seen as the central point where the vertical and horizontal planes meet. The vertical axis represents spirituality, our relationship to God, the cosmos and the underworld. The horizontal axis represents daily life and communications...we are reminded to keep connection with this central point, with our body on the earth in the here and now..." (1986)

Prapto sometimes refers to that central point as *the empty axis*. More a state of being than a physical place, its emptiness is characterised by that deep connectedness to the natural world which has led some to describe him as a modern day shaman. It's not an inappropriate description: the radical openness and reframing implied by shamanism, challenges habituated responses and ways of seeing.

In the same way that photography's new way of seeing at the end of the nineteenth century led to a letting go of some deeply held visual preconceptions, and at the end of the twentieth century digital cameras invited us to continue that journey, for filmmakers Prapto's *empty axis* suggests a letting go on both physical and cultural levels, with many implications for narrative and structure, the physical use of the body in filming, and the place of mind.[3] Together, these require a

---

[3] Nuanced discussions of what 'physical and cultural letting go' implies can be found in Pitty (2005), Reeve (2011), and, in specifically Javanese terms, Hughes-Freeland (2008, 21). A radical perspective, going beyond the human to embrace animals and spirits, can be found in Vilaça (2005).

radical openness that remains physically connected but is not seduced by the visual sense or intellectualised. Prapto's suggestion as to how we might begin to realise this is quite simple:

> *"You know this concept? Resting, re-lease, inter-resting? I am resting. They are resting. I will develop from the earth, lying, sitting, crawling on the earth, create the wind."*

The Frame: Moving in Not Moving

> *It is late in the afternoon by the time the 3m group makes its way out of the house and across the fields. A few hundred metres along the higher path, we stop. This will do. From here, the fields fall away in wide, curved terraces toward the valley. Wooded hills rise on either side, and in the distance La Garrotxa's mountains shimmer in the heat. I set the camera up, pointing it more or less at random across the fields, and flip open the monitor.*

"Where there is attention, reality is." (Krishnamurti)

The frame is about attention, focus and boundary. The body is a frame. The mind is a frame. The bodymind... What is contained within the frame, and how we view it, is the subject of much writing about film[4]; how it is achieved technically, the subject of much writing about cinematography; and the concepts involved much discussed in media and cultural studies. But as we study the monitor, none of these much concern the 3m group. A busy, strenuous, physical day behind them, they settle slowly.

Prapto sometimes begins to work with *frame as window* at a very simple physical level. Melinda Buckwalter describes such a session:

> "Prapto asks his students to use their arms to make windows to look through by opening and closing the shoulder, elbow, wrist, and finger joints as they move in space. Later the legs, the back, and the whole body are included in the activity. The windows open and close as the body moves, giving different views." (2010)

Before walking out across the fields the 3m group had begun to work with frame by using metre-long lengths of strong blue nylon cord. If you try to hold it up, the cord routinely frustrates any attempt to

---

4 E.g., 'Cinema as Window and Frame' in Elsaesser & Hagener (2010, 13-34).

create a static frame. Letting it – and preconceptions about frame – go produces quite different results. New frames emerge, boundaries are re-defined, bodies, and minds, relax.

Although the frame in our camera is far more rigidly defined, its 4:3 aspect ratio reflects the visual angle of human eyesight. As the film group contemplates the view it presents of the landscape, questions arise as new perceptions form. Had I deliberately sought to create this picture? No, not really. Then, as attention settles, a more subtle awareness of what is happening within the frame emerges: changing light, wind in the trees, people moving through the frame: arising, abiding and passing away.

As the group quietens, stillness deepens and other senses come to the fore: hearing seems more subtle and acute, birdsong and distant voices come into focus, we feel the heat on our skin. Some say that meditation has its roots in the quiet gaze into the fire in the cave, or in the kind of focused awareness, stillness and patience of the hunter on the plain, sitting quietly and watching as we are. We shift our weight, move around the camera, look out, beyond and around the frame. There's no attempt to move the camera, but any attempt to change the frame – perhaps to zoom in or out – immediately reveals the state of the body, illustrating, as Vivian Sobchack puts it, how "the art of seeing is entwined intimately with the act of being" (1992).

In both still and movie photography, digital cameras, iPhones and many other devices have radically changed the relationship of the body, and especially the eyes, to the frame. Liberated from the viewfinder, it's common for movers to use cameras and frames in increasingly free ways, responding, expressing and following – embodying, in fact – their movement, reconnecting us with a truth that Xenophanes, one of the very earliest Greek philosophers, understood: "it is the whole that sees, the whole that thinks, the whole that hears" (Ihde, 1976: 8-9).

Dusk begins to settle. We fold the viewfinder, pack up the camera and walk back to the house. Freeze frame. As at the end of *Butch Cassidy and the Sundance Kid*, we leave the scene with one image. It's another illusion. Even as the frame on the screen freezes, the film still runs through the projector, and our thoughts run wide: *moving in not moving*.[5]

---

[5] For Prapto's own use of these terms, in diagrammatic form, see 'The Idea of Joged Amerta' (Suryodarmo 2013).

The Shot: Moving in Moving

The 3m group assembles on the steps of an old Victorian hall in the English countryside. Few have much, if any, experience of movie making. Each person will take the camera, shoot whatever they want for a minute, and hand it back to me. I then shoot something and pass it to the next person, and so on. All of this loosely framed by a walk down the long, tree-lined drive that runs from the house to the road. It's a ragged journey. Some take the camera and describe what they are shooting as if in a documentary, others move around, shooting trees, sky, leaves and track, some frame the journey as if we were in a road movie. At the close we have about thirty minutes of footage – Tim Ingold, theorist of lines, might call it 'the alongly integrated knowledge of the wayfarers' (2011).

"The shot is the movement-image." (Gilles Deleuze)

If the frame in some way holds or defines the contemplative space of the film, the porous and shifting boundary between frame and action – mover and movement – is the shot. It reflects both what occurs in movement and is in and of itself movement: it has direction, angle, attitude, duration and revelation. The moment when the camera and its operator move, reveals both the physical and the mental state of the mover, where attention is, and where and how the body is: the embodied reality. If axis and frame ask questions about who we are, where we are coming from, and from where we look, the shot invites us to find answers in movement, and, especially when we take the camera in hand, reveals them to us. As Alva Noë says, "Perception is not something that happens to us. It is something that we do" (2004).

At the start of the walk, the nervousness of those of the 3m group who had never handled a movie camera before was palpable. Despite its ease of use, their shots were hesitant, jagged and uncertain. Prapto has sometimes said his practice arises "from the Buddha walking, rather than from the Buddha sitting" (Reeve 2009). As the 3m group walk down the track and let go of what they thought they should do, an ease and fluidity begin to emerge: a meditation that puts them into the stream.

The shot itself – its physicality, duration, staying and letting go, and the sense of what is happening outside the camera – intimately involves breath, touch, posture, attention and sensitivity. As they move down the track, the 3m group also come to understand something about moving in and moving through, and how the difference between observing or participating changes one's relationship to the world. 'Holding that shot' becomes, to use Prapto's words, an exercise in *active/passive*.

The end of a shot – and the end of the shoot – represents a closing with the world through which embodied information about posture, relaxation and attention is revealed: the world, of course, goes on. Back in our bodies, and at the bottom of the track, we turn back toward the house, noticing the difference.

The shot is: *moving in moving.*

Editing: Finding Your Stopping

"Prapto says 'composing while dancing' is like recognizing ourselves in the dancing. 'Find your stoppings!,' he reminds us, 'then you can recognize your composition.'"
Melinda Buckwalter (2010)

I am sitting in my office, listening intently to Prapto – is that 'axis,' or 'access', or 'excess' – as he moves through a fast running Spanish river, trying to edit video shot more than six months before. The sound of the river rises and finally drowns out his words. I get up, go outside, reconnect with trees and my own riverbank, then email Paul, my editor – who is either 200 or 4,000 miles away – and get better versions of the sound files sent from Devon. I send Paul marked up transcripts, he sends back cut sequences. It's always a startlingly revelatory, emotional process, this letting go and reformulating. From the confusion and incoherence of hours of footage something that works begins to emerge, flickering across the computer screen.

As John Cage said, "we really need a structure, so we can see we are nowhere."

Editing is as much a letting go as a putting together. It begins not just after you've stopped recording, but at the very beginning, from the first moment the idea of a film arises. The stopping of editing, in Prapto's words, is an opportunity to *recognise your composition*. And although it might seem to represent a big step away from the embodied experience of filming toward the disembodied manipulation of information, it is increasingly recognised that abstract and decontextualised thought is both rooted in and grows out of embodied cognition.⁶ Artists have long been ahead of this curve: "thinking" as Bill Viola puts it, "is a form of movement... art itself has always been a whole body experience" (1995).

Experimental filmmaker Maya Deren's notebook reflects her own more visceral take on the embodied realities of film editing in the mechanical, celluloid age:

> "The minute I began to put the Balinese footage
> through the viewer, the fever began... The immediate
> physical contact with the film, the nearness of the image
> – the fact that as I wound, my impulses and reactions
> towards the film translated themselves into muscular
> impulses and so to the film directly... All this seemed
> for me very important... this physical contact creates a
> sense of intimacy... (the film) is not an
> image independent of me, of which I am a spectator....
> It comes to life out of the energy of my muscles... this
> ultimate copulation between me and the film must take
> place, and out of it will be born the independent child..."
> (1947)

Deren's physicality is echoed elsewhere. Bergman said that film is "inhalation and exhalation in continuous sequence"; Eisenstein, that "montage is the nerve of the cinema"; Bresson, that "film is born three times": film's body has a history as long as the medium. And though it is sometimes argued that video and digital have lessened or damaged the physical and artistic relationship of editor to image, emotional, felt responses remain fundamental to the process whatever medium is used.

Emotion, like much else in editing, is often thought of in pictorial terms, but it is at least as strongly triggered by sound. And here editing returns us to an often overlooked aspect of Prapto's work: his purposive use of sound. Prapto commonly sings, chants and drums in workshops and performance, and that carries with it a psychophysical charge.⁷ For all that film is a visual medium, the brain is said to

---

6 See, for example, Wilson (1997).

7 Prapto's use of sound is too complex a subject to be gone into in any detail here, embracing as it does the sacred traditions of Hindu chant, Buddhist mantra, and drumming that both echoes the gamelan and sometimes carries with it a shamanic force. He often asks that 'Someone to Play' be invited to his workshops, and has worked extensively with musicians. Elsewhere in this volume, Tim Jones and Sean Williams discuss examples of his practice.

process sounds a thousand times faster than images, and register sound even while we are asleep. In the womb, it is one of the first of our senses to be switched on, but at birth, as Walter Murch, who has won Oscars for both picture and sound editing, poetically puts it, "sound pulls a veil of oblivion across her reign and withdraws into the shadows" (2000). For 3m groups, whose access to editing is usually constrained by time and technology, the truth of Murch's observation that "King Sight still sits on his throne (whilst) Queen Sound haunts the corridors of the palace", is usually brought home by the often startling consequences of adding music to the films they have shot.

With Prapto's words, and the sounds of the river, ringing in my ears, a structure emerges. His observation that in "Western culture they have more linear time... I really had culture shock with that" (Morgan 2011) now somehow seems in unexpected agreement with Jean-Luc Godard's, that "a story should have a beginning, a middle and an end, but not necessarily in that order" (Grøngaard 2001).

Endings: Blossoming in the Blessing

> "As soon as we see other seers... henceforth, through other eyes we are for ourselves fully visible... For the first time, the seeing that I am is for me really visible; for the first time I appear to myself completely turned inside out under my own eyes." Maurice Merleau-Ponty, *The Visible and the Invisible*[8]

> *I am sitting in a large hall with the 3m group at the end of a movement workshop. Roughly projected on a big, drop-down screen, the movie they have made unwinds before us. For most, it is the first time they have seen themselves in a film, let alone one they have made. Around us, another audience – the rest of the workshop – is gathered. I'm nervous that they won't like the result, be bored or offended, but there's no reason to be. As the movie plays out, gasps, sighs, laughter, shy looking away and, finally, applause. Just like it always is at the movies. "Films", as Truffaut put it, "resemble the people who make them."*

Whether viewed intimately and informally on an iPhone, or publicly in a cinema, film's intimate disclosing and sharing with an audience

---

8 Quoted in Sobchack (2004, 149).

of self and others is anything from as odd and subtle as catching a glimpse of yourself in a mirror to a transformative engagement. Laura Marks calls it 'embodied contemplation', and talks of 'haptic visuality': "a way of seeing and knowing which calls upon multiple senses without depending upon the presence of literal touch, smell or taste" (2000). Neurobiologists tell us mirror neurons show that the process is embodied. Vivian Sobchack writes that "the moving picture is a visible representation not of activity finished or past, but of activity coming into being and being... the very moment of vision itself" (2004).

However framed, viewing is a deeply embodied response. It also allows us, as Sharon Salzberg says of mindfulness, "to get better at seeing the difference between what's happening and the stories we tell ourselves about what's happening" (2010). In Prapto's terms, film allows us to inhabit *"the space between the wind".*

In *True Perception: The Path of Dharma Art*, Chögyam Trungpa writes that "the basic problem in artistic endeavor is the tendency to split the artist from the audience and then try to send a message from one to the other. When this happens, art becomes exhibitionism... In meditative art, the artist embodies the viewer as well as the creator of the works. Vision is not separate from operation, and there is no fear of being clumsy or failing to achieve his aspiration" (2008). In the end, embodied filmmaking is not about doing something, or about being something: it is about being. As Prapto says: *"So I think the main how to be enjoy pleasure, perceiving, breathing, melody, rhythm. Blossoming in the blessing."*

~ ~ ~

References

Abram, D. (2010) *Becoming Animal: An Earthly Cosmology*, Pantheon

Biro, Y. (1992) *Profane Mythology: The Savage Mind of the Cinema*, Indiana University Press

Brakhage, S. (1963) Metaphors on Vision, *Film Culture*, No.30, unpaginated; extracts available http://bit.ly/ELtp01

Buckwalter, M. (2010) *Composing While Dancing: An Improviser's Companion*, University of Wisconsin Press

Deleuze, G. (1986) *Cinema 1: The Movement Image*, Trans. H. Tomlinson and B. Habberjam. University of Minnesota Press

Deren, M. (1947) Notebook, February 16, 1947, published in *October*, Vol. 14, (Autumn, 1980), pp.21-46; preview online http://bit.ly/ELtp02

Elsaesser, T. & Hagener, M. (2010) *Film Theory: An Introduction Through The Senses*, Routledge

Gendlin, E.T. (1992) The primacy of the body, not the primacy of perception [Excerpt from pages 343-353, slightly revised]. *Man and World*, 25(3-4), 341-353. Online at http://bit.ly/ELtp03

Grøngaard, P. (2001) 'For Ever Godard. Two or three things I know about European and American Cinema,' p.o.v. 12, online at http://bit.ly/ELtp04

Hughes-Freeland, F. (2008) *Embodied Communities: Dance Traditions and Change in Java*, Berghahn Books

Ihde, D. (1976) *Listening and Voice: A Phenomenology of Sound*, Ohio University Press

Ingold, T. (2011) *Being Alive: Essays on Movement, Knowledge and Description*, Routledge

Marks, Laura U. (2000) *The Skin of the Film – Intercultural Cinema, Embodiment, and the Senses*, Duke University Press; quoted in Ilona Hongisto, 'Towards Embodied Knowledge?', Wider Screen 2/2004, online at http://bit.ly/ELtp05

Marks, Laura U. (2004) Haptic Visuality: Touching With the Eyes, *Framework: The Finnish Art Review*, No 2, pp 78-82; online at: http://bit.ly/ELtp06

Morgan, K. T. (ed.) (2011) An Improvised Conversation with Bonnie Bainbridge Cohen and Suprapto Suryodarmo, 26th Annual Body-Mind Centering Association Conference, online at: http://bit.ly/ELtp07

Murch, W. (2000) Stretching Sound to Help the Mind See, FilmSound.org, online at http://bit.ly/ELtp08

Noë, A. (2004) *Action in Perception*, The MIT Press

Pitty, A. (2005) *Rituals of Chaos*, online at http://bit.ly/ELtp09

Poynor, H. (1986) 'The Walk of Life', quoted in Stange, P. 'Silences in Solonese Dance Production', *Southeast Asian Journal of Social Science*, vol 22 (1994), p 220

Reeve, S. (2009) *The Ecological Body*, PhD thesis, University of Exeter, extracts online at http://bit.ly/ELtp10

Reeve, S. (2011) *Nine Ways of Seeing A Body*, Triarchy Press

Salzberg, S. (2010) *Real Happiness: The Power of Meditation*, Workman

Sobchack, V. (1992) *The Address of the Eye: A Phenomenology of Film Experience*, Princeton University Press

Sobchack, V. (2004) *Carnal Thoughts: Embodiment and Moving Image Culture*, University of California Press

Suryodarmo, S. (2013). 'The Idea of Joged Amerta', online at http://bit.ly/ELtp11

Trungpa, C. (2008) *True Perception, The Path of Dharma Art*, Shambhala

Vilaça, A. (2005) 'Chronically Unstable Bodies: Reflections on Amazonian Corporalities', *Journal of the Royal Anthropological Institute*, vol. 11, no. 3, September, pp.445-464

Viola, B. (1995) *Reasons for Knocking at an Empty House*, Thames and Hudson

Wilson, M. (2008) 'How did we get from there to here? An evolutionary perspective on embodied cognition', in Calvo, P. & Gomila, T. (eds.) *Directions for an Embodied Cognitive Science: Towards an Integrated Approach*, Elsevier. Online at http://bit.ly/ELtp12

Steve Hopkins has worked with Prapto for around 20 years. He has organised movement workshops in the UK and Spain, and is a recognised teacher. He has also studied Tai chi, meditation and Zen brushwork, and works as a professional documentary maker, mainly in television. His love affair with the movies began at a matinee screening of *20,000 Leagues Under the Sea* at the Uxbridge Odeon and has continued ever since. He made *Human Nature Spirit*, a film with Prapto, in Spain in 2011.

stephen.hopkins198@btinternet.com

6. A DOG PRACTICING 'TALKING BODY'

José Mulder van de Graaf (Bolivia)

While our puppy Princesa was growing up, she behaved like other dogs, but later, as she began getting closer to us, she developed astonishing peculiarities in her way of adapting to human circumstances. Her amazing way of taking part in the movement practice of 'Talking Body' is an anecdote worth telling.

Princesa jumped into the car whenever I traveled to Santa Cruz to teach at the Art School. There she was not only present at the Anthropology and the Pre-Hispanic Art classes, mostly sitting on a chair like the students, but was actively involved in the 'Talking Body' workshops I used to offer to them as well. I will include in this peculiar story reflections about my practice, which is based on how I understood Amerta Movement, which I had the opportunity to learn in Indonesia under the guidance of Prapto about 24 years ago.

I met Prapto at a time when I was involved with shamanism and studying methods to achieve extra-sensorial perceptions and altered states of consciousness. My research included body and movement-centred methods like Gurdjieff's sacred dance, but also Asian methods that I felt would give a disciplining frame for me, such as yoga and Tai chi. Later I came into contact with Amerta Movement, the method created by Prapto with a strong background in Buddhism and traditional Javanese culture. This attracted my special interest as a method that seemingly did fit me best. I was amazed by the practice, because both sources, the inner feeling and the outer reading that I practiced as a child – a story I will tell in the next section – could be embodied and expressed while we move in the way it is meant in this practice: with absolute freedom of action, not performing defined movement patterns or structures, not applying pre-determined rhythms and developing a priori postures or attitudes that we supposedly 'should' achieve.

~ ~ ~

As a young boy I lived for part of the year in the southern Andean countryside of Bolivia, where my father used to work as an engineer for the state mining company. I loved to walk around these places with my father's dogs, across nearby slopes and through the valleys, often spending the whole day and even the night with my animal companions. At the age of twelve, while traveling along a newly made road with my father driving the car, we found ceramics and bones spread on the ground. My father was sure that this place was an ancient Indian burial ground that was actually being destroyed by the bulldozer as it removed the earth. He encouraged me to start digging the next day to save what was left in the partially-destroyed graveyards. This event marked the beginning of a fascination of mine for old Indian settlements, for doing my rounds looking for items that once belonged to people of ancient cultures, for going on foot through the Andean landscape in search of ritual sites and graveyards. 'Reading' the landscape, as I would today call what I started doing, became a big passion to me, as well as a skill that I needed to continue exploring. An outcome of these experiences was my interest in archeology and a large collection of ceramics and other items: skulls, toys for children made out of clay, etc., which I later handed over to the national museum. The passion of my childhood changed later into an interest in ethnological topics, anthropology, shamanism, and so on, and was finally the power within that gave me the impulse to get to know Amerta Movement and meet Prapto.

Princesa's behavior used to leave everybody astonished. Almost as soon as a 'Talking Body' practice had started, she would begin to 'perform' naturally and easily; she walked smoothly through the midst of the participants, lay down on the floor, sat down and stood up again. Everything she did was done in harmony with the movement done by the people performing 'following the line of the movement' – this is an important part of the practice in which the mover comprehends a dynamic balancing of the body through space and time in accordance with his feelings, his personal needs, and the requirements of the group that is practicing. The body positions that Princesa assumed were of course ones that dogs are able to do, but they were remarkable because her bodily expressions would fit into the practice situation she and the students were in. She

6. A DOG PRACTICING 'TALKING BODY'

would walk from one place to another balancing and weighing the space, or would walk in between two people affecting the direction of their movement, or would influence their speed or intensity while communicating bodily with them. Her facial expressions, ear positions and her gaze used to change while she embraced physical contact, either by letting other people pet her or by being touched by accident, and she too succeeded in indicating, even with a dog's 'smile,' her satisfaction at being part of the practice situation. Remaining in the process, she often contributed actively to creating the group's next steps and managed to let the participants know that she was to be considered part of the ongoing quest to find personal and group dynamic balance in movement, just as the other participants did. The impulse for all these actions was exclusively hers; I didn't intervene in any way, neither suggesting she change her position or place, nor animating her to do this or that; there was nothing that she hadn't decided by herself.

The experiences with Princesa led me to formulate questions like: "How could a dog practice 'Talking Body' together with humans?" "Was her participation unintended and casual, or did she take part simply because she 'thought' it was clever to act similarly to the other participants, maybe hoping she would get rewarded for her smartness?"

Princesa's performance made me recognize that 'instinct' was the main trait she had for adapting to the circumstances of the practice, and that this 'instinct' is a major resource we humans also apply in doing this practice. I realized that 'instinct' could be considered a more important resource than others, like the ones we usually call awareness and consciousness and which I formerly thought of as being more relevant. Princesa's action in the 'Talking Body' sessions was the result of a dynamic condition inherent to the practice, one that enables animals and humans to better adapt to changing circumstances; this quality being to me pure instinct, which I understand to be not only an inherent behavioral action, but also an adaptation to the environment, often emerging from instantaneous impulses, regardless of whether they are a conscious adaptation or not. Consequently, the phenomenon of her participation in the practice of 'Talking Body' could be understood to be a result of nature's intelligence in its 'instinctive' manifestations, emerged from the essential consciousness all creatures have in common. It also illustrates to me that there is no need for a human intelligence or human thinking to participate in this practice, but it shows also that humans are needed to create a situation where a practice of this kind can be carried out, because it needs a special framing. Both instinct and intuition are not only manifestations of an innate intelligence, but are evolving attributes that are being developed while we practice 'Talking Body'. We can gain additional abilities when we incorporate intelligence that works not only on the rational level but also embraces our 'feeling' capability. This 'feeling' is focused on the organism itself, on the soul, and on practicing as collective involvement. The experience we share while we practice could be likened to us weaving a carpet in collaboration with other entities: with humans, animals, elements of nature, etc. None of these entities have to perceive this weaving as their 'personal' achievement; everyone participating recognizes that the weaving is a common effort, as our (individual) input into the interweaving is itself part of nature's interdependent work.

It is common sense that humans and animals differ. Animals have qualities we don't have and lack attributes humans are able to develop – for example, our reflective intelligence, our rationalizing and thinking capabilities, and our awareness and our consciousness of the self, which is the realm people try to develop by following paths of personal and spiritual growth. I am not at all sure if animals really lack the attribute considered by anthropologists to most accurately define the difference between humans and other animals: our capacity for symbolic abstraction. Nevertheless, it would be too reductionist to say that Princesa's involvement was solely a result of instinct, or intuition, without considering the quality of 'feeling' she had in common with the students. This aspect we often forget when we think about the differences and similarities among the human, animal, and plant kingdoms. Princesa clearly 'felt' a sense of belonging to the class, because she had a close affinity with the students taking part in the practice. She often would look at me as if to say: "I'm not a common dog," at least I imagined it that way, receiving her message through her body and her facial gestures. Other dogs I have had didn't behave in the same way, even though they maintained a very close relation to me as well. They didn't look forward to going to the city or to the classes, and they preferred to stay at home and spend their day hunting, behaving like dogs that live within the social characteristics of a dog pack.

6. A DOG PRACTICING 'TALKING BODY'

To develop a more accurate sense for understanding Princesa's conduct, I will introduce the concept of 'lingua franca' – used by the philosopher and biologist Andreas Weber in his book *Alles Fühlt* – which I consider to be another basic condition for practicing Amerta Movement and 'Talking Body'.

According to Weber, all creatures and all bodies on earth possess a language, the 'language of feelings.' This 'true tongue', as he calls this language as well, is considered to be always present and in continuous activity within beings and their communication systems. It is, therefore, the 'true tongue' of feelings that allows humans, animals, and plants to perceive external phenomena in a direct way, before the differentiation produced by hearing, smelling, sight, and touch start to interpret a given situation. This 'true tongue' doesn't refer to an abstract code, which spoken language can be, but rather to a direct expression of our feelings through our body, through neuronal dynamics, through excitement of the circulatory system, and through mimicry and the expression of gestures. If the heart is excited, regardless of the situation and regardless of whether it belongs to a human or an animal, even to a frog or to an insect, it will always mean that this being is excited – in a state of high emotion and emergency. Weber explains that humans and animals are able to read feelings, because there is no differentiation between external and internal feelings, they are one. The feeling being shown by a certain body is the feeling itself and not merely a symbol of it.

Our mind has the ability to deduce what we 'are supposed to do', if we want to achieve something we deserve in a certain situation. This process, which we call 'thinking', is one that we commonly carry out using our rational faculties. Our 'feeling' capacities are rarely consulted to find out what we 'are supposed to do.' We often seem to lose access to resources that are available to us besides the 'thinking' one: resources that are also capable of deducing what we should do in certain moments, while carrying out actions, and so on. From my point of view one of the main resources is the 'true tongue' mentioned above, the 'language of feelings' that enables us to understand and to express, even to enhance knowledge in another way. The 'true tongue' can also expand through the dynamics of the movement practice. Feeling and emotional qualities can increase the depth of a dialog, and the extended language can intensify the lucidity of timing while bodies meet. They can increase our abilities to listen, to smell, and to look. They can enable us to 'comprehend' the space, to 'acknowledge' nature while it constantly changes, and, last but not least, to recognize our self. A special outcome of these processes is that we become able to recognize that the motives and causes that evolve during the practice aren't 'casual.' It is rather that we humans initiate them on purpose by practicing and developing skills, by cultivating our sensitivity. This cultivating capability is a gift that humans have, one that may point to a remarkable difference between ourselves and other species.

Years ago, while practicing Amerta Movement in Indonesia, I entered into a space that was not totally unknown to me but, until this practice, had never been really filled with a bodily expression. I am referring to a 'feeling' of being profoundly touched by the impulse to pray and to its expression of gathering and folding both hands. Of course I had seen other people fold hands and I had done it myself, especially as a child, when an attitude of praying came more from a 'religious' and a 'cultural' background and not from the attitude of 'nature expressing through my body.' My body, not the mind, found the right expression for the feelings that arose in me while my body was 'following the line of the movement' of which I spoke above. This letting the self, together with the body, follow the line of the movement is to me one of the more substantial practices we do in 'Body Talking' and in Amerta Movement. It means to understand that this movement is itself 'feelings in movement,' it is also a way of 'dialoguing in feeling,' and it is 'accepting guidance that is provided by our body,' because we use our body for experiencing all of it. 'Following the line of the movement' can become a skill, one that is 'felt' and not (only) 'thought.' This skill can become an attitude supported by the laws of nature, as it is an attitude that doesn't follow moral codes or social positions that evolved in our cultural and social backgrounds, but rather follows the skill of moving the feeling-self. If we are open-minded and have an open heart, letting our feelings be fluent, our movement will be fluent as well.

As I said before, 'Talking Body' and Amerta Movement are not structured practices; unlike many other methods, there are no movement patterns. Doing the non-designed and non-arranged practice we are able to stay attuned to the needs of our bodies and attuned to the genuine emotions that arise and become integrated in our bodily expressions while shaping our movement. We follow the line of movement that is tailored by our self, according to our individual needs, according to our body's state, and according to our mental and emotional condition. Practicing it we are people seeking for 'truthfulness,' while 'truthfulness' here means authenticity, sincerity, and being steady. In this way, the practice connects to the honest and frank feelings that our hearts can create while we move. It is astonishing that all these wonders happen during the practice, way before we become mentally conscious of their existence.

Taking part in the movement workshops must have been an outstanding opportunity for Princesa to share a unique relationship with her human friends. She simply did the same things the students did when they started talking bodily to one another, moving mostly slowly, but sometimes also fast, more softly, more harmoniously, with more gentleness and care than normally. She spoke through the 'natural' language of her body, using the same language of feelings they used, not solely a language for expression, but also for receiving, for reading the laws of nature and for experiencing what nature's intelligence intends. It is to me not at all common that she, being a dog, grabbed the chance to communicate with others in this way, becoming transformed into one more student.

People know that body and verbal languages don't match in many ways, one reason being that underlying motivations and stimuli are expressed differently in each language. Another one is that the body language of 'Talking Body,' articulating through three-dimensional expressions, does not follow rational and logical structures, and as I said before, 'Talking Body' becomes a receiving and expressing organ, receiving feelings rather than rational thoughts, and it receives and expresses with the 'whole body,' without the 'filter' of reasoning. 'Talking Body' and similar practices are based on procedures in which our reasoning isn't asked to intervene because the actions are done in a pre-reflexive state of mind. There might be thinking or reasoning at times, but these won't dominate our action and will mostly arise after the practice's sequence has finished. Moving the way we move – expressing and receiving, embracing rhythms by giving continuum and fluency to our movement, actually being present with all our senses and emotions – we inevitably get ourselves into a different state of mind than the one we usually adopt in daily life. It is an altered state similar to the state of being that we access in meditation or in prayer, or even in relaxing, which is very different to the daily one and to the dynamics of verbal communication, in which the emphasis is mostly placed on the content and not on the tone, not on the cadence and not on the rhythm of our speech.

Summary and Concluding Thoughts

The practice described in this chapter can be considered one that merges into a systemic perspective of natural laws that govern life.[1]

To summarize, during the movement practice of 'Talking Body' we transmit feelings through bodily signs and gestures; we do this automatically and implicitly, not as a narration of something that did or should happen. The transfer of feelings is the language we share with all living entities. We express through it 'natural' attitudes, cultural norms, and even spiritual perceptions. All of this occurs basically through the moving body's self-organization and dynamic regulations.

We know from life praxis that not every human chooses to self-organize. Humans are free *not* to agree with self-organization of any kind, not to agree with social or cultural norms, not to agree with an attitude of conserving the planet for future generations, living peacefully and not killing each other, etc. We commonly say that these are human options due to the condition of 'free will' that supposedly characterizes the species. Therefore, 'free will' stands for an innate differentiation between humans and animals, which supposedly don't have this capability. Humans do obviously have the freedom to choose what they want to perceive or how they want to act, but the attempt to remain outside the schema of interdependence that nature provides to all entities is never really successful. It is clear that a person can never be freed from creating interdependent

---

[1] Life has given me the opportunity to watch plants and animals, earth and sun, wind and rain, to follow nature's rhythms and to share with her day-to-day life in the midst of the rainforest in the Bolivian Amazon region for the last 18 years. For this reason, even though I am not a biologist, I allowed myself to refer to biological concepts in this chapter.
The term 'systemic' concerns a view of life and natural laws, whose main argument relies on the interdependence of all phenomena. It acknowledges a single cell as the most primitive form of life, the organized bunch of them becoming an organism, then a species and in turn, an ecosystem. An ecosystem can be considered a big organism, and the global ecosystem formed by the earth is an organized, intertwined, self-organizing system.
Joachim Bauer and Andreas Weber acknowledge in their books the systemic issue for explaining nature. They inspired me by embracing views about life phenomena that rely on cooperation and resonance instead of relying on selfishness and competition.

relations with nature and society. If someone does anything against the existing suggestions of nature, then life will become difficult for him; it will become unbalanced as he is breaking the fluent movement-line of his own life. Nature will inevitably re-establish a balance, as it does all the time, with all entities. Nature doesn't decide to act this way or that way; she is the process itself, she is life living, and she is biology, chemistry and physics proceeding.

People who believe in the existence of nature's consciousness understand evolution as steps in the transformation of consciousness. I am referring to people like Pierre Teilhard de Chardin, the French philosopher, paleontologist, geologist and Jesuit priest, and Erwin László, the Hungarian philosopher of science, systems theorist, integral theorist and originally a classical pianist. Thinkers like these believe that as the species with 'reflexive intelligence' and a developed 'symbolic capacity,' humans are not necessarily superior to other animals, nor necessarily the highest species in evolution, but rather the species that must assume a special responsibility for life on earth as they are a unique species, and this uniqueness provides an option to mature, to evolve the capacity to feel, to access altruism, benevolence, charity, mercy, kindness, detachment, nobility, chivalry, and other qualities that humans are capable of developing. Today we know that the phenomena of life are organized in intertwined systems that are integrated in wider self-organizing structures, and we know that observing nature and its fluctuations seems to be a good way to understand life's dynamics. The 'Talking Body' practice, which to me is a path of self-development, can help us improve our awareness for it. It can help to raise our consciousness as well, by acknowledging the interactive mechanisms that govern natural and social life. Last, but not least, it is a practice that supports an understanding of nature's magnificence by recognizing our self as being part of nature.

Princesa helped us find balance during practice, but the most outstanding part of her intervening was that it was pure and gratifying 'feeling,' freed from thinking based on 'right or wrong.' It was nature acting through her, healing and nourishing. The small dog that inspired me to write the present text died in 2009 from lung cancer. She lived with us, me and my wife, horses, donkeys, dogs and cats, as well as forest animals, for eight years in our 'jungle-house' in the lowlands of Bolivia.

References

Bauer, J. (2006) *Prinzip Menschlichkeit, warum wir von Natur aus kooperieren.* Hoffmann und Campe

Weber, A. (2008) *Alles Fühlt. Mensch, Natur und die Revolution der Lebenswissenschaften.* Berliner Taschenbuch Verlag

José Mulder van de Graaf was born in 1946 in Bolivia. From 1964 on he lived in Germany and graduated in Economy and Ethnology. Prapto invited him to Indonesia in 1985/86 to be part of a small group he had started practicing with, for developing the movement method he later named Amerta Movement. Today he lives once again in Bolivia, in the Amazon region of the country.

joseanita@web.de

7. "MAKE LESS THE HOPING"

Sandra Reeve (UK)

Following several warm, thoughtful and funny speeches and some musical offerings, I stood up with a smile and moved out into a space between the tables. Momentarily my gaze travelled across a sea of faces: faces that I love; faces that I hardly knew but would come to love; joyful, generous faces looking up at me with expressions that were expectant, amused, quizzical, knowing. In that moment my inner eye also saw the faces of absent loved ones who couldn't be there for our wedding.

Traditionally, a bride in England does not give a speech at her own wedding.

"The passion of my life is the art of movement. I would like to move for Andrew and for you all to celebrate today."

My legs were shaking slightly and I was worried that my dress might slip if the dance became somewhat wild. I had no way of knowing in advance where this movement might take me. Gently I breathed, and as I raised my arms in the air with a swooping movement, I turned my back towards the audience. The movement was familiar to me. It is one that allows me to pay attention to the sensations of my being-in-movement and to cross the threshold into a dynamic world – a world of movement perceived from movement rather than from stasis.

As I continued the turn and faced my friends once more, I remembered that I had adopted or amplified this habitual turning movement as a way of giving myself an embodied moment to relax my fear. I had practised for many years allowing **Abhaya-mudra** (the Buddha's hand mudra of 'making less the fear' seen on the north side of Borobudur temple)[1] to inform my movement and, through it, my attitude. Just now I understood that this particular habitual, almost

---

[1] See images of each mudra in the Additional Resources: http://bit.ly/ELtp17

ritual, shaping-in-motion [was it a movement mudra?] had arisen directly out of the quality of the Abhaya-mudra in my body.

> *This was it. This was the moment. No preparation – just readiness. Movement had been, and is, a lifelong practice. I relaxed and followed my movement as it evolved in that particular place and context. I just let myself move without a plan and tried to stay present and alive to each movement as it happened, feeling the sensations in my body and the sensations in the environment, responding to those sensations and gradually 'reading' the situation as I moved.*

For me, the process is like reading a book – the book of that wedding moment. It isn't helpful to stop after each movement or sequence, each word or each sentence to ask what it all means, but if I pay attention somatically to a situation, meaning may become apparent as I reach the end of the improvisation, just as it does when I reach the end of a chapter.

Or I may need to wait until the end of the book.

The meaning *I* find won't, of course, be the same as the meaning *you* find. The meaning and the reading are personally and culturally specific and my position during the moving will have been that of involved-witness-within-the-story rather than detached reader or observer. As I move, I can receive a reflection of my own contribution to the situation; this helps me to feel the impact that I am having on that situation and to take responsibility for co-creating the moment as it unfolds.

The joy of movement, in my experience, is that bodily impressions and expressions can be so multilayered, so vectored and textured: lateral, horizontal, vertical, sagittal, inner, outer, cyclical. In one moment so much happens. The strata of an embodied situation and the paradoxes or conflicting interests within that situation or within myself can be received and acknowledged in such a short space of time, each overlaying the other. Acceptance and transformation take longer! My experience is that, over time, movement reading in daily life cultivates a positive flexibility of attitude and expands my capacity to tolerate paradox and difference. It also offers me a broader, more systemic view of the moment of which I am a part – I can be aware of more of the layers and folds.

Movement reading as a performer allows me to be aware in each moment of my own constellation and of my part within the group constellation. Active and passive both have a part to play in movement reading. I am 'active' when I initiate choices for my own constellation and 'passive' as I receive my position within the group constellation. I use the word 'constellation' as it carries a sense of three dimensions and textures for me, while 'composition' creates a two-dimensional image in my mind. Maintaining an awareness of constellation gives me the opportunity to create a fresh and refreshed response in the improvisation by following a different impulse or by moving differently.

Just as I may choose to break a verbal habit and say something different or in a new way to a friend in a conversation that seems to be entering a grindingly familiar and unhelpful impasse, so too I can choose to move differently, to play with time and space through my use of rhythm (moving faster) or my direction/position in the space (moving into the centre for a moment if I normally hover on the edges, or walking backwards…). This opens up a whole new vocabulary of possible relationships in that moment.

> *I moved, receiving the atmosphere of friendship and love, my hands briefly taking the shape of **Dhyana-mudra**, the west-facing mudra of meditation at Borobudur, which I also associate with receiving and accepting. I shaped my body in relation to the wonderful wooden lattice work of the yurt, and felt the texture of the canvas all around me, with the wind outside on the clifftop. I smelt the fragrance of my Javanese perfume and of the carpets and matting, I remembered to breathe, feeling the fluidity of letting go as I breathed out and consciously released my elbow and wrist joints, often points of tension in my own movement patterns. I entered the sensory fullness of the situation, literally seeing, hearing and sensing the situation from many angles, perspectives and points of view.*

A sense of context seems to be key to an awareness that recognises both myself and my present circumstances. This is the threshold of awareness between my inner landscape and the external landscape, as they mutually attract one another. It offers the space, literally, in terms of movement practice, to become momentarily less attached to the experience of myself as being at the centre of things, and to feel myself simply as a part of the life around me. This, in turn, with practice, can lead to a movement, an action that is as appropriate to the context as it is to my personal needs. So I practise being 'among' and giving equal value to my own movement, to the movement in the environment and to the movement of others I am with.

> *At one point, I stepped gently backwards, little steps releasing the tension in my ankles, and I remembered one of my very first lessons on my first trip to Java. I had plucked up the courage to ask Prapto why he had hardly given me any verbal feedback or encouragement*

> over the six weeks or so, when I had been so longing to hear a "bagus" (good) or "bagus sekali" (very good) from him, which he often said as others were moving. By then I had exhausted my entire movement repertoire in an attempt to elicit some praise – Grotowski-based physical theatre, mindfulness pacing and meditation, relaxation exercises, moving meridians... – Prapto asked me to stand, to walk backwards and to pay attention to the feeling in my ankles: "Please make less the hoping". His invitation has stayed with me all my life.
>
> In that moment on my wedding day, I relaxed my hoping once more and touched a feeling of utter satisfaction with, and groundedness in, the present moment. I was present in the presence of the wedding gathering, surefooted and free. We were all part of this traditional situation called 'wedding' and I had dared to offer my dance.

Perhaps, just possibly, one day I could create a movement so appropriate to my being-in-context and so in time or in tune with the needs of the situation, that I create no *kamma*[2] for myself or for the others. I leave no reaction behind me and thus create no history to condition a possible future. There I go, hoping again...

Although my intention had been to dance briefly for my new husband, suddenly, in the process of letting go into the movement, I needed to give thanks and to acknowledge the new constellation of our family: his son and daughter and their partners, my brother and my mother. I looked at each of them, one by one, attuning to my sense of their being in that moment and entering a dialogue with that quality through my movement. The rhythm and the quality of my movement shifted each time, my gestures and facial expressions adapted in response to a change of wavelength, a different resonance. Somewhere my brain was chattering away: "For heaven's sake! don't forget anyone, now you've started this", but my embodied self was assured and consistent as she danced this ritual of the wedding dancer. Letting go or offering is the sense of the south-facing **Wara-mudra** at Borobudur and I allowed that sense of release to permeate my body as I danced, entering different landscapes of being without losing the 'fact' of the yurt on the cliff.

I don't perceive the body and the mind as a duality and I don't

---

2 **Kamma** or **karma**: *kamma*: "causes which are the life-affirming activities produced by body, speech and mind (...) The Process of Becoming (*bhava*) consists of an active and conditioning *kamma* process (*kamma-bhava*), and of its result, the Rebirth Process (*upapatti-bhava*)". (Nyanatiloka Mahathera 1967, 21) In this case I mean that I would I leave no reaction behind me and thus create no history to condition a possible future.

experience the body as a medium for expressing psychological realities; it is – and expresses – the very fabric of our being. Tim Ingold refers to a similar experience of self:

> "when you yell in anger, the yell **is** your anger, it is not a vehicle that carries your anger [..] the echoes of the yell are the reverberations of your own being as it pours forth into the environment."

In the same way, each person's movement *is* who they are. It isn't a vehicle to *carry* who they are or a *representation* of who they are. So, the more clearly I can receive someone's condition through movement, the more clearly I can receive who they are in that moment. (I say 'receive' not 'see' – Prapto uses the Indonesian word *menerima* – as it leaves room for perception through any of the senses and for passive as well as active awareness.)

> "The Buddha could not see a lasting indestructible soul. In other words, he could locate no abiding soul in this ever-changing being." (Piyadassi Thera 1981, 28)

According to this belief, the person present in any given moment is, in fact, the only one that there is to receive or be received. This doesn't ignore the reality of repetition, habits and characteristic tendencies in each of us – things that give the impression of a fixed self. But it bears witness to each of us as a constantly evolving being with the potential both for making infinite choices and for transformation in the present moment.

Just as the environment is as it is at any given moment, containing both traces of the past and seeds of the future within its present 'presencing', so the present movement of each of us is as it is, embodying past conditionings within present circumstances. How each movement evolves in the present moment will condition each person's possible futures. It is this attitude to the moving 'organism-in-the-environment' that informs my practice of ecological movement. Implicit in this view is the idea of transformation as an ongoing process.

> *When it came to my mother, I found myself moving down to the ground and offering a deep bow in a moment of public thanks to her for bringing me into this world and for all her care and nourishment over the years. I remembered some of my father's last words to me: "Look after your mother" and inwardly acknowledged his being*

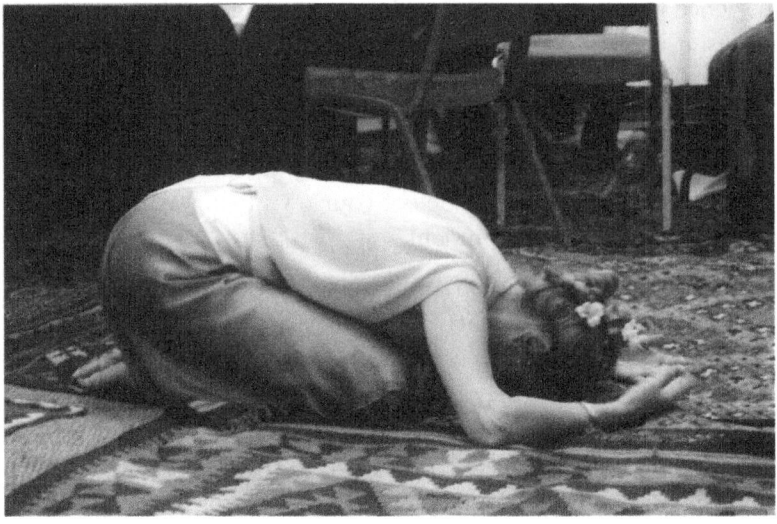

within my bow. At the same time my body remembered touching the earth as my witness, which is the sense of **Bhumisparca-mudra,** *the east-facing mudra at Borobudur that I had spent many hours moving with.*

Finally, I turned to face Andrew and could offer him my embodied vows, held in the crucible of our family and friends. To have and to hold, from this day forward, for better, for worse, for richer, for poorer, in sickness and in health, to love and to cherish, 'till death do us part...the traditional vows stretching back through time.

Epilogue

In my wedding dance I found two intertwined threads of practice arising out of my encounter with Amerta Movement. One is an ongoing research into the relationship of movement to Theravadan Buddhist philosophy and practice, articulated here through the embodiment of a mudra practice, which Prapto has shared with many of us at Borobudur over the years. The other is the practice of 'guiding through movement', be it guiding myself in a life situation or a student in a workshop setting. I've talked about the mudras and want to say a little more about guiding to close this chapter.

Around 1987, when I did my first workshop with one of Prapto's early student/colleagues, Susanka Christmann, I was astonished by her capacity to stimulate sustained transformation in the movement patterns of myself and other participants by moving with them rather than through verbal instruction.

This *guiding* of movement through movement made utter sense to me the moment I experienced it, although terms like somatic, kinaesthetic empathy and mirror neurons were as yet unknown to me. Guiding is a dynamic, somatic mode of attention[3] that attends to a situation in motion, acknowledging time and context. For that reason I talk about an 'ecological body' as a 'body-in-movement-in-a-changing-environment'. The emphasis is on viewing the world through a lens of transition or flux, from movement and constant change rather than viewing/receiving movement through a static lens.

As a movement guide, I am trained to perceive through my senses (including my kinaesthetic sense) the patterns and tendencies in a person's movement/attitude as well as to notice the phenomenon of change itself by practising frequently in nature and at times in the bustle of the marketplace or urban settings. The changing of the light, the rhythm of the waves, the rustling of bamboo, the blinking eyes of a goat, the coming and goings of pedestrians…

'Moving with' someone, whether in direct physical contact with them or not, I pay profound attention to the other's being-in-movement within the environment and I move with my whole body's response to that experience (instinctively, intuitively and empathically), without forgetting my own movement or my own tendencies and needs in the evolving situation. Bringing my professional and creative skills with me into the situation, I enter the process of 'movement reading'.

I don't 'do anything to' the other; rather I offer my sequence of movements into the space, so that, if useful they can be a stimulus for them. Often, attentive to their own movement, the other mover is not visually aware of the movements that I am making. If I forget my own movement while I am reading the other's movement , pulled by the desire to 'teach' them something, my experience is that I become too focused on a result, my perspective becomes too narrow and I exclude a respect for the unknown. Once again, I enter the realm of hoping rather than just being with what is. By clinging to some idea that may have already passed, I can fall out of presence and of being present. My impression of guiding is of an open-ended, creative conversation with the other as I move to create the conditions for a shared landscape with them in which I can stimulate the growth of their movement life and be stimulated by their responses.

---

[3] **Somatic modes of attention** – "culturally elaborated ways of attending to and with one's body in surroundings that include the embodied presence of others" (Csordas 1993, 138).

Movement is always contextual. In fact, guiding for me connects with the mudras at Borobudur in that the practice demands a cultivation of qualities of perceiving, witnessing, receiving, letting go, offering and making less the fear. It often feels challenging to allow myself to be seen in that emergent process, as, similar to the wedding dance, I never know in advance the form that the movement will take, or whether it will be helpful or congruent. I remember similar feelings when I first opened my practice as a Shiatsu practitioner – despite all the training, all the skills, all the diagnostic tools, when it came to the moment would I really be able to offer something for the other's wellbeing through my being-in-touch?

In my own life, be it in conversation with a friend, at a wedding or at a deathbed, I have come step by step to trust the process of guiding myself (and, at times, others) through a dynamic awareness of movement within the changing moment, as I bow to the unknown.

This role of facilitating an experience of 'involved witness', whether in moving, witnessing, speaking, praying or making music and singing, is now called *gardening* by Prapto, rather than teaching or guiding. For myself, in a Western context, I still refer to 'teaching' and 'guiding' but I am practising to maintain an attitude of 'gardening' in every area of my life.

~ ~ ~

References

Csordas, T. (1993) 'Somatic Modes of Attention', *Cultural Anthropology*, vol. 8, no. 2, May, pp.135-156

Ingold, T. (2000) *The Perception of the Environment: Essays in Livelihood, Dwelling, and Skill*. Routledge

Nyanatiloka Mahathera (1967) *The Word of the Buddha*, Buddhist Publication Society

Piyadassi Thera, Venerable (1981) *The Book of Protection* (2nd ed.) Buddhist Publication Society

Sandra Reeve PhD is a movement artist, facilitator, teacher and psychotherapist in West Dorset. She teaches a programme of autobiographical and environmental movement workshops called 'Move into Life' internationally and creates small-scale ecological performances. An Honorary Fellow at the University of Exeter, she specialises in performance and ecology. She is the author of *Nine Ways of Seeing a Body* and editor of *Body and Performance*. She first studied with Prapto in Java in 1988 and then worked with him intensively for 10 years, based in Java from 1995-98. Their practice together continues to evolve through collaborations in the UK and Java.

www.moveintolife.com

8. TOUCHING FORGOTTEN REALITIES

A Practice of Detecting the Happening

Bettina Mainz (Germany)

Preamble

This chapter investigates **critique, freedom** and **reconciliation** – all of them forces that have proved to be important throughout my life. It draws on my background as somebody in Berlin, Germany in the mid-1960s, who began to study movement and performance in the Netherlands in the 1980s and then got involved with Prapto's practice of Free Movement, which I first encountered whilst travelling in Java in 1990. It also draws on my own evolving movement practice, which I call 'Body of Becoming'.

    Meeting Prapto and his work made me recognize my main life pattern, which was one of 'critique', that is, inner fighting and rejection with an implicit longing for freedom. He helped me to uncover the principles of 'unfreedom' within my own system and put them into a context of 'life possibilities'. Whilst doing this he stayed so close to the inner process of my own understanding and readiness for transformation that it could touch my body on a level which allowed for embodied reconciliation to happen. 'Reconciliation' here means a process of becoming friends with my own being and with life itself.

    My immediate response of saying 'no' to whatever might confront me turned into saying literally 'yes' – even if just for a little while. This happened through my physical being which became a place for my mind to transform. From this seed I am still trying to find ways in which the critical mind – which is still alive – can nurture my living practice and teaching in a way that allows embodied reconciliation to take place in me and in others.

My point of view in this writing is personal. Yet to support and widen my thoughts I draw on a lecture given in Berlin in 1978 by the philosopher Michel Foucault which was published as *Qu'est-ce que la critique?* (What is critique?) in 1990 in Paris. In this lecture Foucault speaks about "this critical attitude as virtue in general" (Foucault 1990, 43) and proposes "as a very first definition of critique, this general characterization: the art of not being governed quite so much". (ibid., 45) I also draw on an essay by Judith Butler on Foucault's notion of virtue. Here Butler writes: "Critique is precisely a practice that not only suspends judgment ... but offers a new practice of values based on that very suspension." (Butler 2001, 1) From this point of view I would say that Prapto is practicing a critical attitude; its virtue is embodied in the art of his responses through which he is supporting *blossoming* in the environment.

Born in the Age of Criticism

The main value I grew up with was being encouraged to openly criticize authorities, parents, teachers, governments and ways of living, achievements and friends without being harmed or being asked to be silent. We did not take anything for granted nor did we believe anything just because an authority said it was true. We were passionately expressing our 'no'. As children, we were also treated largely as equals by the adults. We were respected in our rebellion. No punishment was ever given to us, either when we were children or as young adults, for the act of criticizing and questioning. I even received a lot of support in my environment for being critical.

How then did this attitude become destructive?

Embodying the Right to Criticize and to Be Against

I did not distinguish between critique or judgment, criticism or rejection, fear or condemnation, struggle or inner fighting. It was all the same and resulted in absolutely saying 'no' and excluding myself from my environment. As if to justify my negative attitude, my judgment turned against me, and began to govern my mind's activity. It felt like an avalanche of hammers banging my head, not leaving anything whole. All the 'weapons' and strategies I developed to fight them back just increased this utter confusion in my body and mind, which did not leave any place for me to be.

Still I was proud to have the freedom to 'call into question' the reality of all the phenomena I encountered; I doubted my confusion, all my strategies and perceptions, even the distance that I created between them and everything else that exists, including my own being. But by questioning everything, I was left with no thing, no body and no self to refer back to. Questioning thus became a moving pattern of its own, performed in little variations, never finding a resting place in its endless loops and dispersal. It created its own rules and maps which, when followed meticulously, even seemed to offer some freedom – if I ignored the prison within which it moved.

Dance as refuge

move or die
my house has become uninhabitable
movement the salvation
the dance a pleasurable variation of running,
orbiting the contracted places inside
...I am not this and not that!
no middle and no media
will show me
a way

Such an embodied misunderstanding of criticism led me into a dependency on movement as a means of avoiding the collapse of being 'buried by an avalanche.' There was an ongoing hurry and struggle against my body's need to rest. Ultimately my practice of freedom was to develop the art of 'governing' my body. In 1990 after my third year at the SNDO Theaterschool in Amsterdam I felt the need to pause my studies in this institution which had been containing my struggle so well, and to face this fact. I travelled to China and Indonesia, still not knowing how to find my way.

A Way

My first encounter with Prapto is on his land, Padepokan Lemah Putih, in October 1990.

He moves:

His hands meet and rise – feet noticing stepping back
The bamboo's whispering touches my ear – haste drops away

A sense of peace is meeting my sense of struggle and a sense of touch is meeting my sense of separation.

Later I realized that I did not understand what Prapto was doing, nor did I identify the substance in his movements which enabled me to suddenly feel the present moment. As a result, I started to study on his course.

"Find your way," Prapto says – this is our first practice, which we follow for a few weeks.

> *Every day I am coming with my bike to the place where we practice.*
> *I am sitting there and any direction, all strategies, any possible way I start to move, any attitude I imagine, any reason to move – none of them feels appropriate any more. Insurmountable distances keep me in place – mountains of conflicting impulses.*
> *I stay and wait.*
> *Oh! Here I can catch a point of view on which I can ride — no, no, not this!*
> *I wait and stay still.*
> *Each day I think: today will be the day that I can move.*
> *But nothing links me with my way.*
> *Sometimes I overcome distances, layers, walls, gaps and isolations. I jump over – hop! – and then I run. I run and throw away what I have."*

"Freedom you cannot find in your own rejection," Prapto says.

What is 'freedom'? Where could I possibly find something which exists just as a vague yet all-pervading longing?

~ ~ ~

> *However far a spirit may depart from his host*
> *It needs to come home, if not it will become a ghost.*
> *The body welcomes the return of the spirit by feeling the taste of its presence.*
> *'Oho' feeling says, 'I would like to be with you*
> *however strange your way might be*
> *tell me where you go and what you see and I will show you all my mystery.'*
> *'No,' spirit says, 'if I reveal where I go you as well would fly and say goodbye'*
> *'So I will' feeling says and flies away.*
> *The lonely spirit tries to cry but any impulse dies. Aghast he sets off*

*to commune and to find a common tender tune – with the feeling
for only when together are they revealing
the blue of a sky that will never die.*

In my understanding, Javanese culture contains a developed art of feeling. The Javanese learn to position themselves by feeling, to place it in and around their bodies and have it determine the time and their timing. Feeling is a means for communication which then does not need words to speak. It is a sense that nurtures our immediate insight. There is a natural uniting of what are still commonly treated as two distinct disciplines in our Western culture: the field of knowing and the field of sensing/feeling. Growth for the Javanese can happen whilst being in touch with our surroundings and context through the subtle and complex feeling sense and does not necessarily need reasoning. I myself sensed a dimension which touched my being. I felt no need to reject this – on the contrary, I got a sense of a potential in humans that was worth living for.

I am starting to feel that, as the mind touches body, the spirit touches soul.

Reconciliation:

How two things which have been apart can touch again or become friendly is a concept that recurs frequently in the field of reconciliation work. Any occurrence that releases an isolated or solidified item and reintegrates it into something wider may be seen as reconciliatory.

It feels deeply reconciling if the distance that was created out of fear or shame between ourselves and an object or an aspect, an energy, or a feeling, shrinks, so that the object's energy and feeling can touch us and be felt, be received and be transformed. We can perceive a widening of the space that we are in.

~ ~ ~

*"Please practice Seeing:
from the shadow of the light into the light,
from the light of the shadow the light,
from the light of the light into the shadow.
Seeing the shadow in the shadow, the light in the light."*

From where do I look and see?   Is there any location I am feeling?

"I give you practice," Prapto says, and begins to move with me.

> *The gathering point up in my head relaxes, runs down the back as a relief, runs through the heart and pervades the diaphragm; my heels finally touch the ground. There is space to look from, there is space to look in – a vicious circle in my head has abandoned his hiding.*
>
> *I am amazed.*
>
> *The branches of the tree are building a gateway to the blue sky behind, which in turn comes down to me and touches my eyes – I am calming down. Light paves and organizes the confusion that had been in the shadow for so long.*

Reconciliation:

I am not pointing to the content of 'reconciliation' but more to the very act, the mechanism of release when an ongoing struggle or effort ceases. Basically the struggle is embodied and inscribed in our being and our nervous system. This determines how we see and perceive ourselves in the world we are living in. The nature of reconciliation is that it touches an aspect of this struggle, scratches at its insularity or unties its bindings,

We might get a sense of the enemy. It might be real or unreal, seen or invisible, ancient or young, subjective or objective, existing or non-existing. We might also get a sense of relief. 'Reconciliation' can happen in many layers of our existence.

One Way to Describe How Prapto "gives practice"

What is the practice Prapto is giving and how does it connect to the themes of 'critique,' 'freedom' and 'reconciliation?' Here I offer one possible way of seeing it.

Based on the cultural value attached to communing by feeling, Prapto developed a form of art as a way to respond, by moving, by feeling-in-movement and, in this way, communicating with anyone and anything that would touch his field. The field of feeling connects all kind of phenomena. No fundamental distinction is made between the material and the immaterial, the human or non-human world. Anything, whether recognized or not, has the potential to resonate directly with and in our bodies through a vibrancy transported by the atmosphere, which can be seen as the substance through which feeling communicates itself.

The body that feels can not only track a single point of view but can capture a multidimensional picture of what is. It might recognize its participation in creating an atmosphere in cooperation with anything else which is there, seen and unseen. In Prapto's practice this complexity resonates in his body system and his movement moves all of this in the atmosphere. Because I am part of this atmosphere my body system can follow the subtle suggestions given by this moving frame and find new possibilities or new ways of organizing itself. This can be called 'transmission.'

From my point of view Prapto is sharing an attitude of 'critique.' He is responding by questioning whether what is shown is all that there is to that person. He perceives something of what does not want to be seen or be felt. No distinction is made whether what is hidden relates to our beauty, clarity, confusion or contraction, our dissociation, dispersion and fear. Anything has the potential to offer an anticipation of what the person might become, a discernment of what is moving or standing still and what might be caught in timelessness. This all together is what *positively* constitutes a person and one way through which our being expresses itself. Once this constitution is touched and *discovered* it becomes able to move.

Prapto′s practice here is to find and provide *inter-independency*, meaning a relation that *relies* on but does not *lie* on and that can *stand* on its own, balancing and moving the tumbling as a dynamic in responsiveness. Balancing here becomes a stretch of personality; the *inter-independency* is supported by an attitude of non-identification and a curiosity towards life, seeking to support the *blossoming* of a person.

This relational attitude is critical without being identified with the content of what is formulated – Prapto's responses embody and carry a freedom of choice and a sense of offering possibilities and suggestions; his responses are a mirror and a tool containing truth without being *the* truth. He takes the risk of being wrong. His responses are contextual. They can vary with any new situation. They are built on knowledge and experience which increase with any response given and they follow a strong intuition.

Our way of being is not judged, but also it is not left as it is when Prapto withholds attention from those aspects that would keep our separateness in place – for example the effort, the questioning, the struggle, the identification or the fear associated with actually feeling. These strategies lose their power as their resonances dissolve without receiving feedback. This can trouble our system. Sometimes experienced as a sudden effect it might be too strong, too quick and threatening. At other times the reason to sustain our habit becomes incomprehensible even to us. Often there is a wonder involved as the world looks different and our bodies feel different than they did before.

I am still in the process of understanding how to create the conditions for reconciliation to happen through my own movement and living practice. Conditions that will allow our beings to open into a path of participation, supported by an increasing embodied flexibility, responding to whatever is confronting us, leading to a life that might be less fearful and more free.

Body of Becoming – Forgotten Realities

A practice of detecting the happening

I open a window into my own practice:

This sharing takes place in a little studio called UTOPIA-unbedingt in Berlin. It is white and measures less than 45 square meters. It offers a safe frame for *Forgotten Realities* to appear. 'Forgotten' here does not necessarily refer to something we have known before. It refers to a 'reality' which speaks to us in the moment we touch it but which seemingly ceases to exist if we do not remember its – even unknown – presence from time to time.

There are a few people coming.

We begin without a task, without a suggestion, without warm up, without preparation. Maybe we talk about this and that.

Whatever happens, *I will not judge!* What a relief.

For a moment we are retrieving the absent-minded being into the body so we can rest there together – or not. When we come a little closer to ourselves, the space is not so densely filled.

The work is inclusive, which means people bring their backgrounds, their interest, their style, their emotions, their longing for the supernatural or for the ordinary. They bring thoughts and sorrows, their need to destroy or create. Everything is welcome. We work with what is there. It is what we embody, what can be read in our movements, what creates the characteristic of what is seen and felt. People may also bring what they do not embody. Even a self that once left is welcomed. We might find it somewhere flying, somewhere hidden; we try to enlarge the space of our possible attention so it could be included and could start to move with us. It might return when it is time.

I am still finding out how to attend to what is happening today and how to receive tiny signs in the movement of the movers, in between all of us, in the doing and non-doing, in my feeling and in what is touched. Still there are ways that I don't know.

There is a curiosity, how 'attention' influences the dimension and quality of the space that is opening for us to move within. If we also watch the space in between carefully, we wonder how it is alive and speaking.

The movers follow their paths, their needs, their impulses, receiving and attending in their own way. They respond. We all cannot help but respond. If we train ourselves to be awake to subtle influences, our responses can become conscious or chosen. We try to respond so that we still feel free.

We are carefully adjusting the degree of our activities, and perceiving changes in the density and luminosity of the space. That does not mean that we adapt to an overall atmosphere. We might be creating more layers of attention and memories and levels of feeling as we go.

The respect for, and sustainability of, the individual process that each person is developing provides the ground for the other processes to happen. The changing movements and atmospheres may build a background; sometimes also they are confronting. Their fields touch or interfere, forming the context for the next aspect to appear.

We are moving independently, practicing *inter-independency*, responding in nourishment, nourishing the responses. There is a freedom to be where and who we are. This can be inviting, or sometimes intense and hard to bear. It is a walk on a fine line, specific every time.

The sound of the instruments I am playing reflects the quality of dialogue happening between us. Whilst listening carefully, unheard sounds may appear.

I do not have to break down the complexity of the layers and levels that we are touching into a system that I know or control. This complexity is 'reconciling:' here different layers in our being can touch and exist simultaneously, revealing a richness in life that we, for a few moments, can touch directly. Precisely here I feel I am 'becoming.'

There is no need to understand everything that we touch. No classification is needed yet – just random, soft-edged, felt recognition. When it is time we will know enough. In the resting point that our verbal sharing provides for us, we sometimes find much consilience – much convergence – in our perceptions.

In and through the talk we crystallize the specific before we enter again.

> "Find out how to enter this suggestion, find your way
> to deal with it, find what it means to you!"

Slowly our understanding increases. Sometimes we have to let all the layers drop away into the middle of our being; nothing is left in the space to rely on, no impulse to follow but the movement which in itself reveals. It is here that freedom finds a dimension which suspends our critical attitude for moments. It is a state of 'oneness' with 'oneself' which is 'no other' than 'one's body' and no other than the world we perceive. The reference here is not distinction or reflection, which serve to find identity, but a state of 'reconciliation' expresses itself in which one ceases to question one's own activity in the activity of life. It contains the freedom to 'stay home' whilst moving and provides a delicate state in which to trust the evolving liveliness as an 'embodiment of the path of life.'

Conclusion

> "Critique [..] is an instrument, a means for a future or a
> truth that it will not know nor happen to be [..]."
> (Foucault 1990, 42)

To engage with Foucault again at the end, I can say that this *work* has become an instrument to tune my question with my questioning, and to feel possibility in the rejection. It is a means for a future or a truth that it will not know nor happen to be. Growing with our growing understanding and integrity this work becomes a means for reconciliation as an embodied discernment of the present moment's complexity. This might critically shake our being and build a ground for the yet-unknown to blossom. It might offer the freedom to be as we are in a life that is as it is. If we can touch this, we may move together. This is its virtue.

~ ~ ~

References

Butler, J. (2001) 'What is Critique? An Essay on Foucault's Virtue' (Online), Available: http://bit.ly/ELtp13

Foucault, M.S. (1990). *'Qu'est-ce que la critique?'*, *Bulletin de la Société Française de Philosophie*, 84th year, 2 (April-June 1990), pp, 35-63

Bettina Mainz is an independent movement artist based in Berlin. She originally trained at the SNDO in Amsterdam, went to study with Prapto and completed her teacher training with Adam Bradpiece. Other influences include Vocal Work, Shamanic Healing, Key Movement, BMC, and Somatic Experiencing.

She danced in various formations in Europe and Asia and is developing solo work. She teaches 'Body of Becoming' /Amerta in the studio and in the natural and rural environment in the context of Performance, BMC, Body Therapy, Artistic Research, and *Schule der Bewegung/Köln*. She offers Family workshops and movement for Mothers and Babies.

tina_mainz@web.de

www.bettinamainz.de

9. THE ECHO OF LIFE

Developing Resonance Through Amerta Movement

Daniela Coronelli (Italy/UK)

My journey with Amerta Movement evolved out of my interest in the practices of Mindfulness and Shiatsu, and subsequently in the related practice of Seiki. Right from the start, Prapto's training invited me to embody every aspect of the practices of Mindfulness and Shiatsu, through the language of movement, so I could become familiar with the resonance such embodiment had in myself, in the immediate environment and in the group of people I was sharing this work with. This in turn fed back into and greatly enriched my Shiatsu and Seiki practice, helping me to communicate and respond to clients and students through resonance and guiding, rather than from a position of fixed knowledge and experience. In this chapter I want to describe how all these strands have woven themselves together and how I apply them.

Mindfulness

Mindfulness is a form of meditation that invites practitioners to bring conscious embodied attention to their response to what is happening in their lives, with an attitude of open curiosity, kindness and equanimity. Mindfulness gives the opportunity to transform distressful life tendencies and to embrace ways of living that cultivate wellbeing and health (Kabat-Zinn 1990).

   I was introduced to the practice of Mindfulness initially by my first Shiatsu teacher, Sonia Moriceau, and later by John Garrie Rōshi.

John Garrie had laid a foundation of understanding in me as to how we perpetuate certain patterns that can either lead to wellbeing or reinforce tension and limitation. These patterns then translate to a particular physical posture and behaviour, in daily movement. He presented Mindfulness as a vehicle for transforming these patterns of behaviour, which can lead to illness and involve resistance, holding on to or being apathetic towards the realities of life experience.

In addition to verbal teachings on the way of Mindfulness as first outlined by the Buddha in the Satipatthāna Sutra, and how this approach can give awareness of common human causes of health and disease, John Garrie had devised a 'hara'-based exercise and postural health system that reflected our life tendencies and how to change them through mindful awareness (Garrie, 1998).

Shiatsu

Shiatsu is a touch-based holistic healthcare system originating in Japan. It stimulates the body's vital Ki energy to flow, by applying pressure – deep tissue massage and movement – to specific body areas, acupuncture points and meridians (European Shiatsu Federation 2011). My teacher, Sonia Moriceau, had developed a form of Shiatsu called 'Healing-Shiatsu', which incorporated an extensive training in Mindfulness Meditation.

Through studying the Healing-Shiatsu form I was able to build on my understanding of how types of posture and ways of moving are associated with personal inner and outer perception and attitudes. From this perspective, these physical habituations are indicative factors in a variety of physical and/or mental illnesses.

Proprioception

From both Mindfulness and Healing-Shiatsu trainings, I received an important lesson: how crucial posture and movement (proprioception) are in relation to attitudes held, as well as the health consequences that follow when certain attitudes and ways of embodying them are perpetuated in time. Through Mindfulness practice, this fundamental correlation between proprioceptivity and health development became clear, both in my life and in my work with clients.

Seiki and Resonance

In my work as a Shiatsu practitioner and teacher, the influence of Amerta Movement moved me more in the direction of Seiki, a contemporary Japanese Ki manual therapy, a style of Shiatsu that invites the receiver to recognise and follow their own natural movement towards balance and harmony, through the process of resonance.

The word 'resonance' originates from the Latin verb *resonare*, meaning 'to sound again', as in an echo. Here, I use the term to refer to our ability to 'resonate' with another, to feel empathy with them. In Seiki, as with some other touch-based therapies, resonance plays an important role, and empathic listening is refined and nurtured through training and direct embodied experience. The practitioner develops the ability to sense and feel the key areas where the client's need for touch lies. That touch often initiates the release of long-held tension in the receiver, be it at a physical, emotional or cognitive level. Such release may manifest simply as a change in body temperature and spontaneous movement like sneezing, twitching or crying, along with deeper breathing. In Seiki, these areas are known as 'resonance areas', and can only be recognised through the direct contact between giver and receiver, in the moment-by-moment process of resonance. There are no theoretical or rehearsed bodywork techniques that can point to these areas, as each client's body has its own map. The practitioner, through maintaining an aligned posture, a mindful, empathic presence and an awareness of their client's breathing, invites areas of resonance to emerge in the body, where sensitive touch is then applied, opening up the possibility of a healing change to occur in the client (Kishi & Whieldon 2011).

Our understanding of the phenomenon of resonance has recently been strengthened by discoveries in neuroscience, specifically in the field of mirror neurons, which offers possible neurological evidence of how attunement and resonance take place. It is an evolutionary survival development that enables our awareness to sense and respond to non-verbal messages (Lewis, Amini & Lannon 2000). In my understanding of Seiki and Amerta Movement, both receiver and giver are invited to exchange with each other through resonance, or 'the echo of life', as an expression of both environmental and cultural influences, and to find fulfilment in life, in a spirit of respect, moderation and co-operation.

Amerta Movement and Contact with our Condition

The main difference between the methodologies of both Mindfulness and Shiatsu and the Amerta Movement practice of Prapto is that the former two approaches started and evolved from a centralised form and structure informed by stillness and direct observation, whereas, in Amerta Movement, form and structure are in a continuous process of change. Movement here could start from anywhere: a physical area, a feeling or an idea, and develop from either a source of stillness or movement. Listening to, and following, the inner guidance of the present condition was encouraged; a condition that is always moving with the awareness of direct experience.

In the unfoldment in movement of what appears from moment to moment, there is continual contact with the inner condition and with what is being perceived, staying with what unfolds, gradually lessening the sense of identification and attachment that may arise. With this approach I have found that ingrained habits are often unravelled, and even though they may resurface again and again, their potency lessens in correlation with a decrease in the sense of identification with them. I have also observed this in clients, especially when a strong memory would arise that was connected with a traumatic experience. They have found the movement to be a supportive and safe vehicle for embodying and moving through their condition. So when a memory arose, it would be met with a sense of allowing, in the movement of it, staying present with the feeling of it, with less resistance or clinging. Whilst not based on a fixed form or structure, the movement work enables clients to access and move aspects of themselves that have been frozen in time. I have found this to be an effective and healing approach for my own development and in my Shiatsu and Seiki practices.

Shortly after I encountered Amerta Movement I became aware of how it had the potential to expand the practice of Mindfulness. When Amerta Movement is applied to rigid mental and physical patterns, an opening often unfolds which enables us to explore more deeply the nature of ill health and contracted ways of thinking. This gradually leads to an embodiment of postures, movements and attitudes that inform wellbeing. Amerta Movement is not intended as a solution to any problem, but its practice illuminates many issues.

Amerta Movement training encouraged me to integrate movement work into my life as a Shiatsu practitioner, which greatly enhanced my healing ability, my self-development and enabled me to support others in these processes.

Through Amerta Movement one may also feel more connected, in a fluid way, and there may be less identification or fixedness. From such a position, one may easily enter the form of giving Seiki, whilst also bringing the quality of movement into it, enhancing the ability to work through resonance whilst giving Seiki.

Combining All These Practices

John Garrie Rōshi's work resonated strongly with the origins of Shiatsu, the world of Zen meditation and art, including healing, martial arts, Zen calligraphy, Tea Ceremony, etc. He demonstrated how vitality, wellbeing and creativity can be realised by an experience of life which stems from mindful awareness of movement originating from 'hara' – a Japanese term for a specific location in the abdomen region, considered to be the core of being of the person. Here in this centre, thinking, emotional, as well as physical, processes are being witnessed and experienced in mindfulness as passing life events, rather than cognitive, dis-embodied phenomena that have to be sorted out and accommodated to suit our personal or cultural beliefs. With Amerta Movement (which partly derives from Mindfulness/Vipassana) there was no fixed structure or framework for approaching this, and because of this absence of structure, the doors and windows to Mindfulness were very much left open and were in expansion, able to embrace the bigger picture, the wider environment, free from any self-imposed limitations.

Integrating mindfulness into daily life is one of the greatest gifts shared by both Amerta Movement and Seiki, and this foundation informs both the professional and creative aspects of life. Each action – be it sitting, standing or moving – can be experienced fully, with awareness, as we place ourselves in relation to our kinaesthetic perception and our inner condition. In Seiki, the body landscape of the receiver is no longer sensed through an interpretation of how the meridians feel, as it is in Shiatsu. The ability to observe how movement unfolds in the receiver, in present moment awareness, is essential in Seiki and, through resonant contact, the giver may actually feel where the receiver is in their life and tendencies. With this embodied feeling it is easier to bring attention to where inner movement wants to flow again and to guide their awareness to it, so that transformation can occur.

Whatever arises in the therapeutic space, in Seiki, is felt through direct embodied experience and is shared, through resonance, rather than controlled by mental planning of what should happen to bring about recovery. In Seiki, as in Amerta Movement, there is no aim to correct any distortion or restriction of movement that has caused a particular ailment, although there is a different process of embodied guidance on how to recognise the inner condition that gives rise to such a change.

In Amerta Movement, there is awareness from moment to moment of the internal condition and of how it changes in response to the context and the environment we are moving in. Working with Amerta Movement, a teacher, guide or facilitator can enter a deep resonance with the location where the movement is taking place, with the physical elements or the atmosphere contained within it, and with the people sharing movement, be it an individual or a group of students. Mindful of such resonance, as it unfolds, they can guide a process of change for the individual or the group by embodying a quality of movement that emerges and connects with the interaction of all the elements involved, rather than from an external application of a teaching technique.

In Amerta Movement, we are invited to sense each and every part of our body as being a 'member' of our whole body-mind, and to feel that connection in our movement. We are also very much a 'member' of the environment in which we live and move. Not only do we walk on the earth, but we are supported by the earth, which is a part of what we are. Earth, sun, moon and other people are all a part of the inter-connecting whole – not something that is separate. Amerta Movement is rooted partly in Mindfulness (Vipassana) and Sumarah Meditation (a form of meditation practised in Indonesia). Resonance, in Amerta Movement, is the outcome of 'surrender', in the sense that I surrender any fixed position or attitude I may have; I am open to what arises.

Guiding and Being Guided Through Resonance

The experience of one of my students, Roberta (name changed), serves as a case study of the richness of these practices as they become integrated.

> *Whilst moving with a group outdoors, the interaction with the physical elements of the location and the group process triggered a*

childhood memory in Roberta, which she experienced as physical and emotional pain. Even though her memory was not accurate, she was convinced that her father had attempted to kill her, after an operation on her tonsils at the age of 4, by covering her up so tightly that she could hardly breathe. This memory now manifested with acute pain in the lower back and a strong sense of fear and agitation, as she had a flashback to the original experience. Initially there was a sense of being overwhelmed and she entered a contracted, held-back posture and displayed an anxious facial expression.

Moving with Roberta, in guidance, I first felt a sense of compassion and tenderness towards what was happening in the space and then my attention shifted, as I felt movement coming from my legs. I invited her to sense the contact with the ground with small steps, at first, and then by taking longer steps and lifting her knees, until movement from her legs began to gather its own momentum and shape. Moving from her legs changed the way she was experiencing her back pain and her initial contracted response. This gave Roberta the confidence to engage with what was happening in the front of her body, her present level of vitality and her ability to move through and interact with it. By allowing her condition to be, and shifting her attention to the front of her body, Roberta was able to accept her memory with curiosity and friendship. Afterwards, whilst talking about her experience, the sense of fear had subsided, together with the pain in her lower back, and she continued to fully embody her front as well as her back.

Often, when I work with students in a group or individually, through a process of empathy, I can feel in myself the resonance of a memory that the other is experiencing. Through guidance, when relevant for the other and/or the group, I may invite that person to follow the movement that is arising, consciously, while moving with them, so they can allow the memory to unfold naturally. This has the effect of en-lightening their presence in the space and, as a consequence, the communication taking place amongst those involved. During a Seiki session, resonance with the client's process and observation of their breathing and movement pattern guides me to touch particular areas of their body. Through this contact a spontaneous physical movement is often released. The client remains completely conscious during the movement and aware that the unwinding taking place is releasing a part of themselves that felt stuck or that they were not previously aware of. Afterwards, clients often report feeling more open and present in their body and clearer about where they are in their lives.

For a number of years, I have been facilitating a series of workshops that combine Seiki, Mindfulness Meditation and Movement. These are mainly attended by Shiatsu and other touch-based and movement therapists, who find these skills useful for their personal and/or professional development. On one such recent workshop, I invited a group of Shiatsu and Seiki practitioners to move with what Prapto calls the quality of *Oval* (purification in circulation/language of nature), and afterwards to exchange Seiki with each other. The quality of Oval relates to the natural world, including 'nature within ourselves' – our perception, our body functioning, immune system, respiration, etc. All the elements (earth, water, etc.) are at play within ourselves, and in our physicality there is also a tendency towards objectifying the world as outside of who we are. In seeing all this, we can bring this awareness into our Seiki work, so there is no sense of separation between giver and receiver.

Later, we worked with sound, which comes from the sense of hearing, listening, therefore from the quality Prapto calls *Circle* (bowing in prayer/spiritual language). The quality of Circle relates to our sense of the spiritual, self-enquiry and our purpose in life. It also embraces qualities of compassion and empathy, which are valuable qualities to embody when practising Seiki. In working with sound, in the form of chanting specific vowels, whilst maintaining a 'listening' stance, certain qualities of feeling were awakened. When this was translated into touch, it brought with it quite different effects for those who were receiving, in terms of posture, fluidity of movement, response, breathing and in terms of confidence. The movement work is introduced in this way so that participants may appreciate how movement can happen from any part of the body, from the feeling or from the mind. It is also an opportunity to observe the contrast between this Movement model and Seiki, which comes more from the 'hara'.

In Amerta Movement, the space of 'enquiry' is the quality known by Prapto as *Square* (unity in diversity/human language). It facilitates communication, encourages co-operation and offers the flavour of welcoming new possibilities. There is a sense of communication happening, rather than the controlling of it into a particular direction. It invites an open attitude in which communications flow without hindrance. This quality resonates well with the attitude in Seiki, where the flow of resonance between giver and receiver is of prime importance. Amerta Movement has much enhanced my work with Seiki, supporting as it does the facilitation of resonance.

Conclusion

In conclusion, both Seiki, with its more formal expression deriving from the Shiatsu tradition, and Amerta Movement, involve a commitment to remaining adaptable and mindful of 'what is', in the reality of the present moment. Such commitment creates a resonant and empathic rapport with the people one is working with. It is a commitment to stay aligned and to keep moving through any lassitudinal tendency, keeping alive the ability to sense what others are feeling, so they may also become aware and alive to such possibilities. My experience with Seiki has been much enhanced by my background in Amerta Movement, and my familiarity, through Amerta Movement, with the art of resonance. I will be forever grateful for this.

~ ~ ~

References

European Shiatsu Federation. (2011) What is Shiatsu? (Online at http://bit.ly/ELtp18)

Garrie, Rōshi J. (1998) *The Way is Without Flaw*, Sati Press

Kabat-Zinn, J. (1990) *Full Catastrophe Living – How to cope with stress, pain and illness using mindfulness meditation*, Piatkus Books

Kishi, A. and Whieldon, A. (2011) *Sei-Ki: Life in Resonance – The Secret Art of Shiatsu*, Singing Dragon

Lewis, T., Amini, F. and Lannon, R. (2000) *A General Theory of Love*, Random House

Born in Umbria, Italy, **Daniela Coronelli** is currently living in the UK. She runs a Shiatsu and Seiki complementary therapy practice in Devon, is a Member Teacher of the Shiatsu Society in the UK and has taught in the professional programme for Shiatsu Schools in the UK and Italy. Major influences in her life, creative process and work are Buddhist Meditation, Amerta Movement and Seiki. In 2004 Daniela founded 'Life Healing Arts', an organisation offering a programme of workshops that integrates her own approach to Mindfulness Meditation and Movement with Seiki and Shiatsu therapy as a guide to health and wellbeing.

www.lifehealingarts.org

10. I ALWAYS DO THREE THINGS

Shantam Zohar (Israel)

Two years ago, we all went away to *Nachsholim* to celebrate my father's 85th birthday. We took rooms at the seaside village and, on the day in question, skwooched around a very long table in a secluded area of the public dining room to share our festive meal. We are a merry family, and my father is the merriest of us all. Soon he stood up and, with some effort, we all fell silent to make room for his words.

From his seat at the head of the table, my father looked out over his four children, fourteen grandchildren and six great grandchildren. "I cannot count my blessings," he said. Then, wiping a tear, he added, "Thank you all for coming here today." Yitzchak, for that is his name, said to us, "Perhaps you think that I am an old man of 85, and that I am close to the end of my life. And Agam," he pointed towards my newborn son and his fourteenth grandchild, "is a very young man, close to the beginning of his life. But the truth is," he banged on the table, "that we are both smack in the middle of it." Yitzchak raised his glass of red wine. "To life," he roared, "Lechayim!"

So many airline tickets, I thought, recollecting my fifteen years of lofty spiritual migration.... Had he known this all along, or was it something that dawned on him as he faced his blood at this grand event?

My father's father, Alex, didn't do very well as a self-employed electrician. He moved too slowly, and by the time his state-of-the-art results neared completion, there were inevitably impatient clients breathing down his neck to get the damn job done.

Seeing this, I believe, Yitzchak took a big step away from physical labor, turning to become an engineer. As such, he rested in relative safety at the drawing table, still required to get jobs done, but merrily employed with plenty of pension and time to philosophize over lunch. And if things weren't ready on time, clients could just turn to his boss.

Seeing this, I imagine, and just to take it one step further, my older brother dedicated his career to the refined study of philosophy. He took refuge in the mighty volumes of eternal time so as to be pestered by no one but eager students and wicked members of the academic promotion committee.

And fearing this, yet still seeking an authentic place in my somatically distilled male lineage, I made a grand attempt at the most arduous of all detached careers, that of a Himalayan yogi.

The goal of yoga is disappearance. One *uses*, please note this verb, the body, to attain the sixteen states of *Samadhi*. Just as Lahiri Mahasaya once came home from the Ganges, banged his hand and did not even know it was bleeding, so you, oh great yogi, should be detached from your physical body. In the West, led by the United States of America, this truth has been turned on its head and twisted around to become, quite cunningly, the opposite. The goal has become the body. But my guru was clear on this matter. He said, "Forget about health and wealth at least for a long time." And where do health and wealth reside, if not in the body?

Hence, mind you, this chapter is about the body and what moves within the body during so called 'spiritual practice'. And specifically, it is about a profoundly simple display of acute awareness of states of mind, or attitudes towards being alive in a moving body; what it actually means to habitually inhabit a space in time immediately, at once and always. It is, in fact, about mindfulness, freedom and art, responsibility, celebratory madness, discipline, devotion and full-hearted bliss. For these have all come to conscious manifestation, at least from my own privileged point of view, through the iconic presence of one Indonesian man.

At any rate, after several years of dedicated spiritual practice in the Himalayas, I resurfaced at Naropa University. And at this majestic gateway between the destitute East and the hectic West, I was practically awarded a certificate for being a 'Spiritual – Bypasser' par excellence. For that crowd is well versed in recognizing one who may have transcended, but that certainly did not include the mastery of personal matters. So I had to sign up for therapy and rework my limbic system and it was even suggested that I join an eight day Amerta Movement workshop with Prapto, which is where the following dialogue with another participant took place:

10. I ALWAYS DO THREE THINGS

Q: "Prapto, in thinking about your practice, or discipline, what do you actually do when you enter the space?"

A: *"I always do three things: flowering, channeling and semadi. In semadi, I pay attention to everything, my toe, my foot, the air. Oh,"* (gesturing up towards his moving palm) *"my hand. In channeling, just letting in whatever; and in flowering, expression, emotions, feeling. But most of the time, maybe ninety percent, I am doing semadi."*

Q: "Why do you do *semadi* so much of the time?"

A: *"Well, because in channeling I am afraid what might come in through me; and in flowering, I am thinking: maybe I am not pure enough."*

Thus spoke Prapto at the Arapahoe Campus of Naropa University, in Boulder, CO, USA, 80301, on a date I shall not reconstruct, to avoid the now and then fugue of romantic recollection. Rather, I'd like to tiptoe our way directly towards the essential relationship between the practice of *semadi*, the artistic process of flowering, and the mystical experience of channeling. And I'd like to do so in interview form.

SE (Someone Else): having read what you have written so far, do you think that the words of Prapto need further interpretation, or do they stand alone?

SZ: Both are true. They certainly stand alone, but, as in the case of many great oral texts, there is room for interpretation.

SE: If you had to select one word or concept that would characterize Prapto's above teaching, what would it be?

SZ: Responsibility.

SE: And why is that?

SZ: Though not present in the teaching itself, one may wonder what might happen if, through channeling, something "wrong" came in, or if the buds flowering proved to be "not pure enough." I think that it is safe to assume that the results would entail harm to self or other, which is what we tend to fear and describe as impure.

When Prapto explains that he spends ninety percent of his time in a state of discernment, I think he is doing so out of responsibility towards himself and others; that it might be more fun to just flower and let things flow through.

SE: Prapto is an Indonesian teacher speaking to a primarily Western audience. To what extent does this influence your understanding of his words?

SZ: There are two parts to it. First, Prapto is a teacher. Someone sitting in front of him asked him a question. This person had a body: eyes and ears and a heart, and I believe that Prapto answered, first of all, to the person at hand. As I have no recollection of the questioner, I am no good at ascertaining the inter-subjective nature of the response. But of course it was there. These were Prapto's words to a specific person at a specific moment in time; even given the same question asked, he would have to offer one answer to a recklessly expressive person who gallops around the space slamming into people, and another to a grounded Vipassana practitioner, who rests utterly attentive to nothing but breath and sensation. But I certainly took the words as an encouragement to experience myself through paying acute attention to the basics, before waking up the big cats of emotional expression and uninterrupted flow.

SE: What about the cultural part?

SZ: Right. Here I just translated flowering as emotional expression and channeling as uninterrupted flow. But a student of mine went to Indonesia to practice with Prapto. After two or three nights when the lights were left on until daybreak, he turned to Prapto for an explanation. The master answered quite simply that light scared away the evil spirits. So, I think we might assume that channeling signifies the literal entry or passage of distinct entities through one's body self, as opposed to flowering, where one broadcasts latent personal material.

SE: You mentioned a student; where do you teach, and has Prapto's teaching influenced your own?

SZ: I currently serve as co-founder and director of the Mindfulness Based Therapy program at Tel Aviv's Bar Ilan University, where I teach the practices of movement and meditation.

SE: Would you say that mindfulness and *semadi* are one and the same?

SZ: The Indonesian word *semadi* is translated into English as meditation, or to meditate. Given Prapto's account of what he actually does while meditating (*"this is my hand, this is my finger"*) I would describe *semadi* here as tracking or mental noting, which are the building blocks of mindfulness practice.

This moment-to-moment noticing nourishes a type of attention that lays the ground for the mindful state of sustained awareness. Hence, the *semadi* mindfulness practice cultivates an underlying state of awareness that can be experienced also in the non-conceptual states of flowering or channeling, where the fruits of discernment are present, though the practice itself is temporarily tuned down, shut off, or abandoned; however you choose to think about it.

SE: In the dialogue above, the questioner asks Prapto about what he does in 'the space,' and you have mentioned the word 'practice.' In what way are 'the space' and 'practice' related?

SZ: The space, in this context, is where movement practice occurs. But the real space is the world, where, on a daily basis, our miserably heroic and uniquely distinct paths of life intersect and overlap; waking and awakening, together and alone, we sniff to see if practice has stood the test of translation from the precious culture of encapsulated spaces to the all-embracing, messy, breadth and scope of life.

My yoga guru once told me that all people are born as originals, but most people die as copies. I love that sentence, and paradoxically feel that the flowering of this innate originality frequently involves an uninterrupted sharing of meditative space with another human. Prapto has used the word *initiation* to describe such interactions. And initiation kicks off practice within and beyond the boundaries of space, energizing attention and perpetuating the human, 'being signature' through breath and gesture.

SE: Thank you

SZ: Thank you. And, thank you, Prapto.

My father once told me that it is impossible to learn from somebody else's experience, and it is practically impossible to learn from one's own experience. How encouraging, I thought, that it IS somehow possible. But, how?

Once confronted with this 'how' question, Krishnamurti replied, "All you have to do is take the first step, and the first step is the last step and the last step is the only step there is." And by this, I think, K wished to protect us against the useless temptation to follow other people's experience; for the truly risky business of real education is frequently hedged around by preordained conclusions. Having toppled over this hedge, which simply decrees the practically impossible to be impossibility itself, many of us may have attempted to engage K's one-step approach. But Amerta Movement has us treading the practical plateau of practice, before leaping off into the unified abyss of trust and joy. And it is this balanced buffer of integrated personal experience that we nourish by noting, "this is my hand, this is my finger." For here we keep the responsible 'I' in the picture, at least for a long time.

~ ~ ~

Shantam Zohar received his BA from Naropa University and MA in English Literature and Creative Writing from Bar Ilan University, Tel Aviv, where he currently serves as co-founder and director of the Mindfulness Based Therapy Program. He is the award-winning author of *Kabatiye*, (2002) and *Mideast Tango* (2010). Shantam teaches Authentic Movement as a relational awareness practice and is also co-founder and owner of Green Genius, a social platform designed to create transformative living circumstances fit for the 21st century.

shantamazing@gmail.com

11. A PRESENCING DIAL

Margit Galanter (USA)

In my preparation for writing this chapter, I decided to choose a thread of Amerta that was a simple and specific practice. I have found that it can be quite challenging to express the impact of this work, as its coherence is astounding, pervasive, and elusive, like mist or the movement of *qi*. What revealed itself through this process was that even to express a 'simple' practice was to open into a mosaic of possibilities. So, in following a line, I found that there is not only the line itself, but also the lines that cross through it, as well as the spaces between, the navigation through, and the bigger living composition made. In this chapter, I include my earlier (and more simple) understandings of the practice, later syntheses, and an excerpt from a conversation that further articulates and enriches the original view, which developed through the writing process.

~ ~ ~

In 2000, I came to meet Prapto on his land in Java through the recommendation of dance mentors and years of interest in his work. From the first encounter, I began to land into a contemporary and culturally-rooted movement conversation that bridged more facets of life than I imagined possible. After years of movement and cultural studies in Indonesia up until that time, through this work I found a new kind of integration; in Amerta, I found a rich movement world and a living constellation of practices that continue to unfold through my life today.

Practicing Presences, Presencing

The practices of Amerta Movement affect many aspects of living. One powerful element has to do with 'presence', which is a basis, filter, and medium for how one enacts in the subtle currents of a situation. Our quality of presence in a given environment affects how we experience it, and while certain movement, somatic, contemplative, and performance research forms access this awareness, in my experience these tools are uniquely developed in this work. Amerta invites participants to relate with multiple realms of experience – in interaction with one another, the environment, and the subtle qualities of felt sensation. In doing so, our inheritance of ideas and beliefs is often revealed through the movement and conversation, and this invisible context becomes an element of the dance as well. The communication amongst these various realms of experience invokes what I think of as a 'mobility in presence.'

With practice, one can navigate presences and experience consciousness of their changes, ranging from being as loud as a brightness that enjoys being seen, to as quiet as a *happy shadow*,[1] with multiple tones along a full spectrum. Presence is not just something to have or achieve, but rather is a continual process of presenc*ing* that can shift in relation to varied elements as they arise, including being present within one's own center. In this way, presencing is a medium and filter; both. The practices of Amerta can take years to integrate, and over time I have slowly developed in my ability to experience a greater range of qualities of presencing. Through movement and attention, I can broaden my focus while simultaneously attuning to both the subtle elements of the environment and the spaces and movement between. I can be less self-conscious in my own actions, and come from a 'dialogue view.' This encompassing perspective has helped me tremendously in my work as a movement artist, practitioner, student, and teacher. It brings forth a vividness of experience and has an effect in my artistic practices, vocation, and daily life.

In the first month I worked with Prapto, I was introduced to a particular movement practice that has had a huge impact since. The following skeletal description of the teaching is translated through the vagaries of memory and sparse notes.

> *With a partner, move with three different intentions: first 'hooking,' then 'leaving,' and finally 'catching.' Practice with various combinations of the three within the duet.*

As I remember from what we did at the time, with hooking, the mover continually intends to get the other person into their game,

---

[1] In 2008, Prapto mentioned *happy shadow*, which I translate most concisely as a joyful and quiet presence in a mover. This image was strongly evocative, and would take me years to recognize I could access it experientially.

to draw their focus; with leaving, the mover is really anywhere else attentionally than where their duet happens to be, perpetually running away; and finally with catching, the mover does their own thing in the presence of the other, noticing when they are in flow. While in action, movers may happen to slip from one mode to the other, but through practice, they begin to feel the nature of each, so much so that these qualities become accessible and recognizable.

There are paradoxes that emerge through this practice, and when I experience the felt sense of paradox in an embodied context, there is often some potent seed of an idea present. Some of the experiential mysteries I have encountered are that:

- 'leaving' can actually keep you stuck in a process, even though you want to run away

- 'hooking' can keep you separate from your own coherence and felt presence of action

- with 'catching,' despite your focus in your 'own' movement, you may experience a kind of communion in the flow of shared actions, which I have come to call a state of 'dancing-with.'

For years I have practiced these three states – they have become signposts in my own improvising, and at times I have facilitated them with students and colleagues, to communicate and share these fine distinctions in presencing.

As I prepared this chapter for publication, I was in contact with Prapto with Diane Butler's aid in translating. I was trying to understand if my definitions of 'hooking,' 'leaving,' and particularly 'catching' were even close to their originally intended use, since I had encountered them so long ago. Through the email conversation, I found that the terms, of course, have a great deal more to them than I had originally understood. Here is an excerpt:

> *"Actually, 'leaving' is because the being of dance changes and, as it turns out, that is leaving the space and time. In a sense, we want things to be in eternity because we are afraid of changing – because that changing will give a feeling of losing something.*
>
> *We have a tendency of 'hooking' so that something is continually in our network for giving a feeling of safety. Or we want to add to our existence by 'absorbing.'*

> *'Catching' is actually the same as 'hooking', but catching has a gradation that is more momentary.*
>
> *For this, actually the practice of Joged Amerta is a study that emphasizes more toward how we can study movement while conscious of changing in the changes of movement itself."*

While I had not caught the full meanings of these practices entirely, they expanded and found applications throughout the next ten years, both as specific practices, and in the doors of presencing they opened up.

2004, Brooklyn, NY

Several years after that first encounter with Amerta, I began working with people in new ways. With a colleague who is a choreographer, we did a series of 'embodied dramaturgy' sessions. For this, we worked on a regular basis in movement and other creative experiments to access, develop, and articulate the substance of his dance performance piece. Interestingly, I never went to a rehearsal nor met with his dancers; rather we chose for the process to take place in duet in the privacy of his studio, a space for him to anchor his public project with his own discoveries.

In one session, after he took some time to speak about the current state of his piece, we did some hands-on Feldenkrais practice to facilitate an integrated state of body-mind. Then what unfolded was a series of movement practices that ended with him in free movement, 'digesting.'[2] After witnessing his movement for some time from sitting, I rose and joined in, dancing near him. The desire to join and the term 'dancing-with' both arose through an inner voice at that time, making new language. There was something about the clarity of his state (being in his own action-flow, or what I thought of at the time as 'catching') and my role as both witness and participant in that moment that I felt I could more actively support and sense him through moving. The particular state of presence I found had roots in the Amerta practices.

Later we discussed how that movement practice made the day's

---

2 Often in sessions, I will make sure there is time provided for integration. In the context of a dramaturgical session, this is particularly important, since composition requires space to sense and synthesize (this is also valuable in somatic arenas, as well). It is this time and space, and the alternation between composition, sensation, and integration, that facilitates cultivating mobility in presence. This term 'digestion' developed through my collaborations with Josiah Hincks.

session more vibrant for the both of us, that it clarified the work we had been doing up until then. From my own perspective, in dancing-with him, I found a new way to commune not only with the content of his process and this process between us as it was unfolding, but also a new intimacy and vividness arose, which was a third thing, as if I could touch into his movement and empathize from some kind of shifting sense-feeling; it is this felt sense that remains with me most strongly today. I don't think I would have accessed a sense of his work so clearly had I not danced with him and it. It is as if finding him through the movement helped me indeed sense myself, which created something novel and mobile between us, that in turn provided mutual enrichment.

Many aspects of this potent time in Brooklyn became stitches on a thread that I continue with students, collaborators, and clients today. It turns out that this kind of creative enquiry with people gives me great satisfaction, and it developed on its own, as a new quality of presencing opened up. So, a state of presence itself was a basis for future unfolding and change.

2004-2006, New York

I did graduate work on 'permeability' as a phenomenal state in movement, but did not specifically attribute this to Amerta, since other movement forms were more in my focus at the time[3]. Amerta is so pervasive that at times I have not been able to grasp or articulate its effect on me. This particular state of 'permeable' presencing tends to manifest as quieting down self-consciousness, attuning to the various elements in interaction, as a whole and living constellation. The interconnectivity amongst and through is somehow the substrate of mobility. With permeability, there is a palpable shift in the space between whoever is 'we' at a given moment, which in turn affects 'our' actions together.

Now, years later, I see how my understanding of the state of permeability is inextricably linked to practicing presences with Prapto; as I have experienced more measures on an increasingly sensitive 'presencing dial,' it has become clear how the earlier practices set up a foundational palette of states for navigation.

Through the influences of Amerta and other movement forms,

---

3 My thesis addressed permeability as a state that arises in the context of dance – Lisa Nelson's Tuning Scores, somatics – the Feldenkrais Method, and in my own movement and performance practice.

I began to practice my communication in ways that were creative, receptive, interactive, humanizing, and broadening. In certain moments I have become less self-identified and more interested in the conversation and ambience of which I am part. The phenomenon of permeability is perhaps a medium through which I can understand how I am engaging in this dialogical presence. For example, when I am focused on movement, form, and muscularity in dancing, I can recognize that my receptivity is low and there is physical tension – becoming aware of this can help me access a more permeable state. From the experience of permeability, I can more easefully listen to other elements than those on the surface. So, different degrees of permeability are measures on a presencing dial, eliciting specific qualities of interactivity.

The Garden

The aspect of Amerta that I described earlier as 'dialogue view' opens up our cultural inheritance of enclosures and categories. Amerta practices have helped me to understand the ways that movement can have an affect not just on things we have categorized, such as a 'body' or 'art,' but also on the multiplicities of living a vivid life. This sense of interconnectivity had been a pursuit of mine before I encountered Prapto, yet before Amerta (and living in Java) I had only experienced hunches and tastes – what now is the tracing of a thread was then more like a succession of dots, knots and clumps. My own limitations had tended to get in the way: for example, the loudness of my presence – an inherited and learned materiality – is consonant with the culture I live in, my family upbringing, my heritage, and my personality tendencies. Movement practice has the power to create change.

The image of a garden is used in Amerta Movement to imply the rich web of relations that one experiences through moving, developed through the lives of people who share in the Amerta practices. In general, gardens are cultivated, and out from this tending, life unfolds. In a garden, there are multiple forms of life in an interconnected arrangement of movements, operations, and flows. There is a spectrum of colors, tones, elements, and frequencies. Creatures serve different functions; all are in relation and have overlapping effects. We can look at the different beings in the garden as individual matter, but in fact, there is something about the 'interactivity' that engenders being part of the garden.

I consider Amerta a living constellation, and that part of what makes it 'living' is that it is a regenerative set of practices; it invites individuation, conversation, and development for all those who participate. In its interactivity it resonates with a garden's nature. The practice unfolds from dialogue, between humans, art, and the natural world; between our consciousness and our bodily sensations; amongst people from diverse cultures, and more. We explore the multiplicitous aspects of life through practice, which has a deep impact on how we are present in the world.

2008, SEEDS Festival[4] Showing, Western Massachusetts

In Prapto's workshop, in the Circle group, where our focus was *"the sense of bowing and praying,"* he proposed we each dance with a flower or leaf. With the flower, my movement changed. I was caring for something. It mediated my dancing and my movement communication. I did not need to focus on myself, the actions, how I was doing, nor how I appeared. I experienced a kind of suppleness that only comes from the whole being's actions in a dynamic mobility. I danced with another person while feeling my own hand holding the flower…. 'Dancing-with' in a performance-type setting, the flower mediated the duet, allowing for a sense of calm presence in flow. At the time I understood it as a kind of catching, but now with these new understandings of the terms, perhaps the best term would be simply 'presencing,' a kind of dancing-in-the-garden experience, *inter-independently*, from my own shifting position.

2011, Subterranean Arthouse, Berkeley, California

More than a decade after I had begun to study with Prapto, I heard him use the term *inter-independence* as an approach for communication. Instantly, it clicked, giving name to my own experience – not the lonely objecthood and power of 'independence', nor the stickiness of 'interdependence', but something much more fitting the experience of how I had earlier understood 'catching.' *Inter-independence* is imbued with implicit dialogue, sharing space

---

[4] Somatic Experiments in Earth, Dance, + Science (SEEDS) Festival was a multi-year experiment. The international gathering and investigations of ecology and interdisciplinary arts was co-founded by Olive Bieringa and myself in 2008. It was produced at a rural dance center, called Earthdance, in Western Massachusetts. At the first SEEDS, we invited Prapto as one of the main teachers, which set a powerful tone for the whole project. The garden was present as an image for the Festival, as well as being a theme in the dialogues throughout.

in a garden, in which all beings are conversing from their own flow of action. This is an interactivity where one dances from one's own mobile axis, sensing oneself and the other aspects present, be they people or atmosphere.

By tracing a thread of the Amerta work, I am faced with some of my own complex and disjunctive ways of thinking and absorbing. I am not sure if the threads of this chapter are being woven so clearly. The propensity towards multiplicity is a part of my heritage – I have been educated in post-structuralist, post-modern perspectives that utilize a morass of images accessible in the U.S.; my thinking is informed by an understanding of movement and energy that is spirallic and organic; and I was raised on the Jewish habituation of questioning and layering. My complex perspectives at best have a propensity toward the feltedness and entanglement of experience.[5] I am inspired by images that enrich the tension and reductiveness of a binary, opening to include the majestic image of an embroidered brocade – both interwoven, and coherent. With this, the circuitous pathway of thread and lines finds clarity and inter-independence through its navigation.

Dialing in to multiple presences enables a flexibility as it filters, so we can commune with the very basic senses of everyday living right through to the kinds of conceptual complexities that can open up, as seen above. In my own understandings of harmonizing energy, primarily through Qigong and Chinese energetics, I have found complex energetic presences can also be transformed over time and enriched through intentional and practice-based shifts, through the interaction of movement, breath, and attention. We can loosen tangles, following lines to feel the clarity and space through things. These physical processes of aligning can be a doorway to coherent, felt spaces. For example, in Qigong, there are a series of exercises called 'reeling silk,' through which the practitioner cultivates energetic lines, threads, and space within by doing physical movements to gently follow imaginary silken lines in the immediate space in front of her, so as not to break the delicate threads. Tracing

---

5 By placing 'felt' in this paragraph and chapter in two different meanings, I am making a comment on the relationship between felt, the spirallic woollen substance, and felt, as in felt sense, or a feeling-state more primary than emotions, embodied. The former is articulated comprehensively in the book *Felt*, and the latter is a term developed by Eugene Gendlin in 'Focusing,' which is a process where one finds the implicit language through accessing a felt sense by pausing in an ongoing situation and listening, creating space to bring it forth. Often in this chapter, the word implies the ranges of these meanings.

threads can be an integrative, embodied, and conceptual practice, encompassing a multiplicity and invoking flow both within and through the garden of attention and experience.

2013, East Bay, California

Currently, I am working on a long-term dance poetry project called *Relay*. One summer, I took walks with people who are practitioners from diverse fields, audio recorded our conversations, and we made maps of the walks. The encounters took place in a nexus of several neighborhoods where I have spent much time and has personal and geomantic power. In the project I was literally felting dialogue and place, and 'catching' moments where the language embodied vibrantly, so much so that it inscribed itself into our imagined sense of the path. These moments where something living 'shines' is a felt space, and it arises through the interaction of the conversation in flow.

In one of my *Relay* encounters, I realized that I am finally in a performance process where I can access the *happy shadow*. Rather than wanting to be seen, to express with an undercurrent to prove my persona through art, I am enjoying being with people, dancing-with, and letting a larger environment guide me, quietly, accessing new modulations on the presencing dial. I am beginning to more fully follow the line of the inquiry itself, attuning to the thing that makes it *It*, unfolding through the wisdom that shows up through conversation. This is a cultivation of a state of not knowing yet watching things grow. As I have taken the conversations into the next phase of the project, making performance, I have a range of presences to work with, multiple tones on the dial, a whole spectrum.

2010-2013, Ellen Webb Studio, Oakland

I was working with a client who is an artist and has a unique facility in creative process, yet at the time he was not dancing as he would have liked to, and had some medical issues that were affecting his life and art. We found it especially potent when I offered gentle prompts that provided atmosphere, focus, and trust. On this day, we were working with the reciprocity of language and embodiment. At first, we did some 'Focusing' to help him access his felt sense and the words implicit in this state, as a base step. Then I led him through three phases of a process I have developed, called 'inscriptions,' where he could access ideas through speaking and drawing, then embody the ideas through movement in space. Inscribing often ends with witnessed movement, with time after for digesting.

Recently, this client and now friend remarked that the session a few years before had been a breakthrough moment for his art life process, that the way he had found language for that particular constellation of ideas offered him a clear imagistic foundation that was supportive for his art-making until today. I couldn't help but think about the influence of Prapto in our work and in my development. We used a variety of practices from the view of art in daily life. We did not segment out the body, nor the person, from the bigger picture. And through the practices, we helped him find connections between the various aspects of himself in the world. We found an atmosphere of discovery, a field where he could rediscover his whole self.

Through the process, as practitioner, I became aware that what we had done 'for him,' I had also experienced for myself, and that we were in the garden, together.

~ ~ ~

References

Galanter, M. (2004) *Practice Makes Permeable: Movement as a Basis for Research*, Master's Thesis, unpublished

Gendlin, E. http://bit.ly/ELtp19

Hincks, J. (2003) Personal Communication

Suryodarmo, S. (2013). Personal Communication

Thompson, C. (2011) *Felt: Fluxus, Joseph Beuys, and the Dalai Lama*. University of Minnesota Press

Margit Galanter is a movement investigator and dance poet living in Oakland, California. Her practice, 'Physical Intelligence,' encompasses her unique research perspective, helping people experience the innate clarity and vitality one can uncover through the potency of movement. Margit is trained as a movement artist, Guild Certified Feldenkrais Practitioner, and Chinese energetic practitioner, and her fascination regarding the construction and value of movement has drawn her to collaborative embodied research for decades. Margit has lived in Indonesia several times since 1991. She is thrilled to be a co-editor and contributor for this book, honoring the paths inspired by Amerta.

Art Site: www.margitg.wordpress.com

PI Practice: www.physicalintelligence.org

12. AMERTA MOVEMENT AND SOMATIC COSTUME

Sourcing the Ecological Image

Sally E. Dean (USA/UK)

"Amerta Movement is the nectar of life of the movement – or the movement of the nectar of life. So that means how we can find the position – it's like the source of life – how to be in the source of life." (Prapto Interview, Solo – April 2008)

The approach and the methodologies of the *Somatic Movement and Costume Project* led by me, in collaboration with costume designers and visual artists, Sandra Arroniz Lacunza and Carolina Rieckhof, have been influenced in different ways by Amerta Movement. In this chapter, I will focus on one key influence: Amerta Movement's relationship to image/metaphor/symbol, in particular the worlds of *Fact/Fiction* or *Reality/Dream* and the impact of that approach on my somatic movement and performance practice.

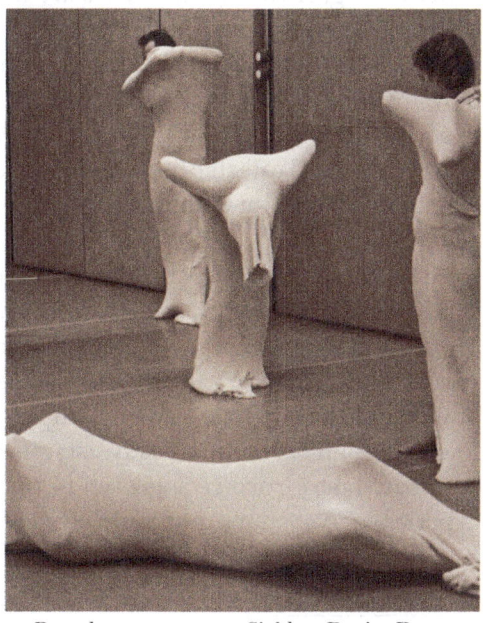

Boundary costumes at Siobhan Davies Dance Studios, Independent Dance Improvisation Class, London taught by Sally E. Dean. Photo: Sandra Arroniz Lacunza. Feb. 2014.

Description and Aim of the Project

The aim of the *Somatic Movement and Costume Project* is to create a praxis whereby costumes act as a somatic resource for moving, creating, teaching, performing and being, a resource that leads into multi-sensorial experiences. The original key research questions were: how can we create and design costumes that generate specific body-mind experiences and support new and enhanced kinaesthetic awareness? How can these 'somatic costumes' shed new light on socio-culturally informed psychophysical habits? And how can they offer new ways of moving, being and performing?

Over the past three years, the *Somatic Movement and Costume Project* has included a series of workshops, performances, lecture/demonstrations, and a published article. Twelve prototype costumes were created and performances were often site-specific with the audience becoming active participants through wearing the costumes themselves. I use the term 'somatic' following Thomas Hanna (1988), to refer to bodily practices and perspectives on embodiment that give attention and value to the subjective experiencing of the whole self and its perceptions, and emphasise the role of the body in that experiencing. Although all senses are important, we have typically started our work from the kinaesthetic sense or kinaesthetic body consciousness.[1] For example, the material, texture, weight, form and movement of the costume itself typically create a direct and tactile experience for the wearer. In our daily life, what we wear (a heavy coat, high heels) affects the way we move and how we are perceived. The basis for our interactions with the environment and with others also changes.

Although costume has been incorporated in performance for centuries, the *Somatic Movement and Costume Project*'s approach differs in the following way: the aesthetic and movement of the performance work comes from the somatic experiences (kinaesthetic and sensorial) of wearing the costume, rather than the costumes being designed to enhance an aesthetic already established in advance. The visually dominated performance approach to costume is replaced by an experience of costume as a multi-sensorial experience.

---

1 "**Kinesthetic body consciousness** is awareness of the body's movement, position, and level of muscular tension. It is achieved through perception of muscle and joint movements and through the senses, primarily the tactual; the auditory is also frequently involved, and all of the senses can play a part" (Storm 1987, 306).

Project Background

The initial impetus for this project came from my experience of living in Java in 2007-08, practising Amerta Movement and witnessing and learning traditional Javanese dance forms. I noticed a quality of 'containment' in the movement of many Javanese people, both in daily life and in dancing and performing, which I could clearly see and sense, but found I was unable to embody for myself – until I tried on the traditional Javanese dance costume. The costume itself created a kinaesthetic experience of 'containment' in the mid to lower body: a *sarong* tightly wrapped around my legs and pelvis, held in place by a *stagen* (sash). The costume helped me to find an experiential understanding of the feeling state of 'containment' inherent in the movement I was seeing around me.

Prapto also uses the term *clothing* as part of his movement practice – as both a functional and symbolic element to his work. This planted seeds, in my own practice, of how one's clothing affects one's movement.

I began to wonder how costumes could act as 'portals of perception' – supporting people to find gestures and movement qualities that might otherwise be missing from their repertoire.

What is a Somatic Costume?

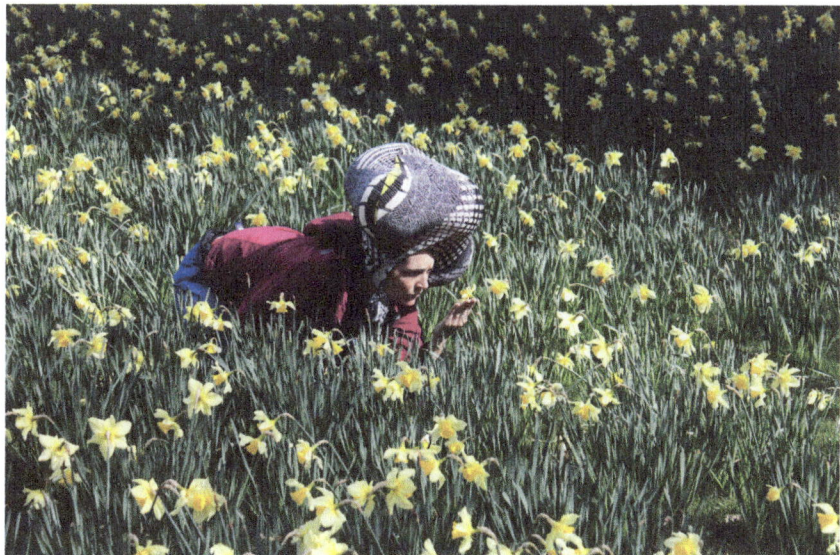

'Balloon Hat' worn by Sally E. Dean. Middlesex University Artist Residency, Trent Park Campus, London. Photo: Sandra Arroniz Lacunza. April 2012

Somatic costumes typically begin with what often gets overshadowed in the performance and costume world – the kinaesthetic sensation and experience that the costume generates while wearing it. They are designed specifically to bring awareness to different areas and qualities of movement in the body – offering intentional sensorial experiences. For example, we created two prototype somatic costumes for the head: the Balloon Hat to give the experience of the buoyancy and volume of the skull and the Pointy Hat (see the final image in this chapter) to give an experience of the direction of the skull in space as a development of the spine as an axis. These multi-sensorial experiences are costume-specific, person-specific and site-specific. They aim to access, integrate and reprogram body schema and body image[2]. The somatic costumes not only have the potential to change our relationship to ourselves (by including body schema and body image) but also to change our relationship with others and with the environment.

Somatic costumes are worn before, during, and after somatic exercises[3]. The experience of wearing somatic costumes is intentionally influenced and enhanced by working with somatic movement in different sensorial capacities, which include the adding, working with or removing of a sensorial experience (e.g. by introducing music or removing sight with a blindfold).

Somatic Costumes and Amerta Imagery

The somatic costumes and exercises arose out of the process of translating many of the changes I had experienced – in relationship to my own body, to the environment and to others, while practising Amerta Movement – into an approach or method for others to experience.

---

2 **Body schema** is the physiological construct that your brain creates "from the interaction of touch, vision, proprioception, balance, and hearing. It even extends it out into the space around your body. You use it to help locate objects in space or on your body" (Blakeslee & Blakeslee 2007, 32). The costumes become part of your body schema. By wearing a Tall Pointy Hat, over time, you will unconsciously begin to develop an awareness of how tall and wide it is, and your body will bend and adapt when going through doorways as if it is part of you. **Body image** is the psychological construct that includes learned attitudes, expectations, assumptions and beliefs about yourself, your body, others, the environment and the world (ibid, 42). It is highly influenced by your social and cultural context.

3 Key somatic exercises applied to the *Somatic Movement and Costume Project* are from my background in some of the following practices: Skinner Releasing Technique (to include the teachings of Stephanie Skura), Amerta Movement (to include the teachings of Helen Poynor) and Scaravelli Yoga (as taught by Giovanni Felicioni).

12. AMERTA MOVEMENT AND SOMATIC COSTUME

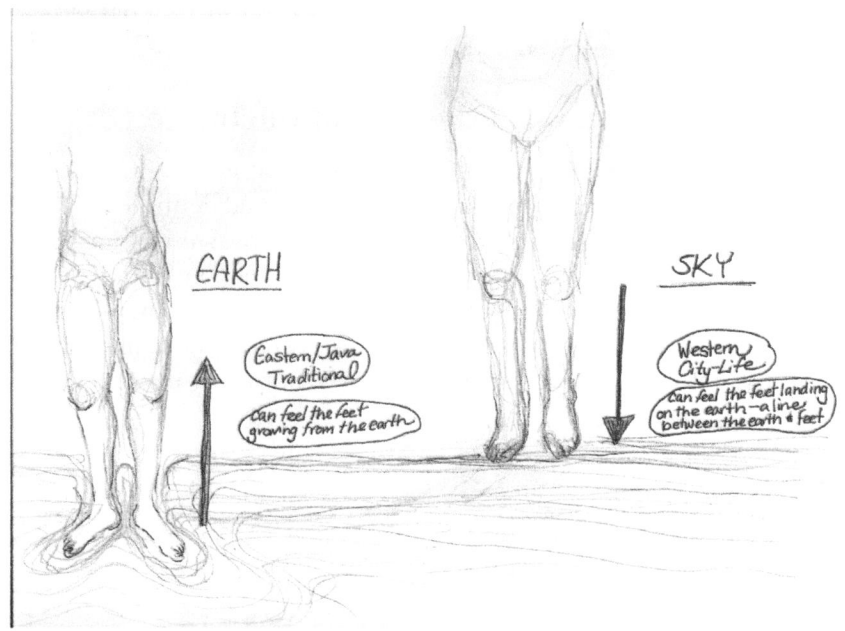

Drawing sketch with support from Carolina Rieckhof

For example, Amerta Movement imagery and my experiences in Java changed my relationship to my feet and the earth. In my journal there are two images of feet drawn: one of feet resting on the top of the earth, and the second of feet coming from underneath the earth.

The latter experience was new for me. Prapto's movement imagery and instructions often invited us to awaken the sense of our feet to what is underneath the earth: *"Feel the sole of your feet – the soul of the earth"*. This supported me to drop into my body – especially the lower half. As I describe in my journal: "I can feel the feet growing from the earth – feel what is underneath – connected to the earth – merging?"[4]

During an artist residency in Java, I made clay with colleagues by standing in mud up to my shins and kneading it with my feet. I sensed kinaesthetically (and literally) my feet underneath the earth – further solidifying my earlier experience.

The "Lentil Socks" were created to support the experience of the feet coming from underneath the earth rather than resting on top

---

[4] Here and elsewhere, unless otherwise stated, Prapto's words and my responses are quoted from the movement journals and interview cited in the References.

of the earth – a direct example of how the imagery arising out of Amerta Movement evolved and became a somatic costume.

Amerta Movement and the Role of the Image

An important aspect of Amerta Movement is that it inter-weaves images, metaphors and symbols – and the roles and definitions of each can overlap and intertwine in the work. Prapto's use of image may represent something literal (to include its function), or it may act like a metaphor and symbol and represent something non-literal. The image may act to represent something specific (like a metaphor) or it may act to represent something more abstract – without a fixed or inherent meaning (like a symbol).

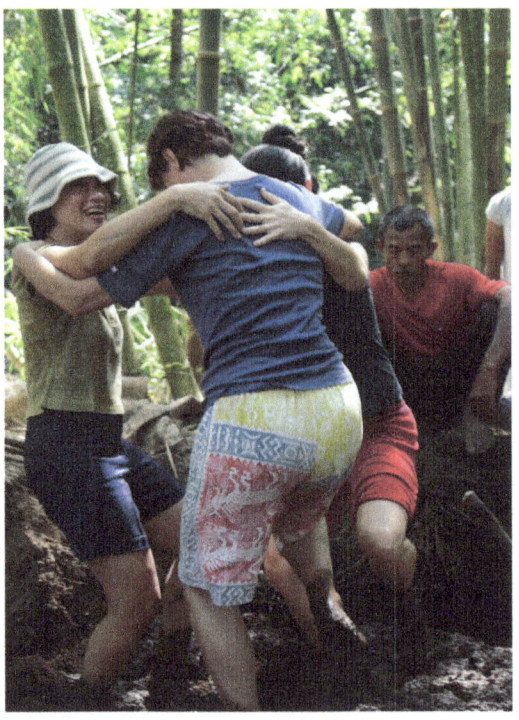

Bedhog Artist Residency as part of the Kemanapun project in Java. Artists shown: Susana Miranti Kröber, Sally E. Dean and Koniherawati, Aug 2008. Photo: Emilia Javanica

For example, one of Prapto's movement instructions was, to be *"aware of your clothing – what clothing you are wearing"* – a literal/functional approach. Clothing also took on metaphorical properties: *"opening and closing is the clothing"*[5], or *"function and relation are types of clothing"* or *"the boundaries or clothing of the heart"*. From this experience, clothing became both a literal boundary between my body and the world, as well as a metaphorical one – a 'second skin' – a living and breathing membrane between 'inner world' (inside the body) and 'outer world' (outside the body).

Amerta Movement's *clothing* made me not only question the role clothing plays in our movement, but also led me to explore both the literal/functional and metaphorical methods of approaching costume through an exercise I devised called 'Second Skin'. Participants are invited to sense their everyday clothing, how it affects their movement, as well the relationship between the clothing and their body:

> *"the skin is touching your clothing and your clothing is touching your skin"* and *"moving with this sense"* –
> The literal/functional, 'Reality/Fact' approach.

> *"as you move, your clothing becomes a second skin... slowly a duet between your two skins emerges – sliding over each other... sliding skin... sometimes meeting, resting on each other, sometimes having space between each other. Finding moments of movement and moments of stillness. A dance between the two skins"* – The metaphorical, 'Dream/Fiction' approach. (Workshop notes: March 2012, December 2012).

Amerta Imagery – The Ecological Image

One characteristic of a symbol, according to its definition, is that an image, as well as one's relationship to it, can change over time and be influenced by the culture, society and context from which it comes.

Prapto's Central Javanese roots and background in Javanese mysticism are very much interwoven into the Amerta imagery he uses – and his symbols often are in a state of flux. These symbols interweave the environment and the body into multi-faceted metaphors.

For example, in one of Prapto's movement exercises, we practise simply moving from pillar to pillar in the *pendopo*[6] site – a literal/

---

[5] This metaphor refers to "the places in-between open and close – how much you open and how much you close, in the movement".

[6] A *pendopo* is an architectural structure that has a roof, but no walls, held up by pillars running from floor to roof. They are common ritual spaces in Solo, Java and many of the classical Javanese dances are performed in *pendopos*.

functional exercise. But, in Javanese culture, the *pendopo* site is resonant with meaning:

The central *saka guru*[7] typically has four pillars[8] or 'brothers'. In the centre of these four pillars is the axis or 'fifth brother', which Prapto calls *"The source… the nectar"*.

The term 'brother' also connects to the body – in Central Javanese culture, the umbilical cord is called 'the little brother' and the 'brothers', according to Prapto, represent the four elements while *"the fifth is the 'jangkar' [anchor] means like a pillar like the axis"*. So a 'brother' can be an umbilical cord, an element, a pillar or axis.

In the *pendopo*, pillars and the spaces between them can be taken literally, metaphorically or symbolically – existing in a 'state of flux', where site and the body are interwoven into the symbol.

If we draw on Sandra Reeve's (2011, 51) definition – "An ecological body is situated in flux, participation, and change" – then Amerta imagery, by encompassing the values of an ecological view, acts as an 'ecological image': an image that embodies the roles and definitions of the literal, the metaphorical and the symbolic, connecting body, movement, environment/site and others through "embodied states of 'interbeing'" (ibid.) in a state of flux.

Somatic Costume and the Ecological Image

The somatic costumes themselves embody the elements of the ecological image – they can be approached literally, metaphorically or symbolically, are often in a 'state of flux' and connect the body with the environment. Somatic costumes act in a similar capacity to Prapto's *pendopo* site – embedded symbols yet dependent upon context.

Wearing somatic costumes can connect and change the performers' relationship to their bodies, movement and the environment. For example, in the *Myth of the Porter's Mess Room* – a site-specific, promenade performance in which the audience was taken on a journey through particular environments wearing the Pointy Hats at the Battersea Arts Centre in 2010 – the hats changed the audience's kinaesthetic relationship with the environment. As they passed through low doorways and narrow corridors, their Pointy Hats would run into the environment, creating

---

7 '*Saka*' means 'wood vertical' and 'coming from' in Javanese, according to Prapto. 'Guru' means teacher in Indonesian.

8 The **pillar** is made from a tree trunk. 'Tree' is '*wit*' in Javanese and 'begin' is '*wiwit*'. Prapto says it's like 'the tree of life' idea that many other cultures have. According to Prapto, the word 'brother' can be interchanged with the word 'sister'.

new limitations and requiring them to move in new ways. Like an ecological image, the somatic costumes acted as gateways – interlinking body and environment in a state of flux.

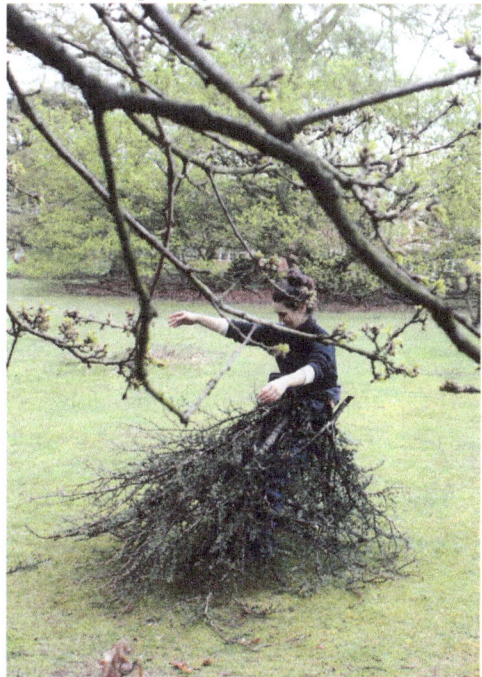

'Tree Skirt' worn by Sally E. Dean. Middlesex University Artist Residency, Trent Park Campus, London. Photo: Sandra Arroniz Lacunza. May 2012

The somatic costumes themselves are also in a state of flux – some becoming 'site-specific' costumes. For example, during our *Middlesex Artist Residency* in 2012, after taking our prototype somatic costume called the Hula Hoop Skirt into the natural environment on the Trent Park Campus at Middlesex University, the costume changed: we took the frame of the Hula Hoop skirt and covered it with found tree branches. This shifted the mover's sense of an embodied relationship with the forest environment, and stimulated new movement qualities that reflected this new relationship. The tree branches attached to the costume had a shaking and shuddering quality, which began to translate to the moving body as well. The somatic costume was mediating a two-way dialogue of influence and exchange between body and environment.

Amerta Movement's Approach: "Dream/Reality" or "Fiction/Fact"

One of Amerta Movement's key practices in relation to imagery is called *Fact/Fiction* or *Reality world/Dream world*.

Fiction/Dream refers to "the imagination, the symbol" while Fact/Reality refers to "the concrete". Fact/Reality typically encompasses objective experiences while Fiction/Dream does not mean that the experiences are untrue, but instead, enters the terrain of the subjective. In general, when approaching an image, symbol or metaphor (or even an object or person) we can consider both its Facts (the function, colours, texture, orientation, location, weight, shape, etc.) as well as its Fictions (associations, meanings, metaphors, feelings, characters, etc.).

A Somatic Costume affects the wearer directly through the kinaesthetic sense – the material, texture, weight, form, movement (Facts) of the costume itself typically create a direct and tactile experience, similar for all wearers. But the subjective experiences and associations (Fictions) are different and unique for each person. For example, one person associates the Bin Bag skirt with "flying" and feels a sense of freedom, while another associates it with the feeling of "suffocation".

In creating and performing *The Myth of the Porter's Mess Room*, both approaches, Fact and Fiction, were applied. For example, if I move with the Pointy Hat costume following its sense of weight and direction in space, I am following the Fact. If I move with the costume of the Pointy Hat, beginning by following my associations with it of the Ku Klux Klan or Dunce Cap, I am following the Fiction.

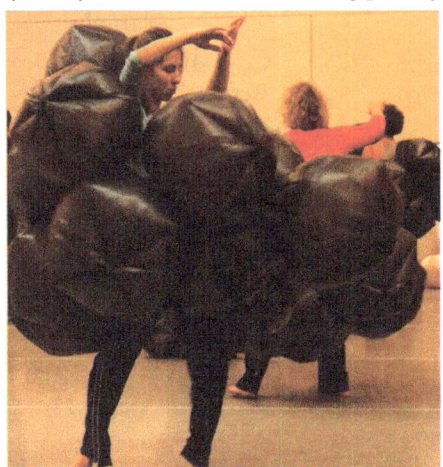

'Bin Bag Skirt' worn by dancer Mariana Camiloti, at Siobhan Davies Dance Studios, Independent Dance Improvisation workshop, London taught by Sally E. Dean. Photo: Sandra Arroniz Lacunza. March 2012

In working with costume in this Fact and Fiction framework, we literally create a meeting or a dance between body schema and body image.

According to Prapto, there are four approaches when working with Fact/Fiction:

- Starting with the Fact to create the Fiction: I find a tree branch and I create an imaginary monster from it.

- Starting with the Fiction to create the Fact: I imagine a cup and then I create that cup.

- Starting with the Fiction and this is the Fact: I start with the symbol of a bird, and then approach it as though it were a fact

– finding out as much as possible what this symbol means. Prapto would call this approach *The Life of the Symbol.*

- Starting with the Fact to find more Facts: like a scientist, I would start with water and then find out all the facts about it – its chemical make-up, its properties, and what it can be turned into, etc. Prapto would call this approach *The Life of the Fact.*

Amerta Movement and My Shifting Relationship to Image

Before I practised Amerta Movement intensively, my performance work typically started with Fiction to create the Fact (Approach 2). Images in my mind would often translate to imagery with movement on stage. I would also place images inside and outside of the body to move to – very much inspired by my training in Skinner Releasing Technique and Butoh. After leaving Java at the end of 2008, my relationship to imagery came to exist even more in the concrete world, starting with Facts: objects, costumes, sites and the physicality of my body. I began to shift from the "view of the mind" to the "view of the body" (Reeve 2011). Images began to come from facts.

Amerta Movement changed my relationship to image and this then translated into the *Somatic Movement and Costume Project.* Although the somatic costume can be approached either by starting with Fact or Fiction, serving dual roles as an ecological image, typically in the *Somatic Movement and Costume* workshops or performances, I begin with the Fact of the somatic costume. Fictions are often created from there – either by myself or the participants.

The Image and the Audience

The somatic costume is translated to the audience by inviting them to wear the costume. For example, in both *The Myth of the Porter's Mess Room* and the performances at the Dance and Somatic Practices Conferences at Coventry University in 2011 and 2013, the audiences were invited to wear Pointy Hats. The somatic costume, since it embodies both Facts and Fictions, can serve as a bridge between the inner somatic experiences of performers and the outer form as perceived by an audience. For example, wearing a Pointy Hat creates particular kinaesthetic experiences and generates particular creative material for the performer; but at the same time, aesthetically, Pointy Hats in the space also create a unique spatial relationship to the environment. They tend to create a particular performance 'world'. Thus somatic costumes can allow both the performer and audience to experience, both visually and spatially, reflections of the kinaesthetic experiences a performer is engaged with. For example, choreographically the audience may see the performer making long direct lines with the Pointy Hat in space, an aesthetic manifestation from the visual form of the hat itself. At the same time the Pointy Hat may create the kinaesthetic experience for the performer of the spine extending out of the top of the head through the hat like an axis – an inner experience of the outer form of 'line.'

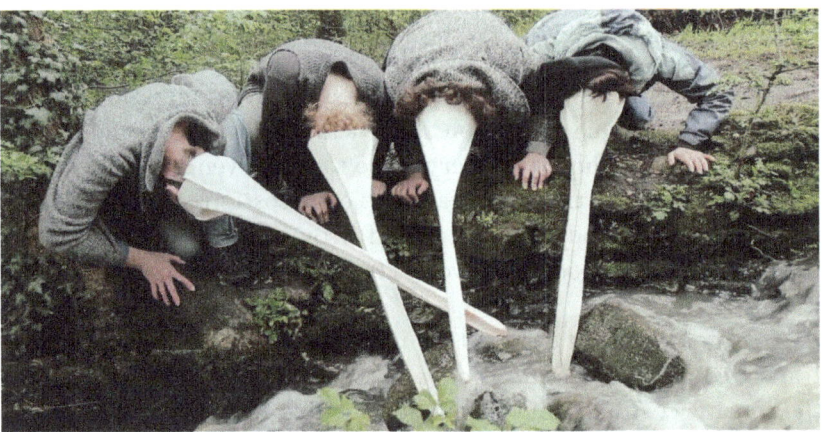

'Pointy Hats' worn by Kate Pyper, Carolina Rieckhof, Shantala Melody Sacco, and Rachel Gildea. Still from *You're Not Supposed To Be Here 2*, filmed and edited by Sergio M. Villar, directed by Sally E. Dean, with idea and concept in collaboration with Sandra Arroniz Lacunza and Carolina Rieckhof

Future Applications

Through my intensive experience with Amerta Movement, my relationship to imagery changed. Images began to embody for me both Facts and Fictions. With the 'ecological image' existing in a 'state of flux', images were able to interweave body, movement, environment/site and others into a value of 'interbeing' where meaning is based on a participating and changing context. This not only changed my body and movement, but also my performance and teaching work – and laid many of the foundations of the *Somatic Movement and Costume Project*.

One of the key aims of the project is to integrate, access and reprogram our physiological and psychological constructs – our body schema and body image. What if our body image was like an 'ecological image'? So that our Facts and Fictions, our learned beliefs, attitudes and assumptions about ourselves, others and the world all existed in a state of flux, participation and change? The 'ecological image' is a gateway into possibility – moving us into the source of life and our greatest potential.

This project has the possibility to bridge many art forms: dance, theatre, visual art, fashion design and live art. In the future, we would like to explore how somatic costume might act as a vehicle for understanding not only the experience of oneself, experience of one's relationship to another, and experience of the environment; but also how these kinds of experiences vary across cultures and across different cultural forms of human embodiment.

Note: Costume designer and visual artist Marta Jiménez Salcedo, joined the 'Boundary Costumes' project (picture p.113) in February 2014 as a collaborator.

~ ~ ~

References

Blakeslee, S. & Blakeslee, M. (2007), *The Body Has a Mind of its Own*, Random House

Dean, S. (2011), 'Somatic movement and costume: A practical, investigative project', *Journal of Dance & Somatic Practices* 3: 1+2, pp.167-182

Hanna, T. (1988), *Somatics*, Addison-Wesley Publishing Company

Reeve, S. (2011), *Nine Ways of Seeing a Body*, Triarchy Press

Storm, P. (1987), *Functions of Dress*, Prentice-Hall, Inc

Notes & Feedback from Workshops, Interviews, and Journals:

- Participant Oral Feedback, Workshop II, 1 July 2011, London, UK

- Teacher's Notes, Independent Dance Improvisation Class, March 2012 & December 2012, London, UK

- Amerta Movement Journal 2007 & 2008, Solo, Java

- Prapto Interview, Prapto's Home, Mojosongo, Java, April 2008

Sally E. Dean has been a performer, performance maker and teacher for over 14 years – in university, professional and community settings. Her work interlinks the fields of health, movement, expression, culture and performance. She is a certified teacher of Skinner Releasing Technique, a teacher of Scaravelli yoga and trained in Amerta Movement with Prapto. Informed by somatic practices, Sally's teaching and performances integrate nature, site, object, sound and costume.

As Artistic Director of Sally E. Dean Performing Arts and the Kolaborasi Project, her mission is to facilitate artistic collaborations and dialogue among American, European and Asian people.

www.sallyedean.com

www.kolaborasi.org

13. CRYSTALLIZATION-PERFORMANCE

A New Expression In Its Own Right

Lise Lavelle (Denmark)

In this chapter about the nature of crystallization-performance I shall refer to my first solo performance, entitled *Healing in Point: A Woman gets her Face*, performed in Java in 1990 at the Padepokan Lemah Putih School.

Within Amerta Movement there are two approaches to movement. One is called *Pribadi Art,* meaning Individual Art in Javanese. It is based on the individual student. Practitioners initiate movement from their inner, felt sense as a basis for their expression, using their personal story as material that is transformed into movement expression in the outside world. The aim is personal development. The other approach is called *Messenger Art.* As I understand it, for this the material embodied in the outside world is based on input from outside the practitioner's own autobiography.

Before proceeding to my performance, I will look first at the background to the performance, at what a crystallization-performance is and at why I see crystallization-performance as an expressive art in its own right.

An incentive for engaging in performance was my passion for practicing movement and awareness in the Amerta manner. This connected with my studies of Sumarah (relaxed) meditation in Solo since 1977. I came to these forms from the perspective of my Danish background, especially my training as a teacher of classical relaxation and movement from the school of Ingrid Prahm, a pioneer in this field in Scandinavia.

In addition, crucial to my process, was the experience of participating in a group dealing with loss and sorrow, called a 'sorrow-group,' following several deaths in my close family. In this group, I learnt that when one has gone through 'the necessary pain,' in connection with parting from persons who have died, it is time to move on. One moves on through learning 'new skills.' How do you know you are on the right track when learning 'new skills' after a major crisis? When your hands are sweaty and your heart is beating strongly you are on the right track. Actually it is a bit like when you learned to ride a bicycle! With practice, the sweaty hands and strong heartbeat will diminish. This to me sounded like crossing a bridge and reaching what Prapto called *the other shore*, thus transcending ways of merely coping that are no longer helpful and moving forward.

Practicing Amerta Movement while developing my 'new skills,' became a journey through all sorts of landscapes, from pain to joy, from humiliation to victory. The practice was a wonderful elixir to get back on the road again; endorphins fill your body and reality your mind!

Prapto's courses are often concluded with public presentations based on Pribadi Art or Messenger Art. They are referred to as *performances* or *crystallization-performances*. I will use the two terms interchangeably. In this chapter I am mainly dealing with performance from the Pribadi Art approach. Crystallization-performances from the Pribadi Art approach are based on one's personal story with the aim of expressing oneself via free, non-stylized, improvised movement. The mover is dancing her/his own steps. The Pribadi Art expression is a personal movement language.

I see a crystallization-performance as an expression in its own right. This is because it takes the form of improvisation within the present moment, in contrast to performances consisting of previously fixed gestures, gaits and rhythms, controlled by a choreographer. Content and form are characteristic of – or specific to – both the person performing (person-specific), and to the site of the performance (site-specific).

This means that the performance makes sense, in terms of content and form, in relation to the individual performer and to the site of the performance (often in the natural environment). Now the performer and the site are, like life, ever-changing; hence a crystallization-performance cannot be incorporated within the confines of a single discipline. Just as one cannot bathe twice in the same river, Amerta crystallization-performances are never the same. Everything relating to these performances is moving and changing from one moment to the next – the performer, the site, and the spectators.

Below, I shall present my building-blocks (or special points) which came to constitute my framework for making the crystallization-performance, *Healing in Point: A Woman gets her Face*. It took place in 1990 after I had completed an initial course with Prapto at the school. I spent three months on this piece.

The making of this crystallization-performance was part of realizing my 'new skills' in relation to my 'sorrow-group.' Moreover, I was on my way towards creating a kind of healing theater. By 'theater,' I simply meant bodily expression and visible form as an externalization of inner impulses.

I was interested in healing in a sense of wholeness, and in letting nature heal us as when a wound heals by itself. I see healing as a blossoming, a liberation of inner stirrings – positive and negative – and as resources and potentials ready to manifest. Hence in my opinion healing is a natural part of human development. The aim of healing and of a 'healing theater' is getting re-connected with lost parts of oneself and, thereby, with the Source of Life.

Growing my Performance in the Valley

It all started in a valley belonging to the school, hereafter referred to as 'the Valley.' That is where the performance took place, as did the process leading to it. This Valley was normally never used during courses because it was isolated from the rest of the school, being hidden from it by vegetation.

The locals considered the Valley to be theirs and used it for grazing their animals. I went there simply because I liked the place.

To the north, the Valley is surrounded by large earthen mounds with bamboo groves and local hamlets. To the south there is a little river and rice paddies. In the east, the volcano Mt. Lawu, famous in the history and mystical practices of Central Java, is visible on the horizon, and to the west is the Padepokan Lemah Putih School.

The Valley was luxuriantly green, with much grassy land, but as a practice space it was a wild place because of its thorny, uneven ground with areas of scrub, liana, insects and poisonous snakes, of which I was afraid.

Prapto called the Valley *the Point* because its bottom was formed as a point rather than as level ground. The practitioner, when starting to move, was restricted to the small confines of the Point.

This dramatically reduced freedom of movement. Thus the student practicing there was in an energy center, i.e. in the center of the forces of nature.

The Valley also has a symbolic meaning according to Prapto. Its theme is receiving. Practitioners receive sensations, feelings and thoughts from inside themselves and happenings in the Valley from outside. The Valley embodies receiving from and communicating with the vertical axis connecting earth and heaven, subconsciousness and higher consciousness.

Through my movement practice, I came to build a whole universe of my own in the Valley and thereby eventually to develop a framework. This consisted of a score based on my building blocks (or special points) as mentioned above.

My movement took place during the dry season, which meant a blue sky, white clouds and a bright sun. In the morning when I arrived, I would place myself on a bamboo mat close to the little bamboo forest that provided shelter from the burning sun. From there I had a view of the whole Valley. My bamboo mat and the area surrounding it became the starting point of my movement every day. It became my 'home' so to speak. I explored the Valley like a scientist: what kind of trees, rocks, bushes and animal life were there and what forms, proportions, levels, colors, smells and sounds did they have? I also tried to decide where exactly things were situated and at what distance from each other. I drew a map of it in order to be in touch with the reality of the Valley and as a help to orientate myself in its landscape.

Sometimes when arriving in the Valley and sitting on my mat I just could not relax or I became bored. What to do today? My body was not yet in tune with the Valley. Then I had to start to get in tune by getting into my body and feelings with awareness. I did so by doing relaxation or Qigong, Tai chi and Kung fu exercises. These exercises had a clear outer form, which helped me relax, instead of having to compose my movements myself as is necessary with Amerta Movement. These exercises also helped me feel myself more clearly and hence helped me warm up so as to start to move freely, now being in tune with myself and the Valley. On other days, performing free, improvised movement, Amerta style, was easy; this was because right away when I arrived I could tune myself in to the Valley and to the present moment and thus I could proceed directly to composing my free movement. This was so easy that it felt like turning on a switch: I sort of 'opened up,' shifting my awareness towards the top of my head and felt that something flowed down from outside, maybe an energy or an inspiration to move. Whatever it was, my body was in tune with it and then knew what to do, i.e. which movements to make and where to go in the Valley.

My mind formed many pictures based on impressions from the Valley; one could say that I projected my life's universe onto the Valley. For example, some trees at the front of the bamboo forest were as big as pillars and formed a majestic arch opening into the forest. To my mind this became an opening into a magical and unknown space. It brought to mind a poem by the French poet Baudelaire:

> *La Nature est un temple où de vivants piliers*
> *Laissent parfois sortir de confuses paroles*
> *L'homme y passe à travers des forêts de symboles*
> *Qui l'observent avec des regards familiers.*[1]

Day in and day out I touched my personal universe, or it touched me. In some ways it was rather like entering the playworld of my childhood or the world of a fairy tale. Gradually I found the special points that appealed to me and upon which I focused as building-blocks or points of support in the natural environment. These building-blocks or points of support, as mentioned above, constituted my framework.

First among these points of support (hereafter just 'points' or 'my special points') was the bamboo forest in front of which I had placed my mat as a kind of home, to which I kept returning, since the bamboo forest provided shelter from sun and rain. At the same time as I projected the poem of Baudelaire onto that forest (a reference from my adult life as a lecturer in French at teachers' college) the child in me was finding that this bamboo forest was 'My Enchanted Forest' with Little Red Riding Hood. Then there was one tree, the only one on the riverbank, jutting out above the river. In my mind's eye, this tree became 'My Tree of Life' from which I looked across the river to the other shore.

---

1 Nature is a temple in which living pillars
  Sometimes give voice to confused words;
  Man passes there through forests of symbols
  Which look at him with understanding eyes.
  (Baudelaire 1954). This is the first verse of the poem, *Correspondances*.

A few other rocks took on a special value; sometimes I would step into the river to move and dance on some rocks there. When returning to the shore, a big rock on the riverbank helped me step back without getting sucked into the mud. This rock became 'My Stepping-up Stone.' This was meant in a concrete sense and in a symbolical one, as in 'stepping-up' from a low energy situation and getting on with it. Finally, there was a rock situated at the far end of the Valley which became 'My Stone of Sorrow.' Hence the points that formed my framework were: 'My Enchanted Forest,' 'My Tree of Life,' 'My Stone of Stepping-up,' and 'My Stone of Sorrow.'

The meanings I attributed to these points were not fantasy. They all made sense to me at the time. By their different physical forms and materials these points woke up stories in me. I saw these points as archetypes in the Jungian sense, as containers of common human factors embodied in nature or projected by me onto nature. The whole Valley came alive to me in an extraordinary manner because I spent every day there for several months with all my senses open.

By finding these points I created my own universe in the Valley. I moved in relation to the points, responded to them physically and worked out a movement vocabulary on that basis. Especially after I had worked through the sensations, emotions, thoughts, memories, and stories that the points represented to me or that I had projected onto them, the points came to provide a structural framework for my free, improvised movement. And later, when I was no longer so overwhelmed or consumed by my subjective experience of what they released in me, these points also took on a more common human value, which I felt would have a broader effect, rather than purely a private one. A transformation happened: 'My Enchanted Forest' with Little Red Riding Hood became 'The Enchanted Forest,' 'My Tree of Life' became 'The Tree of Life,' 'My Stone of Stepping-Up' and 'My Stone of Sorrow' became 'The Stone of Stepping-Up' and 'The Stone of Sorrow.'

The moment I could dialogue with my own universe, including my own pain, and not be overwhelmed by it, the performance was born. Now I could face the world with my story. That explains the second part of the title, *A Woman gets her Face*. The first part, *Healing in Point,* indicates that this healing took place in the Valley, which, as mentioned above, was also called 'the Point.' Moreover, it refers to the fact that by going into the very point of one's pain, one is healed or one finds the treasure, just as the heroine does in fairytales. Personally I felt that through my movement and my

13. CRYSTALLIZATION-PERFORMANCE

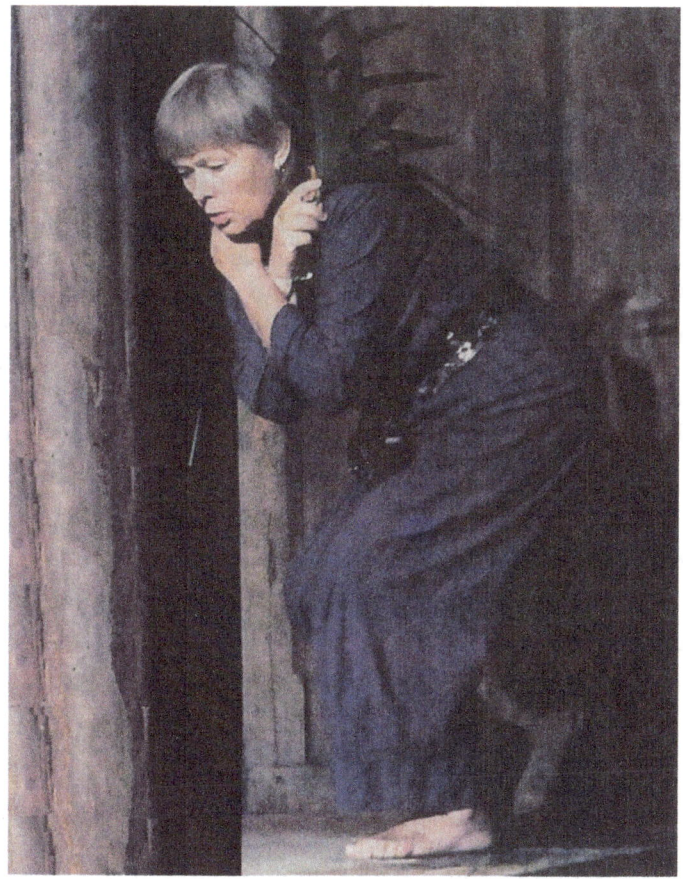

This photo from my performance, *Wings of Flying Mermaid*, on the Open Day at Padepokan Lemah Putih, 12 May, 2009, appeared in *Solo Pos (Solo Post)*, p.12, 14 May, 2009. Photo: Ratna Puspita Dewi.

mindfulness I had recaptured from the underworld an important part of my genuine being and expression, part of my identity, which had been lost for me.

~ ~ ~

When the performance started, the Valley was already shrouded in tropical darkness. I simply came in at the entrance, emerging from the bamboo trees into the light of torches, with a mask on my face. The mask had a neutral expression thereby concealing my 'true face' with my thoughts, feelings and emotions showing on it. I then crossed the Valley at its lowest part moving in improvisation to the top on the other side while visiting 'my' points. Then, at the top of the Valley I took off my mask and showed my new, strong face to the world, now being able to face the world with my thoughts, feelings, and emotions. Finally, I walked down to the river where a fire was built and put the mask high up on that fire. With this fire I drew a connection to my Scandinavian roots, as we have a tradition at the summer solstice of lighting hundreds of fires all over the country with a witch on top to celebrate the longest day of the year. My mask was like the witch. To burn the witch symbolizes the destruction of the forces of evil. I wanted to show the Indonesians this kind of a fire ritual especially as my performance coincided with the solstice.

After placing the mask, I lit the fire and stood there next to it, witnessing the unfolding action: the first flame searching upwards in the dark sky, illuminating it and the mask sitting on top; sparks leapt upward towards the myriad bright stars in the night and the delicately shaped new moon. The many, lit torches placed in the darkness from one end of the Valley to the other looked like a procession of people walking through.

> **Healing in Point: A Woman gets her Face**
> *a solo movement performance by and with Lise Lavelle, Denmark.*
> *Music & voice, Pelok Trisno, puppeteer, Indonesia.*
> *Venue, The Valley of Padepokan Lemah Putih, Central Java.*
> *24 June, at 7 pm, 1990.*

This crystallization was intended as a Pribadi Art performance where one builds on one's private story and transforms oneself on that basis. However one may discuss whether this performance was theater, ritual, healing, therapy, a presentation, or *what*? For me it was a crystallization-performance according to the technique of Amerta Movement, but because of the healing I went through and the way this performance made me learn new skills and discover new ground, both privately and professionally, I also see the performance as a *rite de passage*, a crossing of the bridge, and a stepping onto the other shore to a new phase of my life, the spectators being my witnesses really, as spectators are in rituals, rather than anything else.

My performance was a crystallization-performance in its own right because it came out of my movement practice. Moreover, the performance was not made to entertain but to share my experience, rather like one does after a Sumarah meditation[2]. One does so

---

[2] After having meditated together in a Sumarah meditation the *pamong* (guide) and the participants talk about their experiences during the meditation: could they relax or not? Did their experience come from their thoughts or feelings and emotions, from their physical body or from outside? And they also talk about how this all relates to their daily life..

honestly, but not to entertain. In fact, my whole meditation group was there at the performance to support me. I placed the audience at the very center of the Valley, where normally the performer would be. I did so in order to put them physically right in the performance. I did not anticipate that they would involve themselves physically in the performance; I just wanted them to be there. Moreover, to draw attention to my points, I had placed lit torches around them. To make my performance communicative I had added a few theatrical effects, like adding the mask and enlarging certain gestures. I also chose tools to move with from my practice such as two long bamboo sticks and a big, red dance textile. Although my daily practice had been without music, for the performance my movement was accompanied by the flute, voice and story-telling of a Javanese puppeteer, Pelok Trisno.

The performance itself came out of my practice, as did the message of going into the very point of one's pain to be healed. In contrast to being based on a preconceived form and preconceived contents, my movements were inspired by an inner urge as well as by outer conditions during practice.

Throughout *Healing in Point: A Woman gets her Face*, I had been inspired by Prapto's method which, in a physical sense, is very simple: to understand something you move with it, responding to it physically, be it the white Indian cows grazing in the Valley, a bamboo stick, a flower, a rainy day, a person, an inner chaos or your own body and being. You just move with it. There is nothing mystical in that although surprising events and understandings emerge. According to Prapto his method is not about shamanism nor drawn from religion. All he does, he says, when moving and performing is, *"to smell, to sense, to hear, to see, to touch and so on, because that way one can see much."*[3] One may also categorize that method as what in scholarship is called 'practice-based knowledge' and 'practice-based research.'

It is not necessary to have a concept or a story before starting a movement practice with the intention of making a crystallization-performance. The performance grows out of the process of moving, especially if the improvisation takes place outside in nature where there is much inspiration and input from the vegetation, and from animal and human life.

Moreover, the story, as I felt it, was already there locked up in my muscles and in the Valley, waiting to be found. At a certain

---

3 My fieldnotes, Java, 1990.

point I got the strong impression that it is not I who creates, rather something or someone does it for me. I am just a page in a big book. I believe and have experienced that just as fairy tales come from people's dreams, there are structures and whole dance dramas tied up deep inside our bodies.

~ ~ ~

References

Baudelaire, C. (1954) 'Correspondances' from *Les Fleurs du Mal (The Flowers of Evil)* (1857), trans William Aggeler. Academy Library Guild

In 1988, inspired by Prapto, **Lise Lavelle** PhD initiated her own movement work naming it the 'Dance of Life and Healing Theater,' and in 1997 changed it to 'Em*body*ment, dance of release and transformation.' Broadly speaking, she turned her training in classical Danish relaxation and movement, in Sumarah meditation, as well as in Amerta Movement with Prapto, into a 'holistic' movement practice. Lise also drew on earlier studies and practices of martial arts, Qigong, Tai chi, Kung fu, ritual dance, and Theravada Buddhist walking meditation and mindfulness (studied at the Wat Kiriwong Temple in Thailand), as well as on a Jungian approach to personal development and creativity.

liselavelle@mail.dk

14. BEING AND DOING IN THE WILD GARDEN

Movement Therapy in an East German Psychosomatic Hospital

Susanne Tümpel (Germany)

My experience with Amerta Movement forms an underlying base for my working attitude in general. I will explore the role of Amerta Movement in my movement work in a psychosomatic hospital with patients mostly from an East German background. From the manifold aspects of Amerta Movement I have picked one that is of particular importance in my work. This aspect can be described as the duality of Oneness and Separateness. In Prapto's terminology I connect this to the duality of *organism* and *organisation*.

Setting

I am working as a movement therapist in a clinic for psychosomatic disorders. The hospital is located in a rural, sparsely populated and quite poor part of eastern Germany, in the former German Democratic Republic (GDR).

The common theoretical approach used is psychodynamic psychotherapy, though the clinic does have an integrative attitude towards other approaches to psychotherapeutic work.

Movement therapy is offered in groups (5-8 participants) as well as in individual sessions. Patients stay between 5 and 10 weeks; some of them have an individual movement session once a week; groups meet twice a week for 75 minutes; that means the number of sessions is very limited, 4 to 10 times for the single sessions or 6 to 15 times in a group for the whole duration of their stay.

Patients are often working-class people, many of whom have been unemployed for some years or even since the collapse of the GDR in 1989. Some of them have been multiply traumatised or neglected.

Many of the patients are inhibited about their own being, body and appearance, with feelings of shame or self-hate. This is particularly true for those with eating disorders, for whom there is a special section. Patients have had difficult experiences with their own bodies and movement as well as with important relationships, which have often been harmful or disappointing. As a result of personal and societal experiences (often linked to life in the GDR) they mostly have a deep distrust of any institution and of relationships in general.

Different Cultures in Former East and West Germany?

There is an intense discussion in Germany about whether there are differences between the two German cultures. The head of the psychosomatic department, Dr. J.-F. Buhrmann, estimated that the GDR and its collapse in 1989 is an important life issue for roughly 50% of the patients in our clinic. With some risk of simplification I can say that in my experience of nine years working in western Germany followed by eight years working in eastern Germany, there is still a difference in the way I perceive the two cultures (being from the west myself). In eastern Germany I see more patients who feel severely disabled in living their lives to the full. Shame and feelings of isolation are common. And they even have a deeper distrust of relationships of any kind than patients in western Germany.

One possible explanation may be found in the different ways that society developed in the two Germanies after the Second World War. West Germany (the FRG) slowly changed into a more open society in which it was possible to question authority. In the GDR the Nazi Regime was replaced by another totalitarian regime with all its instruments of repression, which led to deep distrust and anxiety about showing oneself openly.

1989 was also not only a time of liberation but of loss and insecurity. New ways of life, rituals and identities had to be learned and citizens in the East faced all the disorders of post-modern capitalism, including low salaries, short-term contracts and high under-employment.

The Wild Garden

During one group session patients revealed an ambiguity towards me and my work; I imagine this is the same for many of my patients. The situation was as follows:

> *The movement therapy group began to fantasise about me and my upcoming holidays – what I might do, if I was as relaxed at home as they saw me at work, what my garden might look like – and they came up with the image of a wild garden in which weeds would also have a right to grow, a garden in which the paths are not straight and a lot of insects would find good nourishment. It is actually quite close to reality...*
>
> *They liked this, as if it meant for them that their "weedy sides" were also allowed to grow in the work with me. Nevertheless they said they would not create their own gardens like this.*

On one hand they feel fascinated by something that is strange, unorthodox, yet alive; on the other hand it gives them a feeling of shakiness and insecurity, even sometimes shame.

In my movement work, I do not have a specific outcome or result in mind; rather I provide a space where it is possible to sense one's own condition, one's contact to oneself and to the world. My working attitude has a strong parallel to 'evenly suspended attention'[1] as used in psychoanalysis. I maintain this 'evenly suspended attention' not only in the sense of feeling but also with my own psychosomatic body. Just as the analyst goes on the journey with the patient, exploring his own feelings, fantasies and thoughts, so I go into movement together with the patient without knowing how we will move, or what the theme will be.

Alice Pitty (2005) writes about Prapto as follows: "He uses his own body movement as a diagnostic tool, a barometer, to sense what is evolving or trying to emerge in a person's life, or in the interaction between people of different cultures".

I conceive of the patient's movement as their 'free association'[2],

---

1 **Evenly suspended attention** is defined as the "Manner in which, according to Sigmund Freud, the analyst should listen to the analysand: he must give no special, a priori importance to any aspect of the subject's discourse; this implies that he should allow his own unconscious activity to operate as freely as possible and suspend the motives which usually direct his attention. This technical recommendation to the analyst complements the rule of free association laid down for the subject being analysed." Laplanche & Pontalis (1988, 43)

2 In **free association**, the psychoanalyst encourages the patient to say whatever comes to mind during a session without editing or censoring it consciously. With this non-judgemental attitude, patients can bring to awareness and observe thoughts and feelings they might normally repress for fear of exposure or criticism, or because of inner conflicts. Patients make intuitive connections and jumps, through which they may find new understanding and insights. Although neither patient nor analyst knows in advance where their talk might lead, important themes will often appear.

which both of us can explore and 'taste', finding new movements, discovering connections, insights and understanding. In contrast to the psychoanalytic exploration of feelings and thoughts, I am actually moving and relating with the patient in space here and now. The movement dialogue evolves on a conscious, but also on a subconscious, level.

Working as a therapist for 20 years, I am still surprised at the way sessions develop, sometimes leading to very touching contact in spite of the conditions in the hospital with short-stay treatment and with the fears patients have about (movement) therapy.

Process in Individual and in Group Work

The majority of patients have no previous experience in psychotherapy nor with movement therapy. Most would not choose to do movement work. So it is often necessary to address their fears about revealing themselves in this way.

At the beginning of an individual session I usually take some time to hear what the patient is bringing to the session, some current problem from the ward or from home. In the same manner I would normally start the groups with an opening round in which everybody says something about their 'here and now condition'. It gives me a notion of what the atmosphere is, and also everybody's voice is being heard at least once by the group. Sometimes there will also be a longer period of talking.

I then suggest coming into movement, often not with a direct reference to what was said but with the idea of warming up, to feel the body-self. I usually move as well, as it helps me to be in this "bodily-evenly-suspended-attention" if I am moving too. Also if I were only to sit and watch it would often intensify the patients' suspicion of being watched or judged from the outside – this being a sensitive issue especially in former East Germany.

Frequently I start with stretching and yawning: it gives the patients a feeling that the situation is not so formal and serious. If the level of anxiety is high I offer more structure to allay their anxiety by setting a tangible task like "working with the feet, the back, etc.", "working with boundaries, own space", using objects, children's games, rhythm-instruments. In this case the free movement part will be shorter, and my aim is to develop trust, to have a corrective experience like, "being together can be relaxed, warm and joyful".

The free movement part following the warm-up will be daily

life movements, as inspired by Prapto's teaching, such as walking, sitting, lying, rolling, and jumping. While moving with the patient(s) I open myself to sense an underlying current, something with which the person or the group is consciously or unconsciously preoccupied. Often I will sense it in a physical way; it is not a thought or theoretical consideration.

Trying to sense a (common) theme is complex. There will not always be one or sometimes I am not able to feel it. In the first sessions I often put my focus more on a physical theme like 'back', 'feet' or 'using different spatial levels'. For example in working with the back I would propose to move the back in different ways, to touch it while moving, to feel which movements would be comfortable for the back. Later I would progress to themes more related to perception and feeling. This might be an attitude, a perception of the space, a feeling; I may suggest: "putting your feet and placing yourself in the space", "sensing your back and the space behind yourself", "moving and pausing, taking a breath".... The whole time I am very conscious not to be in a sort of 'trance', but on the contrary to be grounded, not spacey or 'mystic'. My hope is that patients can be more present with themselves, with the others and with the space.

Oneness and Separateness

Since my employment in eastern Germany I have found Prapto's themes of *organism* and *organisation* to be useful tools in my work, especially when I link them with similar themes described by the Israeli psychoanalyst, H.S Erlich, which I will discuss.

My first personal feeling for Prapto's use of the words *organism* and *organisation* evolved in a workshop he held in 1995 in Kranichmoor/Hamburg. I was both participant and organiser of this workshop. Prapto referred to a situation where I abruptly jumped from *human relation* to *functional relation*: in the middle of an informal breakfast chat I abruptly checked some financial business with a co-organiser. Prapto had explained how he felt confused and maybe also angry about this cutting of the *being* situation. In the following days we worked intensely with the awareness of *human relation–functional relation*. I got a sense of how it must feel to be more in *human relation*, and still be able to function as an organiser – what Beate Stühm (2012) called to "organise in organism" and how new and precious it was to me. I also felt a sadness knowing how easily it could get lost again in a busy, Western daily life.

This experience impressed me very much and I see a distinct parallel between that which Prapto calls *organism* and *organisation* and the experiential modalities of 'being' and 'doing', as described by H.S. Erlich. Erlich has "developed a conceptual framework, in which the dimensions of 'being' and 'doing' form parallel and complementary tracks, through which experience is processed and organised" (1996).

In Erlich's 'being mode' the experience of self is one of identification, "union and fusion with the other, as well as with the world, nature, universe etc." (1995). Time and space are felt to be non-linear; the overall tendency is one that allows the subject to experience himself fully as ongoing and existing in connectedness, union and oneness with the other. As I understand it, Erlich sees it as a union in which the person is not melting with the other in the sense of losing themselves but more one in which the necessity to emphasise their separateness does not exist. I remember that, in groups, Prapto distinguished between 'group soup' and being together with everybody having their own body.

In the 'doing mode', according to Erlich, self and other are experienced as separate and they have a functional relationship. The central question would be "who is doing what to whom?". There is causality, directionality and chronological experience of time and space. The overall tendency is goal oriented; there is task and accomplishment. "Boundaries are vitally important in this modality..." (1998).

Prapto has repeatedly created images to describe the social-cultural differences between the Javanese and 'Western-European-American' cultures. The concept of *organism*, connected to the Javanese world, is the organic, natural, physical world, with intuitively ascertainable human proportions. This is the field of *human relation*.

Prapto uses the term *organisation* in connection with Western industrialised society, with *functional relation*. Also hopes, fears and dreams are part of *organisation*, because they happen beyond the immediate relationship. *Organism* and *organisation* describe experiences of relating between self and other, and they also include experiences of space and time.

As in Erlich's 'being mode', in 'organic time' everything happening in the same space is interconnected and included. I remember vividly the way Prapto always clearly welcomed everything that happened – it might be a person accidentally passing by, a change of weather, anything that by us Westerners often was felt to be a disturbance, not planned and therefore to be excluded.

Erlich emphasises that both modes – 'being' and 'doing' – exist and function simultaneously; normally one of them will gain ascendancy and dominance at a given moment. He says that from the beginning of life both modes exist and function. The mother's tendency is to adapt herself flexibly to the mode her baby is in. "Gradually, mother and infant acquire the sharing of increasingly finer gradations and combinations of *being/doing* with either the one or the other mode serving as the predominant quality in a given moment of experience or relatedness" (1998).

Erlich also says that psychoanalytic therapy similarly consists in the ability of the therapist to sense the mode the patient is in and to change between two modes according to the needs of the patient. I believe this is similar to what Prapto is doing, having watched and experienced him in many single and group sessions.

In movement therapy I see myself matching the mode the patient is in, as well as modifying it in a way that might be helpful, as illustrated in the case that follows:

Single Session with Mrs. A.

Mrs. A. is a very youthful, attractive woman in her mid-forties. She suffers from extreme exhaustion. Her husband is often absent, working abroad; her daughter is also in clinical psychotherapeutic treatment.

She speaks about the strong pressure she feels to perform, wanting to do everything properly and being disappointed that her efforts are not acknowledged. She has a constant need for approval by the other.

She moves with high tension, creating a hollow back, and putting a lot of effort into moving while at the same time seeming empty, depleted.

Her doing comes from an idea: "I need to do it right", and not from the physical need to do. So she is constantly feeling strained, exhausted and also disappointed if others do not appreciate her efforts. With her I am searching for a way to come into *being*.

My gaze falls on the panorama outside, garden, park and lake, the sun just rising in the fog.

I describe what I see: "Sunlight dropping through the fog onto the lake".

I give this as a movement suggestion, hoping that this more poetic, 'haiku-like' description could help her to come into movement more from a feeling sense as it offers little possibility of knowing how to do it right. The image of light falling through the fog seems to me very fitting, because it gives a sensation of not-doing, of letting it happen.

> *So for about half an hour we both explore. Initially she is trying hard to "do it right", in spite of not knowing what that could be. After a while she begins to move more slowly, in the end she lies down on the floor, resting and feeling her exhaustion, her struggle. She seems to be sad, allowing this feeling to be there at least for a little while.*

I realise how strongly I myself am sometimes stuck in a sort of painful 'doing', and, although being a Westerner, how I have gotten a better sense of the 'being mode' through the movement practice. I believe that this helps me to be open to some 'inner place' of the patient, to be surprised by what wants to emerge, rather than starting from any sort of pre-fixed idea or theory. This openness to being surprised gives space for the unknown, the non-habitual, which can express something more vital and alive, more the real person.

Being honest with oneself is also connected to the 'being mode': not playing a role, not pretending to be a certain way, to be stronger, more powerful, more confident, but also not pretending to be less strong, less confident than one is. Letting oneself be seen, one's body and movement, without going into pre-fixed movement patterns: this has been a core theme all through my own movement experience with Prapto.

The vibrant sensation of being completely present is even perceived by witnesses of the movement situation. I can remember the feeling of the whole space waking up when someone in a movement workshop, after moving 'in the fog' for a long time, suddenly started becoming more in touch with herself/the others/ the space. Even participants who had been dozing at the sides sat up involuntarily.

In working with Prapto I experienced his strong interest in how to *organise in organism*, how the two states of 'being' and 'doing' could nourish each other, how Eastern (Javanese) culture could benefit from the Western attitude and vice versa.

Similarly Erlich says that the task of human development is to integrate the two modes. It seems that in Western society, oriented so much towards performance and achievement, the failure of this process has its roots more in difficulties in the 'being mode' and its integration. "In Western civilisations the *being mode* has been downgraded, and the *doing mode* given exclusive priority and prominence" (2003). Relationship as a value in itself does not count any more; instead there is extreme emphasis on the individual and individual achievements. This opens new opportunities, more freedom on the 'doing side' of life. The drawbacks are more on the 'being side', leading to separation and isolation.

Erlich expresses it clearly, "(being) is involved in and underpins our sense of aliveness as well as connectedness with everything – relationships, nature, life, ideals and values. Without it our psychological life is seriously impoverished and hampered" (ibid).

As mentioned above, the patients I meet often have great difficulties in allowing themselves periods of 'being' states. More often they have feelings of separateness, forlornness, isolation. But at the same time 'doing' is not positively experienced – e.g. under circumstances of being unemployed half a lifetime without any chance of getting a job again.

Being-Doing in My Work - The Wild Garden

The image of the 'Wild Garden' to me implies a balance between *organism* and *organisation*, 'being' and 'doing', a balance that is lost and found again continually. In the garden, I can 'be' and experience the aliveness and diversity of plants and animals, and at the same time I can step in and create an interplay of the wild and the structured. There is no end to this, but cycles of growing and resting.

Amerta Movement for me is a wonderful way to experience this duality of 'being' and 'doing', or *organism* and *organisation* in the therapeutic context. It is not a routine, something I know how to do and master. It is new every time, moment by moment. Thus it is a means to give value to 'being-with-oneself' and 'being-together'. Also 'doing' can grow from self-worth and self-efficacy and not from a feeling of pressure and fulfilling expectations of others. In the best case, this could then become a 'doing-together' or 'doing-in-connectedness'.

~ ~ ~

References

Bloom, K. (2006) *The Embodied Self: movement and psychoanalysis*, Karnac

Erlich, H.S. (1991) 'Die Erlebnisdimensionen "Being" und "Doing" in Psychoanalyse und Psychotherapie', *Zeitschrift fur psychoanalytische Theorie und Praxis*, vol. 4, pp.317-334

Erlich, H.S. (1995) 'Two Kinds of Change Facilitating Factors', *The Israel Journal of Psychiatry and Related Sciences*, vol. 32, no. 3, pp.194-204

Erlich, H.S. (1996) 'Ego and Self in the Group', *Group Analysis* vol. 29, pp.229-243

Erlich, H.S. (1998) 'On loneliness, narcissism and intimacy', *American Journal of Psychoanalysis*, vol. 58, pp.135-162

Erlich, H.S. (2003) 'Experience, what is it?', *International Journal of Psychoanalysis*, vol. 84: pp.1125-1147

Laplanche, J. & Pontalis, J-B. (1988) *The Language of Psychoanalysis*, Karnac

Lavelle, L. (2006): *Amerta Movement of Java 1986-1997, an Asian Movement Improvisation*, PhD thesis, Lund University Centre for Languages and Literature

Pitty, A. (2005) *Rituals of Chaos*, http://bit.ly/ELtp09

Stühm, B. (2012) personal conversation

The support of, and vivid discussion with, friends and colleagues has helped me with the formulation of my thoughts. I owe particular thanks to Anna Budczies (M.D.) and Philipp Kuwert (M.D.) – both specialists in psychosomatic and psychotherapeutic medicine, Sibille Buschert – dance therapist, and Katya Bloom – movement therapist.

And I deeply thank Prapto, working with him has had a strong influence on my life – both professionally and personally.

Susanne Tümpel, born in 1961, works in the psychosomatic department of Helios Kliniken in Schwerin, Mecklenburg-Vorpommern, Germany. Her vocational training includes: Tamalpa Training Program of San Francisco Dancers' Workshop with Anna Halprin; Feldenkrais Training; working with Prapto in Germany since 1984; 2-year Teacher Training with Adam Bradpiece; weekly groups, seminars and single sessions with Susanka Christmann and Adam Bradpiece between 1985 and 1995. She had and still has supervision with the psychoanalysts Gisela Worm, Renate Ritter and Ralph Schindler (M.D.).

susanne.tuempel@web.de

15. 'MANTRA GERAK' / MOVEMENT MANTRA

Agus Bima Prayitna (Indonesia)[1]

I. Personal Background

I was born in Kalang Lor Village in the Wanagiri Region of Central Java, where my father was a primary school teacher and a *dalang* (shadow-puppet master) in the Wayang Purwa style. My mother took care of all the family necessities of which one is the noble task of educating the children.

From the age of two, I was often ill. When I reached adolescence, my father trained me in *laku* (ascetic practices) such as: *kungkum* (submersion in the river), fasting, solitude in sacred places, in caves and on the road without sleeping throughout the night. *Laku* practices for youth, in general, are actually training for adulthood and a way that an adolescent can be close to and learn from nature.

In the 1970s, all adolescent boys in Java still studied mantra from *dukun* (spiritual teachers) and I did too. I learned about the types and functions of Javanese mantra, which are chanted, murmured or recited internally and have the potential to generate energy or strength.

My knowledge was deepened during my research for my undergraduate thesis on 'The Structure and Social-Culture of Javanese Aji-Aji Mantra'. I perceived that Javanese Aji-Aji mantra is a form of oral poetry and learned that, basically, there are three types:

- **Magical** – mantra used to fulfill or obtain something that is wished for with full power and force. In Javanese culture, this is the first level and the first step in a person's journey in the process of life. Usually people at this level are

---

[1] This chapter was translated from the Indonesian by Diane Butler.

still young at heart or not yet mature or old in the sense of *ngelmu* (knowledge). In contrast, a person considered old in Java is someone who already has deep and broad knowledge of, as well as experience of applying, the *ngelmu* they possess.

- **Mystic magical** – mantra practiced by a person after mastering magical mantra and used to fulfill the necessities of life. However, the results depend on the process of nature or of life. Power and force exists, but is not a must. In Javanese culture, this is the second level when a person is stepping into *ngelmu* but is still considering or fulfilling the necessities of life, which is termed *kahanan kadonyan*. At the level of mystic magical mantra, a person is permitted or proven to have control over what they wish for, yet the results are given over to the practitioner's process of life.

- **Mystic religious** – mantra that is used for harmony of life both in relation to other humans and nature. In Javanese culture, this is the third level when a person is already *mungkur kadonyan* (past worldly things). So, although a person still conducts their life in an ordinary manner, they have already let go of any desires and all is surrendered to the process of life or surrounding nature.

II. Chronology Leading to 'Mantra Gerak'

After graduating in 1986, I performed Javanese mantra in the form of a poetry reading in 1987 at the Taman Budaya Jawa Tengah (Central Java Cultural Park) in Solo. Also in 1987, my friend Arja brought me to Padepokan Lemah Putih to introduce me to Mas Prapto. He offered me a program to practice how the mantra that I knew could be transformed or embodied in movement (like the movement I saw that day when he and many Europeans were practicing), even though at that time I had no understanding of what movement was.

For the next six months, I did not respond to Mas Prapto's offer. I was not interested at all as it seemed so very different and distant from my background. In mid-1987, Mas Prapto contacted me again to talk about how the mantra that I knew could be embodied in movement. In his words, *"How about Mas Agus first just try movement practice?"* Starting with no movement resources, I began to practice among the European friends, and also a few Indonesian friends who had already studied dance at the ASKI music academy (now Indonesian Institute of the Arts, Surakarta). My background was in Javanese literature and I had written quite a bit about Javanese *tembang macapat* and *geguritan* (poetry), *cekak* (short stories), drama and critique essays. But I truly had difficulties knowing the language of the body. For sure it would have been different if I had had a background in dance or at least had ever exercised my body.

Starting from knowing nothing, through movement practice with sincere intensity and also spurred on by practicing among European friends, two years later I just knew in an aware way what mantra was and what movement was. From these two different worlds, gradually I was able to embody mantra – the mantra of the universe in Javanese culture – in the form of movement.

I studied Amerta Movement with Mas Prapto regularly and intensively from 1987 to 1997. In this context, my mantra was not in an oral form; rather, it was in the form of body movement. Since 2001, even though I do not take part in workshops any more, I have remained in the weave in the sense of *srawung* (sharing), in friendship and in Java it has even become like kinship.

Since 1997, I have engaged in art practice and art performance of 'Mantra Gerak' with an artistic identity of Teatr Mantra Gerak.

III. 'Mantra Gerak' (Movement Mantra)

1. Mantra

Mantra, in Javanese culture, is pure neutral, natural sound that has the potential to generate energy or strength. By sound, I mean an energy wave or vibration that exists in every human body. This energy wave or vibration is still in a pure and natural form which, as it manifests, can be sensed by one's eardrum. Pure neutral, natural sound includes crying, anger, laughing, as well as serene and satisfied sounds and many other types of manifestations. All of these are *rasa* (feelings) that become a desire. There are several categories of desire such as hunger, thirst, sexual and religious-spiritual desire.

2. Gerak (movement)

Gerak (movement), in my experience and opinion, is the process of change that occurs in all parts of the body that are alive, active and creative in a natural way in every human being. In other words, movement is a process of change in a human body that is living a natural human life. As I see it, a human's existence even just at the minimum level begins with the meeting of sperm and egg until it grows into a human being, which is shaped and influenced by:

- our natural geographic environment
- our culture (including customs and religion, and the social, political, economic, legal, technological, and scientific aspects of life).

3. Embodiment and unification of mantra with movement

'Mantra Gerak' is a unification of two universes or two different subjects, namely the *jagad mantra* (universe of mantra) and the *jagad gerak* (universe of movement). Both clearly exist in every human being, but they are different in nature and form. Though different, both can coalesce into an actual unity in a human being's actions throughout their life. Mantra is not only manifested in an oral form; it is also embodied in movement until our every movement has the potential and quality of energy or strength. The next process is to find how every movement can be meaningful or useful for life. Though mantra is commonly used to obtain inner power, my approach after studying Amerta Movement has been more towards cultivating a condition of relaxation and full participation in the living atmosphere of an environment. This is because, when we return to the origins of 'Mantra Gerak', we find that our sounds and movement come from a pure, neutral, natural potential.

4. The practice process of 'Mantra Gerak'

I practice 'Mantra Gerak' regularly alone and occasionally share the practice with college students, artists, spiritual practitioners, children, and village communities in Indonesia. I have also offered workshops a few times abroad in Germany, the Netherlands, Switzerland and the UK. The process I share is just to help each person to discover the form, manner, and techniques they can use for their own creative innovation.

Preparing oneself

Self-purification means letting go of everything that closes us off from pure, neutral, natural sound and the changes that are within each of us. Purifying here is not copying a stereotypical form associated with some religions. Why do we need to purify ourselves? Because, in the course of our lives, we are colored or shaped by the surrounding natural and cultural environment in its broadest sense.

15. 'MANTRA GERAK' / MOVEMENT MANTRA

Through self-purification a person can more easily practice and ultimately receive what they wish for. Purification in 'Mantra Gerak' does not mean getting rid of, quelling, reducing, stunting or stopping anything in the body. Rather, it is an attitude and actions that stem from the body, which allow us to reach clarity. From this clear atmosphere and condition we can easily see, feel and make pure, neutral, natural sound and physical changes. An analogy for the beginning level is calming, clearing, and cleansing impurities from cloudy water in a neutral glass. At the next level, we transform and apply clarity in our actions or activities.

Practicing for or in nature

As 'Mantra Gerak' prioritizes natural elements, we respect nature, learn from and reflect on it, rather than exploring and investigating nature to exploit it, because human beings are part of the universe and have the same character as nature. These days, virtual global networks have increased communication in the fields of technology, science, politics, and religion. On the one hand, this can help the process of human life. On the other hand, it can cause competition and also reduce the natural role of human beings. 'Mantra Gerak' can help revitalize a person's natural life process in an aware way.

'Mantra Gerak' for, or in, nature can include practicing with:

- Water at a river, spring or water source
- Stones in a river or on a mountaintop or ridge
- Soil, rice field sediment or beach sand
- Wind at the seashore or on a mountain and natural fire on a mountain
- Plants, trees, rice fields, and forests.

I mainly practice 'Mantra Gerak' in nature as it is easier to reflect on the natural elements in my body in order to know, process, and apply them in thought, feeling, and physically. For instance, *kungkum* submersion in a spring or the source of a river while facing the sun's position in the morning, at noon, in the afternoon, in the evening, and in the middle of the night nurtures a sense of fluidity, flowing, and clear spreading. Wind by the sea and natural fire on a mountain connects us with the spirit of life. Practicing on a mountaintop helps us control anger, transform it, and apply the energy in a different way.

A rice field can be a medium to study fertility by various practices such as enriching the soil, choosing and planting seeds, caring for the plants, and harvesting crops. So, fertility is not merely sexual; rather it is the chain of life, which requires mutuality. In 'Mantra Gerak', it emerges from creativity in such a way that it will bring forth innovation in a person with full commitment, playfulness, and productivity. One can share love for the harmony of life.

Practicing for or in society

This practice is very important, especially in Javanese culture. Practicing in society builds on the previous levels in terms of one's ability to be within a community's social environment where individuals may differ in their backgrounds. Each person will be recognized for his or her inner and outer communication skills. In Javanese culture this practice is the final level and termed *tapa ngrame*; meaning that although a person lives an ordinary life, they are always in a condition of being on retreat. This practice can include:

- Practicing in a village

- Practicing in crowded places such as a market or a street

- Practicing for or in a heritage site or a *candi* (temple)

- Practicing together and alone in these places.

5. The function of 'Mantra Gerak'

Based on the understanding that the growth of a human life is affected and shaped by both human and natural systems, in order to become aware of one's existence one can, for instance, use 'Mantra Gerak' as a means for:

- Opening, reading, discovering, analyzing, fertilizing, growing or liberating one's individual being

- Being courageous in bringing forth one's individual being

- Being independent in one's individual being

- *Srawung* (associating) with one's individual being.

The practice can also have beneficial physical, relational, protective, and compassionate effects. For example, since beginning to practice 'Mantra Gerak', I have rarely had flu, exhaustion or a headache. I no longer suffer *buyuten* (trembling fingers) or low self-esteem. It is easier to communicate and dialogue, the feeling of restlessness is less, and it is easier for me to adapt to situations than it was before.

'Mantra Gerak' embodies more than spoken or written language; it is a universal language that all living creatures possess, including human beings. So, in the context of relations both between humans and with other creatures in this world, 'Mantra Gerak' is a bridging language that is not limited to any social, cultural, political or geographical background. In this manner of communication a harmony emerges that respects and maintains the rights and dignity of all beings.

The practice of 'Mantra Gerak' also produces a condition of interpersonal protection so that people do not interfere with, harm, or conquer each other. In this way, individuals feel safe together without creating unnecessary boundaries or closing themselves off.

In 'Mantra Gerak', the source and priority is to explore pure, neutral, natural sound and changes in all parts of the body with sincerity and awareness. This produces a vibration of loving kindness, which manifests in the body as a conscientious heart. In the Javanese understanding, everyone has a conscience that can and will become more clear, luminous and glistening if it is regularly trained through *laku* practices like contemplation, meditation or reciting mantra that have a clear, calm and settled quality. One result is that a person can be more sensitive toward what has happened, is happening, and will happen to them and around them. A conscientious heart surely has a positive value in life or is useful for goodness, which is called *daya hayu* (energy of peace).

6. The embodiment of 'Mantra Gerak' in art

'Mantra Gerak' has as its source Javanese culture, which is heterogeneous, open, and accommodating. I view 'Mantra Gerak' as one of the new embryo elements of culture that still requires a lengthy process to grow and crystallize into a cultural form. Like a tree seed, it needs to be planted in a nursery and it needs fertilizer and care if it is to grow.

Ritual Art

'Mantra Gerak' as ritual art manifests as an offering that has a spiritual nature, as an expression of homage and as a feeling of gratitude for life whether in the past, now or for the future. For instance, at Candi Jago in Malang reading the bas-relief depicting the Arjunawiwaha tale inspired ritual art based on the ascetic ideal. While after the eruption of Mount Merapi in 2010, I created ritual art for nature with the community in East Merapi Village.

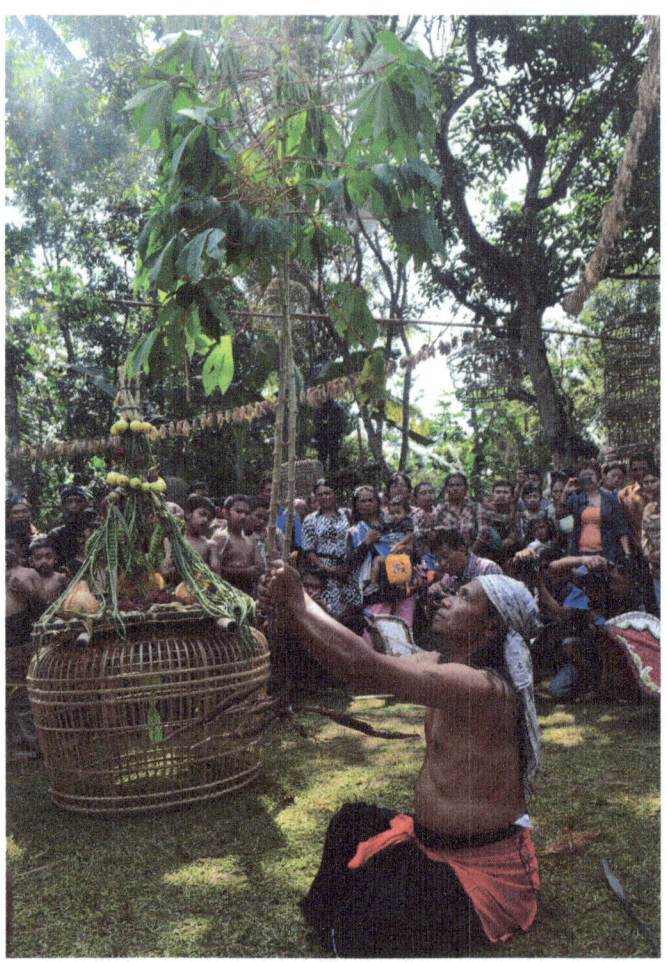

Sembah Ibu Bumi / Offering to Mother Earth by Teatr Mantra Gerak for Banjar Kurungan (hamlet of hand-crafted chicken cages). Photo: Suksma Jati Cahyaningrat

Performing Arts

As a performing art, my art aesthetic in 'Mantra Gerak' is always connected to my feeling of religiosity towards the audience, the setting, and nature. I have performed in communities and heritage sites in Indonesia and Sharing Time events abroad and even collaborated with a jazz organ player. Art practice with children in my village feels very playful and they easily make friends and access creativity. My intention is that any performance will produce a vibration of life together, harmony, and be an ongoing inspiration.

IV. 'Mantra Gerak' and 'Rajah'

A *rajah*, in Javanese culture, is a written or painted mantra. Its functions and characteristics are similar to oral mantra. A *rajah* uses special materials according to its essence and potential such as natural colorants, scents, the cardinal directions, a circular earth shape, triangular mountain shape, and square ocean shape. Sometimes a master artisan will keep the materials or technique for making a *rajah* secret. This is so that the *rajah* is not easily copied, or misused, or used by people who have not fulfilled the required *laku* practices.

Although a *rajah* can be a work of art that stands alone, it can also be combined with 'Mantra Gerak' especially in the form of ritual and performing arts.

V. A 'Mantra Gerak' Perspective on Life Now and in the Future

1. A perspective on Javanese culture as the mother of 'Mantra Gerak'

The role of 'Mantra Gerak' in communication and dialogue or in a *paguyuban* (a social association with a common interest or values), which in Javanese culture stems from communal social patterns, is the main source for placing 'Mantra Gerak' in everyday life. Life in a *paguyuban* society is based on *gotong royong* (mutual cooperation) and tolerance, and almost all decisions are based on togetherness. Any act or attitude of a community member that does not reflect togetherness would be an error. From this perspective, the existence of one's ego or personality is lessened. This lessening of the ego or personal universe is what 'Mantra Gerak' brings forth or encourages.

2. A 'Mantra Gerak' perspective on dialogue and global communication

As globalization and technological modernization is a part of life nowadays, it cannot be rejected or denied. For example, one phenomenon of technology that everyone must have and use is a communication tool. With all the sophistication of telecommunications equipment, we are able to cross all boundaries. This is a gift of modernity in that it generally weaves humans together. Yet it can be a weak point if interpersonal connections become dependent on a device. It can also be dangerous if one person's values are eroded or oppressed by the dominance of another person's values. One example is what has happened to some young Javanese people who have plunged in and followed the currents of other cultures and have become distant from their own culture. One reason for this is easy access to modern communication tools and the influences of other cultures. 'Mantra Gerak' is one way that the quality and potential of one's personal essence can be cared for even in the current of globalization.

VI. Religiosity of 'Mantra Gerak'

Returning to the essence of 'Mantra Gerak', which is the pure sound and movement that every person experiences – by practicing and through a deepening process, one will encounter a sense of the divine. Here, I do not mean in a conventional religious context. A person who cultivates and practices pure natural sound and movement will go beyond the limitations of their thoughts, feelings, and physical ability. They will emit a vibration.

Inner sound that is soft, pure and natural will bring one to a tangible, transcendent, inner atmosphere. Javanese culture as the mother of 'Mantra Gerak' has a mystic, transcendent atmosphere, which practitioners can connect to by themselves when 'Mantra Gerak' comes truly from the inner soul. It is an atmosphere of harmony with nature, the ancestors, one's relatives, friends, and so on. Attainment of a mystic, religious atmosphere is a concrete experience of the sweeping away of one's being. Yet, it does not eliminate one's being as it manifests in pure and natural sound and movement.

~ ~ ~

Agus Bima Prayitna was born in 1959 in Kalang Lor Village, Wanagiri, Central Java, Indonesia. Since the age of 17, he has studied mantra with several Javanese masters. In 1986, he completed his thesis 'Mantra Aji-Aji Jawa' and earned a Bachelor's degree from the Department of Languages and Javanese Literature at Universitas Sebelas Maret, Surakarta. From 1987 to 1997, Agus studied Amerta Movement with Prapto. In 1997, he named his work 'Mantra Gerak' and began to create performances with an artistic identity of Teatr Mantra Gerak.

gigih_sambodo@yahoo.com

16. THE MUSICAL PORTAL

Tim Jones (UK)

I first met Prapto in 1992. It was his first visit to England. As I walked into the room, Prapto, seated on the floor, said directly to me, *"You are wonderful"*. I replied with the well-known English swerve manoeuver, "You're not so bad yourself, Prapto".

Welcome to England!

~ ~ ~

My work as a performer, and voice and singing teacher has the umbrella title 'The Nature of Sound'.

This title brings together two ideas. The first idea incorporates an appreciation of the totality of, and fine discrimination among, nature's sounds – ones we like, ones we perhaps don't: birdsong, the wind in the trees, the natural sounds of human expression (sighing, laughing, singing, heartbeat and nervous system hum), the sounds of traffic.

The second idea approaches the nature of sound as a feeling for sound's own nature.

There is of course a physiology of sound – a sound's frequency, or pitch; its amplitude, or loudness; its timbre, or internal overtone structure; and its morphology, the shape or dynamics of its attack, duration and cessation.

But that doesn't tell the whole story. Perhaps there is also sound's own nature, its soul. From this perspective we can see or hear sound as yet another facet of a totality of being. This may seem an unusual thought.

I take it that my 'own' soul is not an independent entity residing somehow separately inside my body. I take it as the totality of my being, known and unknown, the totality of my expression, conscious and unconscious, and the totality of my attempts to live a life of growing awareness.

But if my own soul is not this independent entity inside me, perhaps neither is my soul, as I have expressed it, an entity that dwells in its own magnificent independence: not independent of the world and the people in my environment and my locality, not independent either, in my movement, speech and song, but more existing in relatedness.

The discrete events in the tapestry of sound outside my window – gardening activity, birdsong, leaf rustle – all relate through stories of season, climate and behaviour, and also in the stories I bring to the identifying and naming of them (the sounds). But they also cohere as an expression of the nature of sound (i.e. not just the sounds of nature). This takes a slight shift in one's relation to the sense of hearing. I remember Prapto calling out to those who might feel words directed to them:

"you do not yet know your hearing has language…"

This recognises that hearing itself *is* a 'language of being', a language whose syntax can be, and initially is, memory, pattern and habit, our relations to objects we hear.

Again that is not the whole story, but perhaps an initial nudge towards letting ourselves be present in and to our own stories. Another kind of hearing can occur in a shift that does not happen by trying to unstick patterns or get rid of habits, but in a space of recognition and kindness, an inclusive widened hearing space. Imagine a room full of people. The atmosphere is still and quiet. We are asked to sense our hearing. I do so, and slowly sense not just my own hearing, but also the hearing sense of all the other people in the room. This is not a listening *to* anything, not to silence, not to our breathing or to any other present sound. It is collective sensing hearing. And then I am aware of hearing hearing itself, which I would term the 'being of hearing', hearing as consciousness present to itself, expressing itself as hearing. This is akin to Rilke's injunction to "learn to forget how you sang… real singing is a different kind of breath, a nothing breath… a ripple in the God". Or expressed in the term '*Nada Brmha*' — Sanskrit words meaning 'the world as sound'. Hearing becomes part of the *speaking being*, as Prapto terms it.

It was an early thought of mine in teaching singing to recognise that to sing you have to know you are heard. Heard at least by yourself (although perhaps that is the most difficult step), or by your

16. THE MUSICAL PORTAL

friend, or your God, or by the wind, birds – it doesn't really matter, the issue at hand is connectedness or relatedness.

Prapto has a movement 'formula' (or perhaps suggestion is a better word). It goes:

dependence ~ independence ~ inter-dependence = inter-independence

Although this can be read as a progression leading to a goal (it can also be that), it is also important to allow that there is no judgement of any state, just recognition of which condition is in action, hence opening a space of movement and change in relation to self, other and to the environment of meeting.

~ ~ ~

In the project *Songworlds*, devised and developed over a period of 12 years by myself and my colleague Michael Dick, and part of the core curriculum of the acting school in Cologne where we both worked, student actors were invited to bring a song from any time in their lives – a lullaby, a children's song, an aria or pop song, any song. They were also asked to bring and be prepared to tell the memory or story of their connection to their song.

A vital part of the process we initiated with them is a Song Circle.

Progressing in a circle from whomsoever starts (basically whoever takes the plunge!), each person, without preamble, sings their song, tells their story and then sings again. The invitation is to inquire into 'now-ness' through their singing and telling, employing what we call vertical memory (as opposed to simply a horizontal, linear re-telling of events). Singing and telling become a way of hearing and sensing where the resonances are for you in your song and in your telling, as you go. Which part of your story is moving in you now? The resonant field of memory evoked for us by our choice of song can act as a doorway to a deeper experience of our own biography and narratives, a doorway allowing permeability, vulnerability and humanity.

The circle is always (and I mean, in my experience of perhaps 50 circles, *always*) a powerful experience of presence for participants: presence both to the self and to others. The circle has the ability to create for participants the dual role, important for trainee actors, of making them both 'actors' and 'audience'. As audience, their own response is clearly just that: watching, listening, enjoying, being moved. And yet each person is also an actor in this, i.e. their turn comes, and their responses to others' stories and the resonances or differences they find from their own offering contribute to the collective offering as well as to their own, individual telling.

Responses after such experiences (I've been part of circles from 2 hours to 5 hours long) often include feelings of shared experience, and of an inter-connected difference of culture, gender, race, experience or story. We commonly hear something like, "I know more about my classmates than I learnt in the whole of the last year".

This is a chance for each participant to be present to their own experience, their experience of themselves and their experience of others, whilst those others are simultaneously engaged in the same process. It is also a chance to learn to negotiate their own tolerance levels within this process – *"to receive the presence of your own story, and how much to let circulate"*, as Prapto once said.

In all this I am reminded of a former Archbishop of Canterbury's thoughts on 'conversation'. Rowan Williams writes extensively about the current debate between 'liberals' and 'communitarians'. On the one hand there is the view that individuals are endowed with intrinsic rights and liberties to be negotiated and protected in the public sphere; on the other hand there is the idea that people "find their dignity, even their sense of 'rights' through identification with values of the community". Williams's interest is in how a meaningful conversation might be effected between these views.

Williams, exploring the concept of 'conversation', quotes the political philosopher Charles Taylor: "A conversation is…a common action in this strong irreducible sense; it is *our* action."

His description goes on to include the 'uh-huhs' and 'mmms' of neighbours chatting over the fence. In this instance subject matter or content isn't the primary purpose. Williams continues by taking up the thought of conversation as a breakthrough into a recognition of common goods, "things we can *only* value and share together". To conclude the quotation: "conversation… in which the positive and participatory enjoyment of some other agent (person) is intrinsic to my own awareness of wellbeing and satisfaction."

This brings me back, full-circle as it were, to the shared space of the Song Circle, or its improvised performance version, *Songworlds*. Here, every circle has its own integrity, its own unveiling of the present for participants.

One group was asked to choose songs with the theme of beauty. Their choices indicated a sense that beauty always lies elsewhere, in another person, another place, another time. Through the month of the project they became aware of beauty as something almost like a scent, an atmosphere 'given off' as they became more and more close, intimate with their own stories and experience.

Another class, culturally very diverse (German, Serbian, Azerbaijani...) worked with themes from *Romeo and Juliet*. Their theme song, 'There's a place for us' (from Bernstein and Sondheim's re-working of the Romeo and Juliet story, *West Side Story*) was reflective of their sense of family fragmentation and cultural displacement. In the final improvised performance, as one of the performers began to sing, the song was taken up by the audience (fellow students at the school) who were also often from displaced and fragmented lives. The audience sang with and to the players in an incredibly moving moment.

In the sharing of songs and the unveiling of our stories and attachments to them, we enter a common ground that reveals both our individual distinctiveness and our mutuality.

I originally chose the quotation from Charles Taylor about the conversation over the garden fence as a link in my own preparation to co-host a workshop project with Prapto with the happy title *Music Garden Chatting*, re-christened *Mu-Ga-Cha*. These were meetings in my garden, in the local village hall, and up on Bulbarrow, a hill fort in Dorset. Williams's take on conversation and the sharing of common humanity made for me a direct link to Prapto's ideas of *Garden* and *Chatting*.

In *Mu-Ga-Cha* the ideas of a common ground of mutuality and distinctiveness were given the added dimension of the idea of garden, the relatedness of being human within the relatedness of human and nature – conversation with the environment, chatting over tea in the garden, musical chats, breakthroughs into the recognition of common goods, things we can only value and share together. The garden becomes the meeting place of human, nature and spirit.

In *Mu-Ga-Cha*, with these themes for moving and sounding within the garden, many 'movers' and 'sounders' would recognise the 'mmms' and 'uh-huhs', gentle signals of presence and engagement in the collective space. The *Garden*, both the collective and shared, my own garden, both the real one and the real one of my soul, is where

I tend my own needs, watering, planting (and in my case eternally mowing), mediated within the needs of the collective, the people with whom I move and sing. *Chatting* is where my own wellbeing is invested also in the wellbeing of other/s. *Music* is where these same intentions and 'listenings' are inherent in the evolving conversation of melody, harmony and rhythm within and around us.

Let's Go Outside!

We are in my garden, in Dorset, in England. It is a hot June day. I am recording a day in the life of *Mu-Ga-Cha*. Prapto and I are there, as are my wife and two friends, one a musician.

Prapto sits by the gently swaying acer tree, at intervals chanting. The musician sits just behind him, to Prapto's left, playing a beautiful repeated pattern on the *siter*, a plucked zither-like instrument from Solo in Java. In Solo, the *siter* is a street instrument, a reminder for Prapto of home……….

16. THE MUSICAL PORTAL

There is bird song   and then
the Doppler effect of an aeroplane lazing at great height
across the sky
   it takes its time
   Sometimes the telephone engineers' conversation drifts down
from their 'perch' up the telephone pole overlooking our garden
And our neighbour wanders down his garden,
turns on the water for his lawn sprinkler
he positions it   so that the water
      hits
the weather-vane-like construction   of his bird-scarer
a rhythmic patter of water on tin
      The siter figure continues
   Prapto   chants
a delivery van arrives
      departs
a bee drones past   hangs in the air
         and   the siter figure continues
         Hangs
   in   the   air
It is beautiful   the sounds of nature   the nature of sound.
   music
   garden
      chatting
"thank you" I hear Prapto say.
No no no,   thank YOU!

References

Cage, J. (1978) *Silence – Lectures and Writings*, Marion Boyars

Rilke, R.M. (trans. D. Young, 1987) *Sonnets to Orpheus*, Wesleyan University Press

Taylor, C. (1995) 'Cross-Purposes: The Liberal-Communitarian Debate', in C. Taylor, *Philosophical Arguments*, pp.181-203. Harvard University Press

Williams, R. (2000) *Lost Icons – Reflections on Cultural Bereavement*, Morehouse Publishing

Williams, R (2012) *Faith in the Public Square*, Bloomsbury

As a singer, storyteller and teacher, **Tim Jones** combines a performing life with a teaching life. He runs a public workshop programme, 'The Nature of Sound', and taught at Arturo Schauspielschule in Cologne, where he co-created the syllabus *Songworlds*, now offered by Tim and Michael Dick as part of their individual public workshop programmes and as a co-led course.

His love of Carnatic music has led to concerts and recordings in the UK, Europe and India. Tim has also collaborated on many performances with gamelan orchestras.

An Amerta Movement practitioner since 1989, Tim studied Carnatic music with Sivasankara Panikkar (1984-2007), has worked as a qualified Craniosacral practitioner since 1994 and is a member of the Ridhwan School.

www.thenatureofsound.com

17. NEAR THE UNKNOWN

Franca Fubini (Italy)

"The more we succeed in letting go of our own
intentions and ideas the better instruments we become
for something to emerge that is more than the sum
of our movements. We are tools and at the same time
witnesses for something that might be shown to us."
(Susana Miranti)

I met Prapto in 1994; from the start his movement work touched a deep chord within, giving voice to something which had always been there, an archaic area of the body and of the being as a whole.

Soon after, I realized that this work had also entered my professional life and that it had had a profound effect both on my Shiatsu and psychotherapy practices and also on my capacity to dream and to remember dreams.

Since the early '90s I had been involved in the development of Social Dreaming (SD), a methodology, discovered by Gordon Lawrence in the 1980s, which allows a collective of people to tap into the cultural knowledge and the thinking embedded in the dreaming of its members. Importantly, it focuses on the dreams and not the dreamer. It stimulates the capacity of the dreamers jointly to find social meaning.

Within the context of SD the meaning of the dreams and of dreaming expands, thoughts circulate more freely so that one and all can hear echoes of thoughts that inhabit the space of the mind where each of us is connected to the social, cultural, and natural environment.

Parallel to that field of discovery, for many years my friend Tim Jones – a voice teacher and performer – and I have offered workshops combining sound and movement. We had worked over the years developing a way of opening to inner and outer sounds, the movement between sounds, the reciprocal support between sound and movement and the connections amongst the people participating as a way of deepening sensitivity, resonance, and artistic production.

The time came when we thought it would be good to introduce SD into our workshops. One hypothesis was that it would accelerate and facilitate the existing process. The other hypothesis was that sounds, free movement, and dreaming would all feed into a common pool of shared connections and resonance.

Our experiment indeed confirmed the initial hypothesis that SD would facilitate and deepen the existing process. Like warp and weft, dreams did provide the language of images to support the movement work. Equally the practice of movement and sound deepened the capacity to connect to both one's own and others' unconscious sources and, by doing so in concert, to foster the potential for transformation of the individuals in the group.

Together both methodologies provided a containing frame to facilitate participants' encounters with unknown parts of reality without feeling paralyzed by them.

A couple of years later favourable circumstances brought the opportunity for Prapto, Tim and myself to work together. Each of us worked in our own specific field, but also as a trio who could share the different languages and who, together, would support the work and the awareness process of the whole group.

In the invitation to the workshop we wrote:

> *"The three of us have worked together for many years and in a variety of contexts. We welcome the opportunity to be in Bolsena once more and host this meeting.*
>
> *The workshop takes place at the beautiful Franciscan monastery in Bolsena. The mineral-rich volcanic Lake Bolsena is a short walk, and nearby are hot springs and Etruscan sites. Our work is supported by this environment.*
>
> *The theme (Sound, dreams and new thoughts), explored through sound, movement and with the stimulus of sharing our dreams, reveals the world of connections: the subtle threads amongst ourselves, the links to our cultural roots, to the roots of our common humanity, to the environment we live in, all expressions of connections to the infinite source."*

Dreamworld and Realityworld

Prapto often introduces his teachings with the concepts of *dreamworld* and *realityworld*. It was not so easy at first to discover what he means by that; however over the years of movement practice with him, my personal understanding of *dreamworld* is that it relates to the world of art, of poetry, of dreams, of shadows and night-life, of hopes and desires and that *realityworld* is more connected to the essence of what reality is about, namely emptiness, as well as to the material level of existence: nature, earth, body, senses.

My own experience of these ideas is that *dreamworld* and *realityworld* are two facets of one interconnected reality, echoing the explanation that is often given in order to explain *the-work-of-dreams* at the level of mental functioning. Borrowing from the theory of quantum mechanics:

> "…it can be said that every atom of our body and mind contains at the sub-atomic level both waves and particles simultaneously. Every elemental event in neurophysiology is related to other elemental events as entities in the cosmos at large through waves and particles. Waves periodically collapse, coalesce or configure as particles. When it is in this form, it becomes a piece of information, a fragment of knowing, a shard of the infinite. We can have the working hypothesis that dream-work, which is continuous for 24/7/365 throughout our lives, is a wave function. When a dream emerges from the 'black hole of the psyche', it is a particle." (Lawrence 1991)

I suggest that, borrowing from the same metaphor, the ultimate truth of *realityworld*, i.e. its emptiness – a concept derived from both Buddhist philosophy and from modern physics – is the wave phenomenon and the infinite manifestations of the world we inhabit are the particles emerging from that emptiness.[1] Through Amerta Movement one can have the experience of the ongoing and infinite dance of life and energy; at the same time it facilitates in the movers an awareness of their own particular way of moving as well as of their connections to the social,

---

[1] Both Buddhist philosophy and quantum physics share the view that the universe is empty, that there is no concrete and objective reality. The mind of the observer creates phenomena. Reality is the inseparability of emptiness and cognition, of calm state and movement. The universe starts empty, but potentially with a huge amount of information. In this respect the words of Buddha expressed in the Prajna Paramita, the empty nature of phenomena, match closely those of the contemporary quantum physicists, like Fritjof Capra, Stephen Hawking, John Wheeler, et al.

cultural and natural context that they move in.

Prapto is deeply involved in observing the web of connections that link humans to the culture they create and the nature that surrounds them. He invites us to observe the connection to God and to the living environment.

Sharing is a word which binds most of his work. 'Sharing Art and Religiosity' has been one of the themes chosen for the work that he offered in Italy during the 'Blossoming in Europe' project[2], where the concept of 'sacred' was explored as the space where humans connect to God, through art, nature, and environment.

My intuition in bringing social dreaming to our joint workshops years later was that dreams in this context would support the work, would accelerate the connecting process and would represent a clear bridge between unconscious contents and the images emerging both from the dreams and from the movement work. Indeed the body is where the unconscious resides.

What is Social Dreaming?

Social Dreaming is a tool of cultural enquiry and evolution: it is a probe that enlarges the field it explores. SD was discovered by Gordon Lawrence in the 1980s while he was working at the Tavistock Institute of Human Relations and it is shaped by anthropology as well as by psychoanalytic and systemic thinking.

SD is a methodology which allows not only a thorough experience of the unconscious processes at work in a group's life, but also taps into its creative and generative core.

SD capitalizes on the power of conscious and unconscious processes to work in concert; it was then a tentative answer to the question of developing an instrument that could mobilize the group potential for accessing its infinite, unknown, collective wisdom and using it to foster change. SD focuses on the nature of the dreaming/thinking that human contexts produce.

Prapto's work is steeped in the unconscious and at the same time it stimulates awareness of the unconscious vision that permeates our lives and that expresses itself through the body and its movements; by doing so, his work develops presence and awareness whilst also tapping into the creative potential of participants.

---

2 *"Blossoming in Europe creates a mandala journey from seven points in Europe. The purpose is to create an exchange of goodness from any place and cultural background. We hope from this process to create purification and crystallization for discovering a new view of human growing in the process of the human art culture."* (Prapto 1996/2002, from the leaflet announcing the events)

Social Dreaming Matrix

A specific setting holds the process of Social Dreaming: the matrix.

> "As a process, the matrix is the system or web of emotions and thinking that is present in every social relationship, but is, for the most part, unattended and not acknowledged. It can be thought of as mirroring, while awake, the infinite, unconscious processes in waking life that give rise to dreaming when asleep…
>
> As a form, the matrix is a configuration of people that provides a unique space, or 'container' (receptacle) for thinking out of the content of dreams to consider and discover their hidden, elusive/infinite meaning."
> (Lawrence 2011)

A matrix, from the Latin word for womb, is a place where something can grow, a mental receptacle for creativity and discovery; it is the net where knowledge and thinking "won from the void and formless infinite" (Lawrence 1991) can be received and brought to consciousness.

At the beginning of each matrix the host/convener states the primary task, like an invocation/act of faith in the existence of an unknown reality. The primary task of the matrix is to transform the thinking of the dream by looking for associations with the dreams offered in the matrix in order to find links and connections, and to discover new thoughts.

In SD, dreams are not interpreted in terms of the individual dreamer so that the potential meanings that are developing do not get saturated by untimely explanations. There should not be any specific expectation about the outcome of the work; the dreams themselves should be set free to work for the members, undisturbed by premature search for meaning. This privileges the non-linear and synchronous mode of thinking and the unconscious/infinite dimension of the mind.

Dreamers should dwell in 'not knowing' until a pattern emerges; they cultivate the capacity of being in uncertainties, mysteries, doubts, without reaching after facts and reason. With its own unique pace, a web of connections amongst the dreams captures and reveals the meaning of the matrix.

This is very close to the mindset which stirs the first movements and the first sounds in Amerta work. Prapto indicates a task, for example: *"work in oval, circle or square"* or *"moving in the garden"* or *"moving in the road"*; movers listen, poise until an impulse emerges, both from within and from without, which prompts them to move, to resonate, even if often unconsciously, with the context they are in. Movers give shape to that innner impulse and by doing so they contribute to the manifestation of collective patterns in space.

The dreaming matrix – like Amerta movement – works as a resonating box for its dreamers/movers; the following dream, once voiced in an SD matrix, captures its resonating essence using language as only dreams and poetry can do:

> "...there is a cobweb, and at each intersection there is a spider in meditation; the web has the same sensitivity of the spider mouth and it resonates with the vibrations of all the other spiders on the web..."

The Workshops

During the two workshops facilitated with Prapto and Tim, unconscious contents that reside in the body manifested themselves as the images of the shared dreams, which quickly became thread and support for the development of the expressive and creative work of the participants.

My experience is that in order to touch the 'unknown', often revealed by the nature of what the three of us were doing, a holding frame made of task and boundaries is needed.

In Tim's work, sound, the seven notes scale, and learning a song all represent the support and the reference point for allowing such exploration through one's own voice.

In a Social Dreaming matrix (SDM) there is a clear task, boundaries of time, rules which regulate interactions amongst the dreamers and make safe and enjoyable the telling of the dreams and the plunge into the unconscious/infinite.

In Prapto's work, there are reference points, but often it is difficult to see them, particularly if you are a beginner. The work is profound, it has an extraordinary capacity to initiate change in the people who practice it, yet it is also difficult to have an idea of what is really happening inside oneself. It is as though the work were bypassing the conceptual mind, in a way that is at the same time extraordinary as well as frightening.

Change is an essential component of being alive, yet it is feared as much as it is desired. Many have tried to capture the inner turmoil and the terror involved both in change and in learning – which are closely connected – due to the difficulty in tolerating the empty space before something new would appear. Both learning and growing are related to allowing change to happen and to the experience of knowing as well as tolerating not-knowing.

Growth, which is the outcome of creativity, is feared because it involves the destruction of the known order on which are based our feelings of safety and the idea of living in a predictable and controllable universe. It can be felt as an impending catastrophe.

Developing awareness and transformation mobilizes these powerful forces; Amerta Movement, SD and the voice work support their emergence and make them visible.

When Amerta Movement and SD were brought together, it was as though the dreams voiced in the matrix provided a light frame of shared images as a support for the movement and, in turn, the movement offered the possibility to take further and into action the trasformation of thinking that emerged through the dreams.

The Evidence

I shall give some evidence of the process even if very partial and short, as a detailed description of the process goes beyond the scope of this chapter.

It will deal mainly with the initial stages of the first workshop which took place in an old and beautiful convent, no longer inhabited by monks, but still owned by the Church, which had given the management of the place to a group of young volunteers.

The atmosphere was extremely laid back and homely, nevertheless one could certainly feel that until a still recent past the place had belonged to a rigorous monastic order.

A SDM would start each morning session. The imagery, the themes and the associations with the dreams offered in the matrix would appear in the movement work and in the free dialogues which would take place during the day.

During the first morning all the dreams and the associations offered in the matrix emerged from the distant past/history of each participant. They were disquieting dreams, speaking of danger and the impossibility of finding a way out:

> *"I am on my own and crucified, I don't know how to save myself"*
> *"I will be sacrificed"*
> *"I am on an ice pack, afloat in the ocean."*

The matrix was followed by a movement session: people seemed weighed down, pulled by gravity and very much on their own. There was still a group that moved, but the impression was that each person had to be alone in order to bear the weight of their feelings. There was neither sound nor music.

Later on during the day, during a time for dialogue, reflections on the day's work pointed to the context of our workshop. A strong connection was made with the Catholic Church, the constrictions of the religious order, and the suffering that monks might have shared within those walls over the centuries. The hierarchy was still visible in the large and luxurious rooms of the bishop and the small cells of the monks. People could easily connect to the dreams, to the feelings and to the atmosphere expressed in the course of the morning. They could pick up the isolated quality of their movement as though the weight did not allow access to a collective dimension nor to the possibility of transforming what was there.

The second matrix brought dreams that picked up other elements from the context, like the beauty of the place, the youthful joy of the people living inside those walls, the pleasure of the group in being there. A process of transformation was taking place and the initial heaviness was giving way to lighter feelings which manifested in a lighter quality in the movement sessions.

The third matrix opened with a dream from the previous night.

> "I am here with this group, we are about our activities, a Swiss man in his forties is with us. He looks incongrous; he tells me that he is in fact about to go on a walking tour in the Alps, he is all dressed for that, from boots to hat. I am surprised because I know we are all in Bolsena near a lake and very far from Switzerland. Then he leans to my ear and says something sexual, that again I feel is incongruous."

A therapist in the group asks about this Swiss man: "What does he look like?" and a detailed description follows. She says: "He is a client of mine! He has not found access to me, I have closed down when I came here. He is very demanding and finds his way in: he has found you."

I didn't doubt these words for a moment; they felt true. Rather, I was in awe as the group had already found the stage where dreams don't belong to the individual and dreams can be dreamt on behalf of somebody else, which is a phenomenon that often appears in the SD matrix, when the boundaries between oneself and the shared context become more porous.

What followed, unplanned, at the end of the matrix was a fluid sequence of movements and sounds. There was surprise and joy, as an extraordinary piece of improvised music was performed, where the quality of what emerged was clearly not produced just from the sum of the sounds made by individuals, but from a different level of music production.

The 'sound of the matrix,' a common womb where something can grow, had become manifest. It came both from each person's source and from something else, well beyond the wish of a personal intention.

The initial hypothesis which brought the three of us together seemed to have been confirmed.

Social dreaming, movement, sound and our joint work brought the group to a level of connection where some deep and beautiful content could be expressed.

SD, movement and sound fed into each other and the whole existing process was enhanced by reaching an area of expression previously unexplored. The group, by connecting deeply to the holding of the dreams, had reached an inner opening where 'something' different could happen and be received.

Conclusions

It is not an easy task to draw conclusions – there were only two workshops with the three of us and the circumstances which brought us together changed, so that we could have no more; the integration of that experience needs still further reflection and development.

However that experience was for me a milestone for the work to come. I often introduce elements of movement and voice work in the context of both my therapeutic and consulting work.

Bridging different languages has proven, over and over, to be a worthwhile effort. Not so much in terms of mixing the languages, which could be confusing, but of finding the terrain where differences can meet and, through the act of meeting and of integration, bring a deeper quality of awareness to the experience of the participants.

I often work in institutions and within pretty rigorous psychoanalytic settings, like supervisions, management teams, leadership development skills, group relations, conferences, etc. Most of the time participants are willing to let the unconscious speak through the sharing of their dreams and for the purpose of finding their collective meaning; when that happens, there is also an openness to letting movement and sound shape the unconscious contents of the dreams, so that a reasonably clear picture of the shared reality of the participants can emerge. Then transformative actions may follow.

I am very grateful for the opportunity to reflect and write about these experiences. As Prapto would often say: *"sharing thoughts and experience helps a process of crystallization."*

~ ~ ~

References

Baglioni L. & Fubini, F. (2013) 'Social Dreaming' in Long S. (ed) *Socioanalytic Methods*, Karnac

Bloom, K. (2006) *The Embodied Self*, Karnac

The Dalai Lama (1997) *Sleeping, Dreaming and Dying. An exploration of consciousness with the Dalai Lama*, Wisdom Publications

The Dalai Lama (2010) 'Emptiness, Relativity and Quantum Physics' in *The Universe in a Single Atom: The Convergence of Science and Spirituality*, Morgan Road Books

Lawrence W.G. (1991) 'The social dreaming phenomenon' in Lawrence W.G. (ed) *Experiences in Social Dreaming*, Karnac

Lawrence W.G. (2005) *Introduction to Social Dreaming*, Karnac

Lawrence W.G. (2011) Unpublished lecture given at the Tavistock Institute, London

Namkhai, N. (1989) *The Mirror*, Shang Shung Editions

Franca Fubini lives in Perugia, Italy and works as a psychoanalytic psychotherapist, group analyst and organizational consultant. She has also studied and practiced Healing Shiatsu for many years. Since 1992 she has been developing and applying the methodology of Social Dreaming in many and diverse contexts. She is a trustee of the Gordon Lawrence Foundation in the UK and co-founded the *socialdreaming.it* association in Italy. In 1994 she met Prapto and studied with him in Europe and in Java. It was a transforming experience which has greatly enriched her life, as it was to organize 'Blossoming in Europe' in Italy. She is a grateful student of Namkhai Norbu Rinpoche, whose teachings are a constant source of learning, compassion and awareness.

franca.fubini@gmail.com

18. FAMILY

The Field of Blossoming

Una Nicholson (UK)

"From you I receive, to you I give
Together we share, by this we live"

Anon (cited in Kumar 2002)

Family is both easy and difficult to define. My immediate family consists of me, my partner Sean and our children Ollie and Vernon, who are 5 and 2. But our family is also much bigger and richer and less easily delineated. It has boundaries that change and that are porous. It includes our parents, siblings and their partners and children, the friends we see every day and friends who live far away but who feel close in heart. And there are times when colleagues and clients feel like family too.

Bronislaw Malinowski, the renowned British anthropologist, tells us that human beings, no matter what the cultural setting, form family groups and ties (1913). The United Nations Declaration of Human Rights states that "the family is the natural and fundamental group unit of society". In recent years, psychiatrist Susan McDaniel has defined family as "any group of people related either biologically, emotionally or legally. That is, the group of people that the patient defines as significant for his or her wellbeing"(2005).

Through Amerta Movement and Prapto's teaching we discover that family is a dynamic and creative vessel. Prapto talks about the family as a dynamic generator, a source of regeneration and a place to practise the art of everyday living and being. Over time we have discovered that adopting an 'attitude of family' can reveal a field in which we are deeply connected and where things get done easily and collaboratively. Without sacrificing anything, the individual and the whole family can flourish.

Sean (who describes his work with children with autism in chapter 21 of this book) introduced me to Prapto and his work at a workshop in London in 2006. Ollie was born in 2007, and Vernon three years later. We found working with Prapto so nourishing and supportive of our growing as a family and as individuals that we attended and organised as many workshops with Prapto as we could.

I would like to share some of what I have learnt. One of the gifts of Amerta Movement is that Prapto offers an idea or a practice and, through use and reflection, we make it our own. The practices always add something, never diminishing us or taking anything away. They broaden the context, offer a new perspective or way to understand ourselves better. Prapto has shared many, many ideas over the years and these are a small sample of those that took root and supported the blossoming of our family.

The first idea is about receiving, how embodying an attitude of family requires being able to receive oneself and the environment. The second idea is about being able to identify and move from a sense of 'we'. The third idea is about the importance of the sense of place. Lastly, once established, 'family sense' is easily extended to include others in a common field of being a human family.

Receiving

Sean and I both work with the art of listening and receiving. Sean works with children as a developmental specialist and I work as a group facilitator using listening, creativity and co-creation in work settings.

For me, receiving starts with stopping. If I stop 'doing', whether that's thinking or sensing or attending to something, and let myself be quiet, I can begin to receive myself. I might notice a tension in my shoulders or behind my eyes or an emotion; but I settle, feel my feet touching the floor, and I wait. Gradually I find that I have a softer and quieter feeling of empty receptiveness and connection. My focus broadens and I am aware of other sounds such as the movement of trees in the wind outside, the quality of the light or the texture of the carpet. I become aware of what I am already receiving and am in connection with. I am not alone, I am part of this place and it bears witness to me as I am its witness.

At a workshop in Balcombe, Sussex, in 2011, Prapto encouraged us to practise receiving being witnessed by the trees in the woodland near the hall where we were working. I like to practise this in the woods near Ollie's school. In the quiet of the morning the trees and foliage feel so benevolent as they witness me. There is a rich diversity of plant life each with its own shape and coloured leaf and they all have the space they need to be and to witness. Receiving nature is a beautiful way to practise receiving. It happens so gracefully and one can practise without the more challenging complexities of receiving another person.

In my second pregnancy, family and work life were full and I felt the need to take time and space to let in and receive the new being growing within. It was puzzlingly difficult and private. The new being was there, there was growth and movement and life but how could I really let it in and receive it?

At a gathering of teachers and workshop organisers in France, Prapto invited us to make a solo moving-dancing piece. I created a haven amongst some bushes, away from everyone else, and sang and danced and prayed for receiving this baby. My father had died when I was pregnant with Ollie and, as I moved, the grief resurfaced. There was a sense of an inextricable link between the love and connection I had enjoyed with my father and the arriving of this new person. Both were blessings and miracles. Both arrived from nowhere and would one day be gone. Life was so beautiful and so, so fragile. I was deeply touched by the beauty and wanted to cry and cry. Images of destruction, forest fire and loss consumed me and I held the beauty in one hand and the loss in the other. I wanted to defend and protect the beauty. But, in the first place, there was nothing to do but allow both to be at the same time.

Exploring receiving the baby in movement enabled the process to be amplified, filled out and embodied. More was brought into awareness. The baby became more present to me and dialogues were begun. I also wanted my new baby to be received by his community. My solo moving-dancing finished with me cutting a melon which Sean and Ollie helped to share with the Amerta Movement community. Before we left we gathered everyone's mobile numbers so that we could let them know when labour started and when baby had arrived. The baby's family had already extended to include friends from all over the world.

The 'I in the We'

The most significant element of my work with Amerta Movement and family has been developing my understanding of the 'I in the we'. As we began our life as a family, I was very much identified with my 'I', my individual needs and wishes and I saw family as a vehicle for fulfilling those. Family was like a car, you put petrol in and it took you somewhere. I put time and energy in and I expected to receive warmth, nourishment and good familial feelings in return. It didn't quite happen like that. There was conflict. Sean and I bickered, competed for support, time off or lie-ins. I would keep a tally in my head of who was working harder, how much time Sean had off, who was doing the most and was due a break. I got angry and resentful if I wasn't getting enough mileage out of my 'car'.

Our culture places great importance on the individual. Since the Enlightenment and Descartes' separation of mind and matter we have a tendency to view the world and its people as objects that can be classified, analysed, compartmentalised and controlled. Darwinism tells us that these people, plants or animal species will compete and the strongest and fittest will thrive and others will not. My view of family was rooted in this culture. I felt I could view relationships objectively and calculate how well they were working for me at any given moment. I would make myself as 'special' and 'important' as possible so others were motivated to do things for me, maximise my return and make sure that 'I' got what 'I' needed.

Prapto's teaching offered an alternative view: we are not alone and nothing is separate. We exist because of other people, because the sky does and trees, grass and the sun do. We can't exist without each other. We are always in relationship. Even an island is only an island because of the water that surrounds it. Seeing something as separate is just choosing to ignore the context and all the relationships and connections it is part of. Gradually and gently practising working in nature and reconnecting, I remembered how we are so much more than our individual selves. I learnt that the 'I' is important but sits within a greater 'we', the 'we' of family, human beings or the natural world. I came to understand through my body that, as Thomas Berry says, "The world is not a collection of objects but a communion of subjects" (2000).

In 2010 in the countryside in Sussex, Prapto asked us to pick a long piece of grass and move with it in a field where the grass was growing. He asked us to watch the way the grass moved in the wind and to move with the grass. This practice really inspired me. Focusing on the grass and its beauty softens and releases my need to stand out and be special. Without taking anything away it offers another way of being. One where my needs aren't distinct and I am one of many, all of which are blessed. As a family we are deeply connected and interdependent. We affect each other and impact on each other. We are one entity and I give for the simple pleasure of giving and being together and I receive because I am here.

One of my first experiences of understanding the 'I' in the 'we' was in a workshop with Prapto in 2008 when Ollie was about 9 months old. Ollie, Sean and I were working as a group and Prapto observed that Sean and I were taking it in turns to be with Ollie and that our three was often a two with one apart. We worked through the week and gradually found ways to be a 'we' rather than individuals taking turns to be with Ollie. We were helped considerably when we practised with a focus on creating lines with movement and a sense of architecture in space. We created the feeling of an external space that contained the three of us. By the end of the week we found a way to be together that was playful, inclusive and allowed all of us space. This was a step towards being the 'I in the we' and of understanding the support that can come from building a sense of place.

Developing a Sense of Place

For Malinowski, family was defined by having a clear sense of who was in and who wasn't, by bonds of love and also by identification with a place (1913). In 2007, when Prapto was teaching a workshop at the Toynbee Studios in London, he said to Sean and me, *"When you have a kitchen you can cook"*. It was some time before we understood that he was saying that to create something you need a place designated and organised for doing it. The act of creation is really supported by having a clear sense of place and a frame.

My experience of having my own family was shaped and framed by the family I grew up in. My mother was a successful costume designer doing work that involved lots of travel whilst my father was our main carer with a family business based near home. At the beginning of our life as a family, when Sean earned the money and I took care of Ollie and the house, I experienced a state of discontent. Just the act of vacuuming or loading the dishwasher could make me angry. I was quietly resentful of Sean's career and needed my own work and time and space away from family. My sense of home was of being trapped.

Around this time in 2009, we went to Prapto's 10-day movement workshop in the stone circle and sites around Avebury. It was beautiful but I had no idea how to move in this place. The stones and the space were so big and overwhelming and I felt lost. I floundered through the week, wafting around the stones. Then we went to work in the Sanctuary, the site of the first circular wooden henge that predates Avebury. The Sanctuary is on top of a tall hill and has 360° views of the countryside all around including Silbury Hill. As we moved there, I felt the enormous solidity of the ground beneath us. The hill was a huge, ancient and timeless mass of earth below us and the sky was an immense, timeless expanse above. I was there but I felt as thin, delicate and translucent as a damselfly's wing. People had built this wooden henge 5,000 years ago and now they were gone. I was here to dance for a moment in time and I too would be gone and the hill and the sky would remain. It was beautiful, humbling and liberating.

In the same week I was working with that feeling of being lost and finding my place; a place from which I could be present. If I was lost, I would stop, look around and then move until I had found 'my place'. This was a place that felt comfortable, that felt good in relationship to others and what they were doing. It was a practice of choosing and being awake and active in being here.

I brought the practice home and in time it helped me to anchor and wake up in my daily life. I needed a sense of myself in the present in my place so that I could really inhabit myself and the choices I was making. I actively stepped into my choice and my love of mothering. It was joyous, creative work and the most important I had ever done. Gradually the habit of living in the frame of tightness and resentment that I had brought with me from the past eased and I found more ease and pleasure being at home.

Since the beginning of our movement practice in Sussex we have been working with a theme of 'home'. We have made homes by moving and creating installations inside and around trees in the woodland. We've explored making our own homes and our sense of home, leaving our home and also going to visit others' homes.

During Prapto's first Sussex workshop, when I was pregnant with Ollie, Sean began practising building 'home' in the woods, in part as preparation to become a father. Intricate installation structures would emerge with branches balanced as boundaries and for decoration.

This practice continues with each trip to the woods. It is about building something whilst maintaining flexibility, movement and artistry using the materials of the environment. In these structures Sean is looking for balance, with a sense of home that resonates within, and which is also functional and beautiful. His exploration of balance and aesthetics helps him cultivate an internal feeling of space and balance whilst being connected to the environment.

As time goes on the structures have developed in their stability and scale and are no longer restricted to woods. They have become more connected to our family life, both being more functional and involving the children as they help out. These 'Living Homes' have been created on Greek beaches and French campsites to shade us from the sun and rain and have become hide-aways for the boys and their friends. The children love to play in them and also to make their own, complete with blankets for snuggling and places for snacks.

Sean's 'homes' have parts that move and balance and through this he explores how he can fulfil his male roles of father and provider in an artful way, not getting stuck or weighed down by the responsibility. How can he be a father with firm boundaries, who can also be flexible and see all the different perspectives?

Extended Family

On the last day of the 2011 Family Workshop, we invited friends, family and colleagues to come and see and share in what we had been doing. We shared some movement in the hall and then we all went to the woods and moved together amongst the trees. There was silence and then song and play. Children played, a father sang loud and strong, the trees witnessed and a community formed for a timeless moment. There was a sense of wonder, possibility and tears as we came together in one circle.

It seems that with the right kind of invitation we can find a sense of being one family quite easily. I see this in my work as a facilitator all the time. When there is space for embodied listening and receiving, differences dissolve and our common humanity reveals itself. This is family sense. When we are aware of the 'we' and how we are connected and interdependent, our 'I' with its unique offerings and needs can live quietly or noisily within our 'we'.

Sean and I have noticed that often, on leaving a workshop, we behold people outside the workshop in a new way. When 'family sense' is embodied we carry it with us so that we feel we're more able to share a joke with a shop-keeper, more able to smile and connect with a child on the street. Spaces we enter feel more friendly and welcoming.

We went to meet Sean at the airport one evening last week and Vernon and Ollie loved the big spaces of the arrival lounge. It was 7pm and there weren't a lot of people around and they ran about the space making big elliptical shapes and then coming together on a spot. They wove around the columns and sailed half-way up and then back down the escalator. Their presence was light and playful. They live in family sense, have little self-consciousness but instead an attitude of open connection with the people they meet. They also really occupy the space they're in. It is contagious, people see them and they smile. Their joyful presence and embodiment of family sense invites people to re-member, that is, to reconnect with being part of an extended human family.

When we experience the world as a "communion of subjects" (Berry 2000), we experience ourselves in the world as part of a living system and not separate from it. We feel ourselves within a web of interconnections. My own experience is that, once in this place, I feel less fear and more joy. It is nourishing, satisfying and light. Awareness is effortless. Rather than feeling onerous or overwhelming it feels full of open possibilities, some, all or none of which could be taken up.

Blossoming

Amerta Movement gives us ways to practise in everyday life so that we can live our lives with greater awareness and more love, creativity and happiness. Applying Amerta Movement to family involves the study of bringing awareness and art to everyday life.

One of the things I have noticed is that I often understand a comment Prapto makes or a practice he suggests long after he has given it. There are some things, such as *"family as a generator"* that I still do not fully understand. I can understand it cognitively but I haven't yet inhabited it and made it my own. I have shared here the things I have used and experienced and lived. They are the importance of receiving, of finding ways to live from the 'we' and to unpeel habits and cultural views that aren't useful anymore. And there is also the importance of place and re-membering ourselves. Amerta Movement offers simple ways that we can practise as we go about our daily life. I still struggle with most of these most days. But I do get better with practice. I have learnt to slow down, listen and give others time and space. I have become quieter within and grown in love and enjoyment of the richness of everyday life. Our family ties and the knowledge that we are together for the long haul provide a kitchen where we can cook each other's souls. Prapto talks about the polishing that happens as we rub up against each other. As we live and share together we can rub old habits away and make each other shine.

~ ~ ~

References

Berry, T. (2000) *The Great Work*, Broadway Books

Kumar, S. (2002) *You Are Therefore I Am*, Green Books

Malinowski, B. (1913) *The Family Among the Australian Aborigines*, University of London Press

McDaniel, S.H., Cambell, T.L., Hepworth, J. & Lorenz, A. (2005) *Family-oriented primary care (2nd ed.)*, Springer

Una Nicholson studied International Relations at the London School of Economics and movement-based theatre at the Jacques Lecoq School in Paris. She has choreographed dance and physical theatre pieces, performed in outdoor theatre and worked in film in costume design. She currently works as a group facilitator specialising in participative leadership and social collaboration. She is a Feldenkrais Practitioner and director of 'Everyday Extraordinary', a business that she and her partner Sean Williams created as a platform for their work in the fields of learning, therapy and facilitation, work that celebrates the art and wonder of everyday life.

19. THE INFANT'S LANGUAGE

Katya Bloom (USA/UK)

"I try to receive the language of the baby. How can we touch this source?" (Prapto)

When I take an overview of the various strands of my involvement with movement over the years, I see that a consistent thread has been my interest in the residual effects of our earliest preverbal experiences on later development. As a therapist, a teacher, a writer and researcher, and even as a performer in years past, that thread has woven its way into all that I do.

The practice of movement, and of movement therapy, can automatically tap into the roots of these elemental bodily communications, which originate before language and verbal thought. In this chapter, I want to consider some relationships between the atmosphere and practice of Amerta Movement and its resonance, conscious and unconscious, with that period of earliest development.

There has been a profusion of research in neuroscience in recent years, through which we have come to recognize that preverbal experiences can have lifelong effects on patterns of perception, including our ways of responding to stress and our expectations of, and beliefs about, others. This early patterning forms the inner landscape of our lives, physical, emotional and mental, affecting the way we interact with the outer world.

Supporting people in recognizing these embedded patterns has been part of my work as a movement therapist with various populations and, more indirectly, as a teacher of movement in different settings. And of course, they also come to light in my own movement practice. The wish to recognize and unravel some of the early patterns and assumptions we don't even know we have, is probably at the root of my enduring attraction to the field of movement, particularly to practices of free movement like Amerta. This unravelling happens, as Prapto often intones, *"slowly, slowly"* and *"layers by layers"*.

Conferring with Infants

During the six-month period prior to writing this chapter, I found a way to study these earliest preverbal experiences firsthand, by 'conferring' with infants in the Neonatal Intensive Care Unit (NICU) of a local hospital one afternoon a week. There, I encountered infants, just hours, days or weeks old, who, through a variety of circumstances, started out in life with vulnerabilities that required close and specialized professional care.

As a volunteer, I was able to hold babies who were in need of soothing; I also observed them, and sang and spoke to them in response to what I sensed and imagined their experience to be. I learned to appreciate their emotional stresses, at times being deeply affected by their pain and fear, as I tried to resonate and share communication with them. They taught me much about my own being, stirring deeply unconscious memories.

Organism/Organization

This preverbal way of speaking and listening, this primary level of shared attention and intuitive responsiveness, seems to strongly echo something of the essence of the Amerta Movement practice. Prapto used the term *organism* to differentiate the realm of sensory-motoric experience, responsive to gravity, from what he calls *organization*, the term he uses to refer to the realm of 'planning', the province of the cognitive mind, well-known to Western cultures. He has explained that his own innate character, shaped by Javanese culture, was embedded in the way of the *organism*, which meant taking his understanding of the world from the materiality of nature, with its flora and fauna. This bodily-centered, instinctive and sensory realm, it seems to me, is dominant in the period of early infancy. It is this 'thread' from Prapto's work that I wish to weave through the material in this chapter.

Choreography in the NICU

Infants in the NICU, encased in their isolettes, whether the tops are open or closed, whether needing assistance with breathing or not, all seem like astronauts in reverse. Having emerged from a dark and weightless universe, they find themselves, often prematurely, in an alien environment with light and shade, shape and color, air, gravity, a cacophony of new sounds, and many other beings; and with their former lifelines abruptly terminated.

They have no names for anything, but their perceptions seem so keen. Though their new world is a complete unknown, research has shown that they will recognize sounds and smells from their previous realm of existence, including parental and sibling voices. Infants have also clearly been shown to recognize their mother's smell.

Like other living organisms they relate and respond to the world through movement. Movement provides the possibility to engage, discover, and express. It stimulates perception and sensation. Watching infants in the NICU, I sensed their movements and sounds were seeking relationship with their world, sometimes desperately – seeking safety, equilibrium, and contact.

Newborn infants' movement is traditionally thought of as a response to random neurological impulses. Though the movements I witnessed may have been in response to raw experience, and not necessarily conscious, they seemed particular, and meaningful. For some babies, movement seemed like a sensory delight. For others it felt like an expression of pain, a plea for help. Like the Amerta practice, I would say, the infants' movement wasn't random; but rather, in response to inner sensations, and also at times, outer stimuli – visual, aural, tactile or motor. Watching the babies move, I sensed the emotional communication embedded in each movement and gesture, and I felt an emotional response.

> *I notice the exquisite sensitivity of each finger, even each joint of each finger as they slowly and so sensitively touch the air. Also each toe explores independently. The little finger and the pointer on the right extend slowly and deliberately toward the torso. They touch the belly and rest, poised there...*
>
> *The second toe extends, leading the foot to twist a little at the ankle joint; the toe touches the rolled blanket. There is a registering of this.*

Then the third finger moves and encounters a thin wire; there is a pause as if registering this...

I am aware of the many possible articulations of fingers, hand and wrist as the infant makes small, mindful movements. I imagine that when gravity is new, air is a new medium, sensation of skin and body are heightened.

When I observe, I wonder if the infant senses that someone is there, being attentive and receptive. Did the atmosphere really change, or was it my imagination? I saw infants who definitely seemed to respond when I, or a nurse, was near, as if they are tuned to respond to movement... as if their body-minds naturally resonate with other body-minds. This was especially clear when I tried to soothe infants with sounds – even though I couldn't be sure they heard outside sounds when completely enclosed in a covered isolette.

I watch the 3-day-old preemie in his covered isolette. Does he orient toward me? When he cries out, I try to soothe him with sound. He seems to settle, as though he hears and feels my presence.

Often, I asked myself, "Did I really see that?" "Did that really happen?"

On another occasion:

I'm asked to hold a fussy baby. She is hiccupping when I am given her to hold. She has her hands to her ears and seems distressed. As I hold her in the rocking chair, she slowly relaxes, her body literally getting heavier; she reaches out toward me. She squeezes my finger, which I sense as her wish to let me know she recognizes my presence. I am amazed, hardly believing my eyes, when her hands both make mudras of thumbs touching forefingers. As if something has resolved, and she has been put back together emotionally... she has settled. She soon falls asleep, making a deep dreaming (it seems to me) 'mmmm' on each exhale.

I came to realize that there was a mutuality to my engagement with the infants, even without touch. Meeting them with an open heart, I allowed something of my own infant self to be reflected back. I could empathize, and we were both changed by the encounter.

I can say that, like the Amerta practice, the NICU taught me to see things freshly, to slow my mind and step back from what is known or expected. In this setting, as in an Amerta workshop, I could appreciate embodied communication and resonance, and savor the moment-to-moment nuances of change, even as the moments of fear, pain or terror of the unknown arose and subsided... arose and subsided...

Organism to Organism

I was often guided by the infants into the realm of preverbal silence – dropping into this silent space brought an experience of gravity and spaciousness at the same time.

> *I feel my three-dimensional bodily form clearly, and my mind is expansive. Settling together in a rocking chair, sensing the rise and fall of my breathing belly against her body, and her rapid breathing against mine, I wonder if this might recapitulate her experience inside her mother's body. We are both weighty organisms, just being together, with no agenda, partaking in an open-hearted, nonverbal, dialogue.*

Measuring in the Unknown

Infants seem capable of self-regulation up to a point, using movement, stillness or sleep to control discomfort, disorientation, fear or pain. I was reminded of Prapto's idea and practice of *living measurement*, in order to keep ourselves within a manageable physical, psychological, and emotional range. Keeping ourselves present, by *measuring* our pace, position, direction, form, would seem to combine the attitudes of *organism* and *organization* described earlier.

Here is a description of measurement in action, as this baby begins to discover her body and her new environment:

> *She moves with gusto inside the covered isolette. Limbs each explore, separately and independently of the others, so many permutations occur, extensions across the body, one side stretching long as an arm reaches up and a leg reaches down, also the same in a cross-lateral fashion. Both arms reach up, a heel reaches up and out into space then twists the torso as it reaches across. Eyes are open and looking. I think she sees me. I show my fingers. She extends a hand toward me. There are lots of yawns in between. She finds her mouth and face with her fingers. Her head rotates, almost seems to lift. Expression in being alive in the world is what I feel. This baby is loving exploring through movement... exploring movement itself. I am following, not only with my eyes but with my whole body; I'm feeling joy and wonder.*

Of course every human organism is unique; each has its own threshold for sustaining homeostasis, and its own strategies for self-regulation. Some infants are more easily overwhelmed than others, and especially if they have had a traumatic birth or other trauma, like one who was born with a substance addiction.

> *She goes through waves of intense terror, loud crying, arching her back, shaking her head, squeezing her eyes shut. As I held her I felt she was having hallucinations, as well as pain... and in between there were lulls of comparative calm, before the next wave. I rocked her and sang her painful song... and settled deeply into being with her. She was able to gradually settle and get some much needed sleep. I still feel the painful ripples of this encounter.*

A less traumatized fellow, two days old, is also working through some distress:

> *As we rock, there are moments of slowly sinking into despair, one moment of crying. It subsides, and his eyes close. As if a memory came and went. Terror and relaxation... I am aware of sensing him through my third eye area, and imagine he's unconsciously remembering his birth. I feel he knows I'm reassuring him with my holding and singing.*

The needs of the babies seem to come and go, in between which they are able to settle and relax, weighty three-dimensional human organisms. Observing them one senses the transience of experience; the present moment is all there is, and it is always changing.

Singing in the NICU

Singing softly to infants in the NICU was something that arose naturally, but unexpectedly: an organic response to another organism. This too was reminiscent of the Amerta practice, in which the play of vocal expression can spontaneously arise out of engagement in movement. In the NICU I would usually find myself creating a 4-8 note chant-like phrase, which arose from my experience of the baby's mood, and would be repeated over and over with variations.

At other times, actual songs sprang to mind – I found myself singing *Here Comes the Sun* and *You'll Never Walk Alone*. Sometimes I was moved to take a cue from the baby's own sounds, to pick up the pitch of a cry, and improvise a melody from that. Sometimes slow, plaintive singing returned us to the realm of silent communication.

> *I noticed the baby was whimpering. I sang to her, a repeating somber phrase. She stopped crying. I thought maybe she slept. I was concentrating on holding her mind with my singing, to help her not feel so alone in her nightmare.*

Sometimes we both emitted sighs of settling, of relief as the rocking chair's soothing motion helped both of us relax. As Prapto proffered, *"remember that the chair is holding you."*

> *I settle into gratitude for the chair, holding me as I hold the baby.*

Time Outs

Over time, I found that I if could take a few minutes of 'time out' between the deeply involving meetings with infants, to sit alone, in a comfortable chair, I could realize the depth of affect I was holding. In the time out, I sensed the full force of the infants' helplessness, the ripples of fear and terror. I started making brief time outs a regular part of my routine. It was then that I fully experienced my inner organism, which called forth something of the infant level of me.

> *I sit rocking my baby self. Sensing much holding… What an opportunity to examine the rigidities, the self-protections of the infant part of myself, I rock and breathe, "receiving my condition," as Prapto often put it.*

Moving in the Studio after being in the NICU

When I moved in the studio after being in the NICU, something of the experience of being with the infants was still tangible. I could sense them with/in my own body. I allowed a deepening into the unknown. Letting go of another layer. Remembering gravity.

> *I start lying down, as the infant does, at least today I do. The movement takes its own time, there are many stops along the way to digest the sensory, affective, visual interrelationships, to sense the whole of me, and then, reengaging with the part that leads me on into the unknown. Organism led. What a relief. To trust this. "Not too deep," I remember Prapto saying. I keep myself open to the outside world, the light, the floor, the color, the textures… to all that is changing in an ongoing process of being.*

I had seen in the NICU that each infant is different from the others, each a unique being. But in the studio, I could more fully sense it.

Also each nurse. I never knew who would come to my body/mind as I moved or lay or sat still – I re-membered and sensed them, not by thinking about them, but by resonating with them, organism to organism. It was a surprising and integrating process, which could open me to new experience, new perceptions and ways of moving. It was a kind of play, in the unknown, following my own curiosity, much like an infant seems to do.

Depth Movement

As a teacher/facilitator and as a movement therapist, I try to develop my capacity to be rooted in my body-self, and from that starting place, to be open to shared experience; that is, the sharing of another's physical, mental and emotional fields, and the co-arising field of our mutual interrelating. This calls forth the same qualities of intuitive attention and 'being with' that were described in my encounters in the NICU. I am interested in supporting people in finding the psychophysical form to tap into their own moving reality, to participate more fully in the process of change and to navigate the unknown with minimal anxiety. I call my work 'Depth Movement'.

Through sharing the development of his practice, Prapto has been an important role model and teacher for me. His ability to engage consciously with others in a process of unconscious-to-unconscious communication, playfully, and without becoming enmeshed, is an invaluable inspiration.

In the following examples, I describe my movement therapy work with two women. With both of them I wondered whether patterns of interaction with me may have reflected expectations and beliefs about others that could be traced, in part, to the interactive qualities of their earliest relationships.

Two Clinical Examples

Molly was a young woman who seemed to have an underdeveloped sense of having her own boundaried body. She liked to sit uncomfortably close to me in the beginning of our work, and to grip me with her eyes. She found it hard to speak or move spontaneously. I imagined she felt like the caretaker to a vulnerable, unpredictable mother/therapist. I felt challenged to maintain a sense of my own three-dimensionality, so both of us could have space for mental as well as physical movement.

19. THE INFANT'S LANGUAGE

A key point of change happened in a session in which Molly picked up the larger of two big balls in the therapy studio and handed me the smaller one. She bounced her ball increasingly forcefully and loudly on the ground, over and over, erupting in tears. I supported this by bouncing my ball, tossing it in the air or strongly stepping on the floor, in a syncopated rhythm to Molly's. I felt that through her action, Molly was standing up for herself, and also finding an outlet for hostile and rivalrous feelings. And as she established her own vertical axis and relationship with gravity, I became a more robust and trustworthy figure in her eyes.

Another young woman, Ann, had an inherently strong vertical axis and connection to gravity. She was the eldest of several siblings, and very self-reliant. But she struggled to know how to make use of therapy. In her movement she liked to explore going up and down, in a rather monotone and symmetrical fashion; her movement had the quality of a self-contained ritual. She had little relationship to the outside world, making it difficult for her to know how to interact with people, including me.

After some time together, as Ann moved in the middle of the space, I started to move on the sidelines. As I 'listened' to her move, I found myself introducing diagonal movement, creating many angles. Sensing new possibilities, Ann's space began to open up, as she was able to appropriate different points of view in her own movement. Gradually, I began to exist for her, no longer as a remote, judgmental and threatening figure, but as someone available for verbal and nonverbal dialogue. She became more playful and imaginative, sometimes spontaneously and sweetly accompanying her movement with songs from her childhood.

Summary

I've come to recognize that our infant needs are never fully overcome – they reside at the core of our beings. However, we can strengthen our capacities to transform them. Like infants, we can practice receiving the sensation of our bodies and experiencing the space and the others, all on what Prapto once called the *carpet of time*, while using our organizational skills, to make *in-formed* decisions that keep us present and safe.

Prapto's work greatly supported my understanding that although our earliest relationships may set certain patterns in motion, we can alter their course through movement practice. We can become more 'organic organizers' / more 'organized organisms' – bringing the instinctive and infant qualities together with our more awakened and developed adult choices and plans. In this way, we can develop greater empathy and common ground with others, and more fully recognize ourselves as part of the 'garden' of all life.

~ ~ ~

Katya Bloom, PhD and Board-Certified Dance/Movement Therapist, is author of *The Embodied Self: Movement and psychoanalysis* (2006: Karnac) and co-author of *MOVES: A sourcebook of ideas for body awareness and creative movement* (1998: Routledge). Since 2010, she lives in Santa Barbara, CA. Her teaching and clinical work in various settings is called 'Depth Movement', and is influenced by her study with Prapto and her training as a Laban Movement Analyst. She lived in London for 27 years, where she worked as a movement psychotherapist, and taught for twenty years at the Royal Academy of Dramatic Art.

kbloom@depthmovement.com

www.depthmovement.com

20. "GOING OUT OF THE SITUATION" AND "STOP, DON'T FOLLOW THAT, WALK!"

Two Movement Themes That Support My Work With Children

Regula Nell (Switzerland)

'Prapto work' (as we used to call it in Switzerland in the 1980s) still influences my daily life as well as my movement practice and professional communication. At the age of 25, in February 1986, eight months after finishing my diploma as a gymnastics teacher, I went off to Java to study movement practice with Prapto. I found myself at the other end of the world, part of an international group of people with no-one else speaking Swiss-German, my mother tongue. At that time there was no internet, nor mobile phones, so there were fewer possibilities for distraction or for finding ways out of the embodied situation that I found myself in: far from home, alone and plunged into an utterly different culture.

Nowadays I work as a movement teacher, a Feldenkrais practitioner and a psychomotor-therapist working mainly with children. My personal way of guiding clients towards an expansion of possibilities and choices for their wellbeing and physical expression is strongly influenced by all that I learned and experienced within the context of Amerta Movement. That practice created for me an important foundation of observing and understanding the physical and energetic aspects of movement within the context of the environment and of personal interaction.

Awareness of one's personal movement is a first step towards change or adjustment of behaviour. My aim is to support individuals to broaden their awareness of movement and their expression and communication skills. My understanding of group dynamics was also clearly influenced by the movement practice in groups with Prapto: moving in small groups, witnessing others in their work, and supporting them by watching without judging and without any applause. These models helped me to find a form of accompanying and understanding people in my work, both in movement and in spoken dialogue.

It is useful for me to cultivate being a 'neutral' observer or a witness with my clients because I want to understand the possible source of the two patterns that I'm going to introduce in this chapter: *"Going out of the situation"* and *"Stop, don't follow that, walk!"*

Going Out of the Situation

The expression *going out of the situation* is one that Prapto used to say at specific moments – and it is still very clear in my mind. *Going out of the situation* offers the possibility of escape. *Going out of the situation* in order to escape happens spontaneously, often unconsciously. It is different from a clearly conscious change in direction or action. It can also be a form of resistance, a way of avoiding, a well known but unhelpful habit, movement pattern or behaviour. When a situation is emotionally too intense or overwhelming, an immediate change of direction is needed. If there is no possibility of expressing with words the need for help and change in such a moment, then *going out of the situation* can be an unconscious reaction, in order to feel safe again. So *going out of the situation* can become a strategy for self preservation: for example when the child has to do something he dislikes, or that he cannot cope with, he might just need to go to the toilet! As with any strategy, it can become an unexamined habit and, once out of date, can become unhelpful.

To give a few more examples: James is building a construction with long cardboard tubes so he can shoot small balls around a track. He suddenly changes everything and starts a completely new construction. There was some difficulty in adapting the construction – instead of asking for help, or finding a way to adjust it, he just started again from scratch. These changes of activity come unexpectedly; I may not know the reason for the sudden change at first. But it doesn't disturb me, as I recognize the pattern of *going out of the situation* that underlies the change. It is important that he learn step by step that he can adjust situations by asking for help or by making small changes too. It is not necessary to knock everything down when a part of the construction needs to be done better.

Another time I worked with a boy (let's call him Mike) who used to say "cha me oo" (translation: "can do too"). Whenever he changed situations, he said that as a commentary on his activity. So he had found a ritualised way to name his *going out of the situation*. With his words he showed that he was somehow aware of the fact that he was about to change his position and/or the situation. When I see this pattern of *going out of the situation* occur, I usually interrupt and speak with the child. I often ask whether he or she is aware of the change there has been in the direction of action. For example I might say: "Do you realise what your feet did just now?" and I might ask whether they are aware of a reason for this: "Do you have any idea, why they did this?" Eventually I ask the child whether I should tell them my opinion about what just happened. To Mike I suggested that, in these moments, he continue with his activity, in the situation as it is, before he changes anything; for example, before he rearranges any material.

Finally, for a child with hyperactivity syndrome it can be essential to recognise the habit of *going out of the situation*. This is an important first step for possible change and more self-control. It can also be helpful for parents to recognise the pattern of *going out of the situation* in their child's behaviour. They can then find different forms of communication and support their child in learning to express through words his embarrassment or difficulty with the actual situation.

For all these conversations with my clients my personal attitude is fundamental to the outcome – it requires from me an observing attitude, no judging, but understanding. Sometimes we talk about different forms of movement or behaviour. In this way, the child can learn to understand himself better. Being guided without being judged is often not a well known situation for the children I work with; it is in fact their (un)conscious judging of their own action which often brings them to *going out of the situation*.

Stop, Don't Follow That, Walk!

In contrast to *going out of the situation*, there is the phrase: *Stop, don't follow that, walk!* This describes moments when a change of momentum is strongly needed and cannot be found because the child is too lost in her own dynamic. The child is losing herself in her way of moving and behaving. Of course, often this is a sign of being lost in thought or emotion, or both. This is different from an authentic expression; it is more a form of constant, choiceless repetition which could (in extremis) lead into some sort of obsessive behaviour.

Prapto once said to me *Stop, don't follow that, walk!* with a clear and demanding voice. It was at a moment when I was rolling continuously on the floor without any possibility of getting up and standing on my own two feet. His advice/command was like an anchor for me. I managed to get up and walk – and as a result my perception of myself and the space changed completely.

Often in my work as a psychomotor-therapist I like to be receptive and to give the children a huge amount of free space to let them follow their impulses and create their 'things'. However my own experience with: *Stop, don't follow that, walk!* helps me to come into a clear and active position of guiding and, if necessary, to be demanding as well. I find that I often need and use the quality of *Stop, don't follow that, walk!* with my clients.

Those children who easily lose themselves in whatever they are doing need clear, strong, boundaried guidance in moments where they have to change direction in their doing, in order to experience a new way of movement and a new form of expression. To adjust and to broaden the possibilities of choice in personal behaviour, it can be necessary to become a clear advocate for change from the outside.

These two expressions of Prapto's: *Going out of the situation* and *Stop, don't follow that, walk!* have proved vital for me in my professional work. Both help me to be able to guide the children through movement dialogue itself and not necessarily with words or fixed exercises. They also describe very clearly some specific mechanisms within movement behaviour. When a child displays certain aspects of these movement behaviours, they are not confusing for me, even if they appear suddenly and unexpectedly, because these two phrases act as a doorway for my understanding of the patterns that underlie the switch or the repetitions. So I can move between the child's present moment, their movement and words without hesitation to access a deeper place in my communication with these children.

As we have seen, both of these forms of behaviour may have been helpful strategies in the child's life. But the difficulty starts when they appear as patterns functioning unconsciously, habitually and continuously. Often a curtain comes down, when something overwhelming is happening, for instance any sort of frustration, and this can create either a sudden shift or repetitive motion. Then the child isn't in a balanced position with the capacity to respond adequately to the actual situation, but is more a victim of held-in behaviour patterns that may be well out of date.

My understanding of the world and of intercultural dialogue and diversity has been strongly influenced by Amerta Movement. I am very grateful for this influence in my life. The combination of physical experience, movement in nature, philosophical talks, communication in groups (including aspects of Javanese life and Sumarah meditation) forms an important line in my biography and still influences my daily life. It broadened my Swiss mode of perception and guided me to become more of who I am. I, in turn, am now committed to offering this potential to my clients.

~ ~ ~

Regula Nell was born in 1961, in Bern, Switzerland. She was first in touch with Prapto in 1985 and went to Java three times: in 1986 and 1990 for trainings with Prapto and in 1996 she visited Solo for a movement project at a school for handicapped children. Currently she works as a psychomotor-therapist at a primary school in a village near Thun and teaches the Feldenkrais Method in Bern.

rnell@bluewin.ch

21. AMERTA MOVEMENT AND AUTISM

Therapy, Communication, Collaboration and Art

Sean Williams (UK)

On a bright and sunny day in a garden in Wales, Prapto asked me about my work with my clients on the autistic spectrum[1], and if I could show him what I did through movement. After several minutes of interacting in movement with a colleague in the group, who wonderfully embodied the fragility of someone on the autistic spectrum, Prapto began to talk with remarkable yet practical insight about my world of being with people on the autistic spectrum. He was able see 'where I was coming from'. He explained how I needed to understand the people I was working with and how I could stimulate growth for them rather than fixing, pacifying or trying to educate them in ways they weren't ready for.

Since 1999 I have been working as a developmental specialist[2],

---

1 The autistic spectrum describes a range of neurodevelopmental conditions that include diagnoses of autism, Asperger syndrome, pervasive developmental disorder, childhood disintegrative disorder, and Rett syndrome, as defined by *The Diagnostic and Statistical Manual of Mental Disorders* 5th ed. in 2013. Those on the autistic spectrum "share a triad of impaired social interaction, communication, and imagination, assoc-iated with a rigid repetitive pattern of behaviour. Onset is usually at birth or during the first three years of life but problems can begin in later childhood." (Wing 1996)

2 Developmental specialists specifically look at the development of an individual from conception to the present day. Developmental specialists do not address one specific area but instead look at a person globally (e.g. cognitive skills, language and communication, social-emotional skills and behaviour, gross and fine motor skills, and self-help skills) and identify areas of need and of strength. They develop activities designed to help the individual overcome their challenges and improve their skills and ability to learn. This enhances functioning in their daily living, education, work, play, leisure, communication and social participation.

educator and play therapist, with the majority of my clients being on the autistic spectrum, commonly ranging between 3 and 18 years old. In that short interchange with Prapto a door to a totally new understanding began to open. Our conversation on the warm wet grass that day began a process that is still enlivening, informing and changing my work with my clients. I feel I have only just begun exploring how working with people on the spectrum is an act of collaborative communication – creating something together that enriches all of our lives.

This writing is an attempt to share some of Prapto's teachings and how they have developed in my work. I give examples that convey the application of this unique approach (names have been changed).

The Meeting of Amerta and Autism

Prapto casually and very generously offered to host a session in London where I and others interested in Amerta could move with people on the autistic spectrum. I leapt at this chance and one month later in August 2006 our small group moved with three families (one at a time) in a dance studio in Islington. The afternoon was a deeply touching and nourishing experience for us all, with therapists and teachers being moved and stimulated into interesting questions about their work. The children who joined us seemed to enjoy it too, dancing around with smiles on their faces and not wanting to leave. I was fortunate to be able to do two more workshops in 2006-7 developing this theme with Prapto, and from this moment on there was ever-present cross-pollination between my personal Amerta practice and my work with my clients.

New Meaning to 'Special Needs'

With his unique insight, Prapto frequently reveals the hidden depths of our English language – for example, the term 'special needs'. He posed the question *"how can we find someone's special needs?"* in order to understand and support them better. We all have special needs, unique requirements that enable us to be ourselves and to blossom. Prapto suggested that understanding the special needs of an individual (whether autistic or not) was an important starting place for collaboration and growth.

The 'special need' of 14-year-old Edward emerged quickly at our first meeting. His conversation was quiet, stilted and rarely spontaneous. Hard working and sensitive, he could overcome his sensory and motor learning challenges with intense focus and manage to speak and, with the support of home tutors, keep up academically with his peers. When under any pressure his face and shoulders would quickly tense. He would hit himself while working and his sleep would be dramatically disrupted if his day had been unsettled.

In free moments he would pace up and down the corridor of their flat or lie on his bed. His favourite activity was brisk walking or roller-skating around his neighbourhood.

He once led his mum and me on a two-hour walk through Paris, determined in his route, and that he would not be persuaded to shorten it. I accepted and treasured this walking, seeing how important it was to his wellbeing. As we walked he answered my questions naturally and spontaneously. His mum was amazed at his sustained conversation. He was normally silent and rarely spoke unless firmly prompted. In those two hours of enjoyment there was more communication and understanding than in the six hours we worked together. The rhythmic movement of the walking was his special need. In it he was calm, and available for interaction.

This leads us to consider the process of how someone finds their own special needs and how we might support this unfolding. Prapto calls this enabling *autistic gardening*.

Collaboration in Autistic Gardening

Exploring this part of his teaching has been fascinating, mysterious and had a huge influence on me. With gentle, persistent nudging from Prapto my emphasis is gradually changing from trying to direct or change the other, to one of "gardening", where we create the atmosphere or possibility of growth and communication together with a sense of enjoyment. The starting place of gardening is attitude. Rather than being focused on affecting change, the gardening approach trusts that the individual will find their own way, and much like a gardener our goal is to help create the conditions by which the seed can grow. The heart of this approach is communication, understanding and the blossoming of those moving together. An added benefit is that every day it becomes less "work that I am doing" and more of a thoroughly enjoyable way of being with people from which discoveries, learning and nourishment emerges for all present.

With 30 years of experience practicing therapeutic approaches, where it was my job to address clients' health issues, changing to this new way of working has not always been an easy or immediate process. It has been supported by how Prapto has also worked with my family (See Chapter 18 by my partner Una).

Children often don't want to do what you want to them to do. This is very familiar to me with my own children and particularly with my clients on the autistic spectrum who often have hypersensitive senses and are very easily overloaded. As a result they are particular about extra, new or unfamiliar input and find it difficult to respond to a request if it is not following their motivation. My brief from educational authorities and parents is often to help their education, like talking more, dressing themselves, being more attentive or stopping certain behaviours. The question I am then faced with is: how can I introduce a stimulus for learning to someone who finds it difficult to connect with a stimulus that is unfamiliar to them? Recently it seems I have been working with more children that are particularly sensitive and quite resistant to having things done to or for them. Combined with the growing emergence of the gardening approach I am being forced to listen to the special needs of the individual –"what is it they really want?" – and something very different and exciting has been happening.

I have begun to explore following the children's interests and the things that they are exploring already as the main route for their development. During a recent visit to my clinic, Andy, who was seven years old, did a few parts of my assessment protocol but spent most of his time playing with a toy train track which is also his passion at home. He was generally inflexible and had been quite resistant to doing things that his parents think might be good for him.

In his play he was both flummoxed and fascinated by the spatial orientation of objects, for example whether a train would fit into a tunnel or not. I noticed how he was beginning to learn problem solving, and when encouraged and left to find his own solutions he spoke more, became more interactive, more flexible and was growing in confidence. Andy generally played alone. The adults around him tended to try to direct him or to be the problem solvers for him, which as well as removing learning opportunities meant that they remained more distant players in 'adult mode,' rather than really playing with him.

I encouraged his family to find toys that presented him with spatial orientation challenges he could enjoy, starting with train tracks and the constructions around them. Andy also had challenges that related to not being fully aware of his body: neither coordinating movement efficiently nor having awareness of his body in space, or its position and orientation relative to things around him. This meant he was anxious in busy places, had difficulty sleeping and tended to be clumsy. He really liked strong pressure on his body. This was when he was able to relax most. We played games that followed his themes of interest, some of which involved going in boxes, and pushing him around on a train track, hiding under futons and pressing on him while looking for him, games with crawling under things, swinging and jumping games, and other games to play at home to help body awareness. The immediate effect was that the whole family (including his 10-year-old sister Izzy) enjoyed and fully engaged in the games and activities. With their new understanding the family began to spontaneously discover and create activities in play that stimulated Andy's learning along with everyone else's. The sense of togetherness and enjoyment was striking. Andy started sleeping better. His attention is better, he is calmer and his language continues to expand rapidly. I am continually delightfully surprised how the special needs of my clients emerge during collaborative play and we just need to nourish them.

The Sensory-Motory

Prapto suggested from his observations of my work that if I was to really understand and interact with people on the autistic spectrum I needed to understand and embody what he refers to as the *Sensory-motory*[3]. It is the integration of the sensory perception and motor systems, which is independent of complex conscious planning and cognitive filtering. Externally it describes a form of movement while internally it is a state of being. It is the foundation of how we experience and relate to the world.

Piaget (1936) first used a similar term to describe the "Sensori-motor developmental stage" from 0-24 months and how the infant relies on seeing, touching, sucking, feeling, and using their senses to learn things about themselves and the environment. He theorised how the early manifestations of intelligence evolve from the interactions of these sensory perceptions and motor activities.

Prapto differs in referring to the *Sensory-motory* as being present in everyday life for everyone regardless of age. He talks about how *"Sensory-motory is movement that has a quality of organism and organization"* or how it has the quality of natural organic processes of the body (organism) and a co-existent quality of structure or

---

3 Also referred to as Sensory-Motoric.

arrangement (organisation). He teaches us to reconnect to this basic level of our movement and how it *"needs to be placed in or linked with awareness so that human beings existing in movement have the ability of being aware, recognizing and understanding"*. This is the foundation of growth.

People on the autistic spectrum often have issues related to the *Sensory-motory*. Some of them have eloquently described how their sensory perception and its integration with the motor systems is disorganised and can dominate their life experience and daily functioning (Bluestone 2004; Grandin 1996; Higashida 2013; Fleischmann). Perseverative behaviours are common with people on the spectrum, often related to disruption in *Sensory-motory* processing. Behaviours such as rocking, watching light move, making sounds or involvement in particular obsessions can each have many different reasons, such as a response to distracting or overwhelming aspects of the environment, an attempt at self-calming, an exploration of a disorganised perception, or a full body unmediated reaction to emotion, whether anxiety or excitement. The stronger the autistic tendency the stronger the presence of these repetitive, and often rhythmic behaviours and the more the individual appears locked into habitually doing them.

The autistic individual is frequently deeply and intermittently involved in the *Sensory-motory*, sometimes to the extent of being an expert in it, such as reproducing visual images, identifying sounds most people don't hear or mastering complex balancing acts. Prapto talked about how at the same time the *"Sensory-motory"* can be *"not so well connected to awareness of (the person's own) mind"* and there is *"less awareness of outside"* or that they are not so clearly distinguishing between internal experiences related to themselves and those from the outside world. Consequently the learning of planning and our culture of 'organisation' can be blocked – such as measuring space and following time or understanding social conventions. This immediately made sense to me, helping me to understand my friends and clients with stronger autistic tendencies and why they often struggled with conventional education systems.

The more relevant idea Prapto suggested is *"how to wake up the Sensory-motory so that it can connect with awareness and planning"*[4]. Or as he was to later say *"how movement can have a quality of organism*

---

[4] During the *Moving with children on the autistic spectrum* workshop, August 2006. Moving Arts Base, London.

having organisation and also organisation having organism".[5] Here he is describing movement that has two cooperative qualities.[6] It is the waking up and interaction of these qualities with awareness that can create growth.

When the *Sensory-motory* is not acknowledged, learning for the autistic individual is likely to be stressful. Education in our society favours and fosters a culture of organisation based on organised abstract "thinking" and for many on the autistic spectrum it is so foreign that they find it difficult to engage with. Conventional teaching of things like social skills, academics, or computer skills takes for granted this particular organised way of seeing the world. We need to first understand the *Sensory-motory* before we can effectively support the learning of people on the autistic spectrum. Education of the autistic individual that ignores the innate and instinctive organisation of the *Sensory-motory* is like trying to build a house without awareness of the ground that you are building it on.

Prapto often talks of true 'understanding' as being able to 'under-stand' or get underneath the matter at hand. Aside from being pleasurable, touching the roots of the *Sensory-motory* experience can help intimate what might be behind apparently mysterious repetitive behaviours, perhaps a different way of perceiving the world or the experience of challenges or even pain. This empathy also makes it easier to 'guess' what similar things might be of interest and the possible next steps in their development. This approach makes us like the best friend who knows what is needed. With this attitude and position we are also better placed to offer tools for learning, growth or healing that match the person's needs. In essence this way of experiencing creates more understanding for all concerned; it promotes greater empathy and social interaction, which are often the very things that we are defining as missing for those on the spectrum.

The Baby Sitter Therapist and Waking Up

During those London sessions in 2007 Prapto used a phrase to describe my work that both enlightened and haunts me – *Baby Sitting*. He described how my unconscious and habitual attitude was one

---

5 Conversation with Prapto via SMS October 2013.

6 Prapto explains these qualities: *"Usually if we say natural movement, it is interpreted as free of structure or form, but actually it is not. Our organism movement in the body has form and structure. Our organism has organisation that is very complex."* He also described the quality of *"organisation has organism"*: *"Like the structure of our body, every joint has space and fluid so that every joint has a life in its structure and form in our existence."* SMS, October 2013.

of looking after my clients in a way that did not stimulate them to grow or *wake up*. It was as if I was subtly focusing on pacifying them, keeping them safe or entertaining them. A crude analogy would be how we might cheer up a baby by making funny faces or putting on the television. He also showed how I put their sense of ease before the authenticity of my own being. I had without realising it become attached to being the nice therapeutic babysitter.

I began to learn how there was an option to stimulate genuine growth and 'waking up' rather than doing 'anaesthetic therapy'. I am still learning about this! Deep set habits like this one are often difficult to change and he encouraged me to play lightly with it and just notice what I was doing. In fact I notice how it is usually a joint habit with both myself doing it and the child willingly receiving it, and how it is remarkably like a play or story that is acting itself out again and again. As I am becoming aware of my part in the play and acting it out more consciously I am able to bring new aspects to my role such as humour, variation of attitude and emotion, pauses and self-reflection. With these qualities it becomes easier to be awake in the "play," step out of repetition and stimulate something new.

Although wanting the habitual and repetitive, people on the spectrum also respond powerfully to appropriate and authentic interaction. I am reminded of a client, Peter, a gentle and quiet 13-year-old who came to our first London session. He was very sound sensitive, wary of and stressed by new environments, especially if they were noisy and busy. His helper Jan had got lost in traffic and Peter was more stressed than usual. Prapto was singing and playing the drums while some of us 'warmed up' ourselves and the room. Peter came to the glass doors and then disappeared with his fingers in his ears. Jan explained that he was finding it too loud and asked Prapto to stop the drums and singing. Peter then drifted into the silent room and we said our hellos. As we began to move Peter joined in by sliding his feet around the room, me chasing him (as requested) and others moving gently in the space. As the atmosphere softened and settled, so too did my nerves at how this meeting would go. A few minutes later my stomach lurched as Prapto began singing and drumming again and very soon at full volume – louder than previously. Didn't he understand Peter was hypersensitive to sound? What could I do next? My next surprise was that Peter did not attempt to leave the room or stick his fingers in his ears. He seemed to enjoy and respond to the music. This was my first lesson in how hypersensitivities can change instantaneously and dramatically. In this case it was influenced by a drop in stress. I learnt how the quality and intent behind the 'noise' is as important as the volume and pitch.

Peter did the opposite of what I had expected – instead of causing him to withdraw from his environment, the music seemed to wake him up and support him having greater awareness of his surroundings. Prapto later described how with his music he had used trance-like repetition to soothe and to create a sense of 'common field' and community in the room. He explained that he hadn't wanted us to become lost in the trance, so with sporadic changes in rhythm he had helped us be more aware in the trance and to create an overview. Or more simply put he was helping us wake up and step out of our repetition. During my play and work with people on the spectrum I had become familiar with how to create a common field, a sense of resonance or comfort with another, but this was my first experience of consciously stimulating awakening, and expanding another's awareness.

Happiness as the Source rather than Healing Illness

Prapto has been talking to me for many years about an idea that has been difficult for me to grasp or to implement. But, ironically, the approach of starting from happiness and wellness rather than from illness, dysfunction or suffering is now one of the most exciting for me. Any helping involves enabling what is wanted, what the individuals are good at and what impassions them, as a starting place, rather than starting from what is seen to be missing or what society wants of them. This approach is more restful, playful and enjoyable for me. It is also more engaging for everyone involved. Cooperation frequently has at its base 'I want you to do my idea' and revolves around 'my needs' being acted on. Children on the autistic spectrum are often viewed as being 'uncooperative'. But how cooperative are we being with them? Our expectations of them can be very challenging if their 'hidden' special needs are not being understood.

Prapto impressed on me how the process of development involves the whole family including the therapist, and that focusing on one person and their problems was somehow limiting their growth and the growth of all concerned. He encouraged an emphasis on sharing and communication.

Sharing time in this way contributes to the mutual understanding and harmony of all involved enabling greater happiness and growth in each person. Something unfolds and is shared that leaves each of us with an impression that lasts well beyond our time together. It is not just an artistic process, it is art that is enriching lives.

Bringing it All Together

These themes have been evolving since that conversation in Wales seven years ago. They have influenced my work, family and personal life and continue to grow in and with me. Gradually I slide into a way of being where work is pleasurable and growth is for all. Enjoyment and collaboration is becoming the source of growth rather than hard work and effort. I am dazzled by the extraordinariness of life, and the treasure of the individual and the family as it unfolds and reveals itself. I feel honoured to be part of these people's lives, their growth and I am touched by what they share with me. Finally I am part of the garden and I can't help but notice that Prapto has been gardening for me too, stimulating and helping me and my work to blossom.

~ ~ ~

References

Bluestone, J. (2004) *The Fabric Of Autism: Weaving the threads into a cogent theory*. The HANDLE Institute

Fleischmann, A. with Fleischmann, C. (2012) *Carly's voice: Breaking Through Autism*. Touchstone

Grandin, T. (1996) *Thinking in Pictures*. Vintage Press

Higashida, N. (2013) *The Reason I Jump: One Boy's Voice from the Silence of Autism*. Sceptre

Piaget, J. (1936) *The Origin of Intelligence in the Child*. Routledge & Kegan Paul

Wing, L. (1996) 'Autistic spectrum disorders', *The British Medical Journal*, vol. 312, issue. 7027, February, pp.327-328

Sean Williams is fortunate to draw together many important themes in his life into his daily work. He is a HANDLE Instructor and Practitioner which is the main influence of his Neuro-developmental practice. He studied Shiatsu with Sonia Moriceau, and later Seiki with Akinobu Kishi. He practises Play therapy and has been inspired by the Special Time and Son-Rise approaches. He studied Ecology at Edinburgh University. His family, Una Nicholson, Ollie and Vernie have immeasurably enriched his life. He combines all these influences along with Amerta, while helping individuals and groups to reach to their potential.

www.seanwilliams.co.uk

22. "FIND YOUR POSITION"

An Embodied Approach to Movement and Daily Life

Susan Bauer (USA)

Passing a leaf back and forth. It started like this: just as I begin moving forward, I get a feeling to turn back around. I do this slowly, just in time to see the leaf Prapto is handing over to me from behind, as he heads off in the opposite direction. I take the leaf and continue to move on my own. We each move separately, yet with the energy of our leaf between us. Later the leaf is passed back to Prapto in some energetic moment of swiftness that is beyond memory, but now he has it.

When we end we are each on the ground, suddenly together again, in stillness and looking up at the cows on the hill, the leaf now on the floor between us.

After a moment of this stillness, we rise and face each other, and Prapto makes a series of gestures like a prayer before bowing with hands together: "Thank you," he says to me simply. Yet in this simple bow I learn a great deal.

Prapto has suddenly pulled back, gone deeply and calmly into him-self, as if returning to neutral. Perhaps this is a way to disengage. As I realize this, I feel very American, in the forward and outgoing way of my own bow: simultaneously nodding and smiling my "thank you."

Later, as I watch this same ritual at the end of each duet, I see each person tacitly learn this way of bowing from their center.[1]
(Bali, Indonesia)

Through this movement interaction, I was able to experience a deep centered presence in Prapto and, by comparison, reflect on the

---
1 (Bauer 2005)

presence or absence of this centeredness in myself. While within the dance of passing the leaf I actually felt myself to have had that inner connection – which I believe contributed to the evolving synchronicity of our interaction in the dance – it then became all the more obvious to me when I had 'lost' that centeredness when observing my way of bowing. For in that moment, in my enthusiasm to acknowledge and thank Prapto, I began to focus outwardly on him without a simultaneous inner connection within myself. The simple phrase, *find your position*, was one that I heard Prapto use many times in his workshops that seemed to represent a rich, multi-layered perspective on practice which includes this sense of centeredness or inner connection. By *finding our position* we stay grounded within ourselves, while we remain aware of and receptive to our surroundings – and open to the creative possibility of the moment. As I have found to be true in both the practice of Amerta Movement as well as in my own life, two aspects are key to *finding my position*: this type of embodied, centered presence, and the development of a non-judgmental inner witness, which together allow me to arrive more fully in the moment. Further, when I enter the present with openness, I also expand my perceptions – leading to deeper ways of knowing that contribute to the inspiring and often synchronistic flow of life – such as was evident in my leaf dance with Prapto.

Yet while the above journal excerpt marks a moment of insight through an actual interaction with Prapto, my own introduction to Prapto's movement work in fact began before I had even met him. I had been very moved by an article about Prapto in *Contact Quarterly*[2], and sensed that his approach was similar in many ways to a form of dance improvisation I had developed years earlier called 'Moving-from-Within.' Therefore on my first trip to Bali in 1995 I also traveled to Java, both to visit Borobudur, the famous Buddhist stupa I had longed to see, and to meet Prapto. After visiting Borobudur, I set off with a friend to Solo to find Prapto. When I arrived at his land a Javanese woman informed me that he was not there but was teaching in America! Seeing my disappointment, she suggested that I visit his outdoor practice area and stay as long as I liked. Bordered by a stream, the land is a 'mosaic' of many separate sections that Prapto designed – earth mounds, a long walkway, a Catholic grotto, a bamboo hut shaded by trees, a Balinese-style tower, an octagonal paved platform, a grassy square in the sunlight – each meant to

---

2 (Morein 1994)

activate specific energies. At each spot, I stopped to feel the presence of the land, subtly different at each place, and began to dance, while my friend responded as well by playing on the small bamboo flute he'd brought from Bali. We stayed several hours, resting here and there as well. After this experience, I felt relaxed and complete in a way I hadn't expected, especially after not even succeeding in meeting Prapto. And yet, it seemed my sense of Prapto as a kind of 'kindred spirit' had been affirmed – by this place and the attention and intention I felt on his land. It would be another five years, when I was again living in Bali, before I would finally meet Prapto, and begin a fascinating and inspirational journey of working with him and performing together.

During our work in Bali that year, I soon discovered ways in which, as I had sensed, his movement practice shared particular philosophical concepts with that of 'Moving-from-Within.' This validated my path in a deep and inspiring way for, while there are significant differences in the actual form and cultural background of these practices, I recognized a core similarity. Each improvisational movement practice consciously provides a container in which to practice developing greater awareness in both 'our way of moving' and 'our way of being,' by encouraging specific inner attitudes – such as compassion and non-attachment – that are seen as essential to the practice, much as we find in various traditions of spiritual practice.

For instance, in my early work with Prapto he introduced us to the type of presence that emerges from internalizing an inner 'witness,' comparing it to the state of 'pure attention' found in the Buddhist practice of Vipassana meditation. While this pure attention can be present in a stationary practice like sitting meditation, it can also be activated in our dancing, as explained here in this excerpt from a journal I kept while working with Prapto:

> **Prapto:** *"We can have this kind of inner awareness in both the active and in the passive. But, to be a witness, actually, we don't need to be active in there. Like at Borobudur, there are so many Buddha [statues], have you been there? The Buddha is always the witness."*
>
> Then, after a pause: *"Also, our father and our mother, always our witness."*
>
> He looks directly at us now: *"...Then of course we also witness each other... [But then] I can get so caught up in the environment around me that it can be like a trap... I must also witness what's going on in the environment in me."*

And he demonstrates, as if at a party: *"What's going on, Prapto?"* he says, leaning forward and looking eagerly all around him. We all laugh and nod in agreement.

Then, stopping himself abruptly and sitting squarely, *"Yeah, what's going on Prapto? You see, then I have to remember to witness for myself. Really to see and be in there."*

Then simply, *"By this you find your position."*

"So you try this with yourself and one other. Two people please come." And we begin this practice of finding our position. (Bauer 2005, 16-17)

This type of more embodied sense of *finding one's position* occurs when I simultaneously become conscious of my own body and open to the present moment. Yet, as Prapto explains – and as I had sensed in my bow with Prapto – often we orient by focusing primarily on the external, rather than the internal, environment.

Exploring this very human dilemma, of how to simultaneously maintain awareness of our internal and external landscape, had actually been my impetus for creating 'Moving-from-Within' back in 1987[3]. As a long-time student of a discipline called Authentic Movement[4], I yearned to bridge the deep inner-connected movement I experienced in this eyes-closed practice with my 'eyes-opened' dancing in a group, community setting – where I felt I experienced many people getting 'lost' in a way similar to what Prapto described. In Authentic Movement, 'movers' move with eyes closed, in the presence of a skilled 'witness,' who sits to the side of the movement space. Movers learn to allow their movement to unfold from within their body, rather than primarily directing it consciously.[5] After

---

3 **'Moving-from-Within'** was developed over a ten-year period in collaboration with musician John Sprague, who provided original improvised music for our classes and workshops.

4 This practice was developed by Mary Whitehouse in the 1960s. While Whitehouse is considered the founder of this form, the formal name 'Authentic Movement' was later chosen from many that Whitehouse used to describe this process, and formalized into a 'discipline' by her student Janet Adler.

5 Mary Whitehouse describes this sense of allowing one's impulses in this way: "The ego learns slowly an attitude toward what wants moving, not to act while the action is going on. Movement, to be experienced, has to be 'found' in the body, not put on like a dress or a coat. There is that in us which has moved from the very beginning; it is that which can liberate us." (Whitehouse 1963, 53). Janet Adler similarly notes that "with an increasing capacity to concentrate, to listen to impulse, the mover learns to recognize the channel within which the creative or authentic energy flows"(Adler 1987, 156).

moving, the mover speaks with the witness as a means of further understanding the movement experience. Over time, movers learn to internalize the witness presence – much as Prapto has described – such that they can maintain an open awareness while moving.

Drawing on the philosophy and form of Authentic Movement, in 'Moving-from-Within' our movement is similarly self-directed, yet in contrast to Authentic Movement, we move primarily with eyes open – and also with a combination of silence and musical accompaniment – during movement sections or 'dances,' each marked at the beginning and end with the sound of a bell. After the dance has ended, we gather as a group and discuss our experience. I also include guided warm-ups before our dances that serve to enliven our proprioceptive senses and discover our inner source of movement. For instance, a movement exercise I call 'Spiraling Inward' guides participants more deeply into connecting with their authentic impulses for movement, while 'Spiraling Outward' allows them to practice maintaining that inner awareness while entering a duet or small group interaction. These exercises provide an avenue to practice staying centered within oneself, while actively participating in the creative group process. After working with Prapto, in addition to my own descriptions of the practice, I often referred to his example of the enthusiastic 'party-goer' described earlier, as well as his use of the phrase *find your position*, to further emphasize this core goal of the practice. As participants come to discover, with such inner awareness we each gain a deep knowing of where to be, which evolves from moment to moment within the creative process. Thus, rather than 'trying to dance together,' we learn to allow the dance to emerge.

This sense of embodied knowing can also be present in everyday life. For example, I still remember an instance when I had arranged to meet a friend at a local mall, but could not find her when I arrived. I soon realized there had been some confusion as to our meeting place, and began to look for her in places I thought she might be waiting. Eventually, after not finding her I left the mall and was about to walk to my car, when I had a thought: *find your position*. I realized I had been looking for her in the environment around me, yet had never taken a moment to feel where *I was* and where I felt drawn to be. I found myself stopping right where I was, and checking in with my body, found there was actually nowhere to go – no impulse to go to my car, nor to go back in the mall. I became curious about this new way of orienting to my situation and stood still, surrendering all agenda to find my friend and just being present to the moment. Perhaps a full five minutes had passed when suddenly I found myself turning around to my right, and realized I was then facing the doors of the mall; in a moment my friend emerged from the exit. Listening more deeply, from this centered place that includes my body sense and my inner observer or witness, I *find my position*. I use this practice in many situations: when choosing where to sit on a bus or plane, who to speak to at a conference or dinner party, or when I am ready to enter or leave a dance.

Through connecting deeply with ourselves in this embodied way, I believe we can likewise begin to reference a field that includes, yet is larger than, our individual selves. Javanese culture shares a similar concept in the term *rasa*, which refers to an inner feeling and associated expanded capacity – often considered a spiritual capacity – such that the embodied Javanese self is best understood as a field of forces and potentials, some of which are more bound to the body than others, rather than as an individual entity (Hughes-Freeland 2008, 80). Prapto likewise referred to such an expanded perceptual field in an interview we did together in 2001 in which he described a *"field of expression in art... made up of human, nature, and the light of God as a field."* He went on to describe how we might access this field of expanded perception:

> *"[But] when we relax... and connect inside and outside our presence, and have awareness in there and – in awareness – surrender, then we become just aware. And slowly we can grow a presence, still aware, but not being in judgment. Witnessing, but at the same time involving. Because in witnessing, we are also melting, surrendering."*

In this passage, Prapto speaks of the need to develop the type of inner and outer awareness necessary to *find one's position* – the key to which is surrendering to the moment, while simultaneously keeping one's inner witness alive. Philosophies of Authentic Movement similarly refer to the importance of "unpremeditated surrender" (Whitehouse 1963, 82), while the witness is often referred to as a compassionate and non-judgmental presence, much as Prapto has articulated above. But what does it really mean to *surrender*, and why is it significant to describe this type of 'letting go' as 'unpremeditated'? As I have found, the quality of surrender necessary ultimately requires that we let go of any attachment to a specific outcome. This includes any pre-conceived or 'premeditated' notion of what will transpire, such as in the previous anecdote about being at the mall, or even in the earlier description of my leaf dance with

Prapto. In this way we allow life to unfold, not by giving up action or intention, but by remaining open and receptive to our inner and outer environment in light of our intentions. For example in the mall, while I held an overall intention of reuniting with my friend, in the moment I was not consciously trying to manipulate the situation toward that end. This requires a certain level of trust not always accessible to us, however, such that we can surrender and follow an internal knowing – without being sure where it will lead. It also requires a non-judgmental presence inside that supports, rather than inhibits, our authentic impulses.

For instance, I remember working with a client who was just beginning to get comfortable with the practice of Authentic Movement. She was a young graduate student, busy working two jobs to pay for her studies. After one of our sessions, she reflected that she felt like going home and sitting on the couch with a cup of tea, rather than working on a paper that was due as she had planned. I suggested that she might consider following that impulse, and offered several possible scenarios: perhaps she would sit for a while and then feel rejuvenated and inspired to begin writing; or realize how tired she actually was and go to bed early, yet wake up earlier to write once refreshed from a night's sleep. Or in resting, she might realize she was beginning to get sick, and get the idea to ask for an extension on the paper. This concept that she might actually follow her impulse to rest, trusting that it would ultimately lead her to a workable solution, was just amazing to her – as she had not yet translated the newfound idea of 'listening to her body' into her practical, daily living.

Such habitual responses that may inhibit our authentic impulses can be quite strong – such as in this case the conditioned response to push ahead despite fatigue – and may also impact our dancing. For example, in the practice of 'Moving-from-Within,' while various qualities of movement emerge over the course of the dance – dances may be celebratory and wild, still and calm, or quite varied in mood from moment to moment – within this freedom, as a dancer I must continuously *find my position*. I may be moving in a way that is quite internal and slow, for instance, when a particularly upbeat, energetic group dance begins to emerge among others in the group. In one instance, I may want to continue with my own movement, but notice an inner judgment that I should join them to 'be where the action is.' Or conversely, I might be suddenly drawn out and discover the desire to participate; or perhaps I want to participate, but hesitate as I imagine that I am unwelcome – thus perhaps projecting my own conditioning or judgments onto others. As another example,

I may be involved in an inspiring duet when I realize I am ready to move on, but stay instead for fear of a perceived tacit agreement that we are now 'dancing together.' By bringing more conscious awareness to the subtleties of these dynamics within ourselves, such as in our discussions after the 'Moving-from-Within' dances, we learn to distinguish between authentic impulses and conditioned responses, between clarity and fear. Rather than being caught in reaction or habit, we can then begin to have more choice in how we respond. While not explicit in Prapto's model of *finding your position*, I have found that adding this layer of conscious awareness of our conditioned responses further liberates us to move with integrity from a more authentic place. Moreover, when each individual moves from this quality of centered openness, we also collectively invoke the creative inspiration and synchronicity of the interconnected whole.

Bonnie Bainbridge Cohen, founder of Body-Mind Centering, describes a similar process: "There is this kind of inner ability to yield into emptiness so that something else pops up into the spaciousness and says, 'This way.'"(2013, 34) Bonnie defines this emptiness – from which inspiration or form emerges as we 'yield' – as "generative space":

> "Another word I like is 'generative.' There is a generative force that actually takes over… I don't think it has been identified as a place; I think it is probably space….
>
> Space has consciousness…When we're inspired and we have this generative power, or when we're creative, we are in space.
>
> …It's not like I'll gradually go from planning… and then going to dancing. No, all of a sudden you are dancing. And it is not a doing process; it's a practice." (ibid.)

Likewise, in both Amerta Movement and 'Moving-from-Within,' we have the opportunity to practice and create within the generative space. Perhaps it was in fact the generative space of Prapto's land that allowed me to experience his practice so profoundly on my first trip there, even in his absence; the land and the space held the essence of his practicing there, alone and with others, over so many years. Yet, to achieve an expanded state of awareness such that we can perceive the information within the generative space requires first and foremost that we *find our position* within – a 'coming home' to our own bodies. As Bonnie describes, our dancing thus becomes not a "doing process," but rather a practice – and I would add, a practice of 'being.' And from this state of beingness – such as in the heightened spiritual capacity of *rasa* – we expand our perceptual base to include the 'generative space' around us.

Such an understanding of what it means to become present and *find one's position* is in fact becoming increasingly relevant and essential in today's fast-paced, technology-obsessed world. Even in small moments of 'down time,' rather than pause to reconnect with ourselves, many people reach for their cell phones or iPads; or, when walking, keep their heads down to attend to their technology in hand. Chances for even momentary 'spontaneous' inner connection, much less moments of intentional conscious awareness, thus increasingly elude us. Simultaneously, we may also miss a moment to view the trees as we pass by, the clear blue sky above, or the eyes of a stranger crossing our path.

Yet these potential moments of awareness live inside and around us, within and without – but they require our attention. They require that we wake up and consider our relationship to self and other, inner and outer awareness, in the ongoing practice of living. In this way we take our position, and allow each person the freedom to do the same, as we live with presence and awareness. I have used Prapto's phrase *find your position* to help remind myself, my students and my clients of this intimate interrelationship of mover and witness, self and other, individual and community. Like a compass, it draws us into ourselves while maintaining an openness to life that invites the fullest breath of life – inspiring greater creativity and grace in our dancing and in our lives.

Afterword

After leaving Bali, it was another 10 years before I saw Prapto again[6], when in 2011 an opportunity arose to work with him in a workshop in Berkeley, CA where I had been living. After the first morning of movement practice together, but not yet having spoken a word, we found ourselves outside during a break. He paused and was just looking at me. "What is it Prapto?," I finally asked, as I sensed he was perceiving something. *"Ahhh, you're very busy, so many projects, Susan!"*

---

6 Immediately upon arriving back in the US in 2001, however, I did do a final workshop with Prapto at Naropa University. Coincidentally, he was teaching a workshop called *Remembering in America* that same month, which seemed a perfect way to 're-member' upon my return from my year abroad.

This was very true; in fact I had planned to come only to that one day out of a five-day workshop as I just couldn't fit it in. *"But now,"* he added slowly, *"ahhhh, now – more being in the doing."* As I took this in, I realized that this was also quite true. While I did have many responsibilities, I was not feeling overwhelmed by them, but rather was inspired and present in a deeper way in many areas of my life. *"Yes, so it's good, very good"* he remarked. I was so very thankful that he had brought this to my attention, as I became aware of how much had changed since I had first worked with him, and how important it has been to integrate this idea of *finding my position* into my daily life.

~ ~ ~

References

Adler, J. (1987) 'Who is the Witness? A Description of Authentic Movement', in P. Pallaro (ed.) (1999), *Authentic Movement, Essays by Mary Starks Whitehouse, Janet Adler and Joan Chodorow*. Jessica Kingsley Publishers, pp.141-159

Bainbridge Cohen, B. (2013) 'On Cellular Imagination and Generative Space, Excerpt from an Interview with Nancy Stark Smith', *Contact Quarterly*, vol. 38, no.1, Winter/Spring, pp.33-34

Bauer, S. (2005) 'Finding the Bone in the Wind: A Journey with Suprapto Suryodarmo in Bali, Indonesia', *A Moving Journal*, vol. 12, no. 3, Fall / Winter, pp.14-20

Bauer, S. (2001) unpublished interview with Suprapto Suryodarmo, Samuan Tiga, Bali, Indonesia, 2001. Used with permission

Hughes-Freeland, F. (2008) *Embodied Communities: Dance Traditions and Change in Java*, Berghahn Books

Morein, A. (1994) 'A Practice Called "Road": studying "movement in meditation" with Suprapto Suryodarmo in Central Java', *Contact Quarterly*, vol. 19, no.1, Winter/Spring, pp.24-35

Whitehouse, M. (1963) 'Physical Movement and Personality', in P. Pallaro (ed.) (1999), *Authentic Movement, Essays by Mary Starks Whitehouse, Janet Adler and Joan Chodorow*. Jessica Kingsley Publishers, pp.51-57

Susan Bauer, (MFA, MA, RSME/T) is a dance/somatics educator who has taught in college and community settings in the US and Asia over the past 30 years. Her work is informed by her extensive background in dance, Authentic Movement, and Body-Mind Centering, as well as dance anthropology and cultural studies. She serves as Adjunct Professor at the University of San Francisco, and has a private practice in the SF Bay area as a Registered Somatic Movement Educator/Therapist. Susan is also a Fulbright Scholar to Bali, Indonesia, where she has studied Balinese dance, mask-making, and ritual since 1995.

www.susanbauer.com

23. "BODY BODY"

A Movement Practitioner's Journey with Amerta Movement

Helen Poynor (UK)

My point of entry to Prapto's work is movement itself. My understanding and my application of the work are from the perspective of a movement practitioner, which includes my practice as a teacher, artist and movement therapist. I run the 'Walk of Life' Workshop and Training Programme in non-stylised and environmental movement.

My intention here is to trace the influence of Prapto's work on the continuing evolution of my approach to non-stylised and environmental movement. This includes my integration and interpretation of the work as a Western feminist and the interweaving of the Eastern and Western lineages of Prapto and Anna Halprin with whom I had trained at the San Francisco Dancers' Workshop/Tamalpa Institute.

I will reference the early stages of Prapto's work with Westerners, specifically his notion of *Body Body*, which was central to his teaching at that time and which provides the ground for this chapter.

I first encountered Prapto's work as an established movement practitioner in the mid 1980s. My background included training in theatre, dance and body-orientated psychotherapy. I attended one of his earliest workshops in Europe in Hamburg in 1985. Prapto said very little, his command of English was limited, the movement tasks were simple and repetitive consisting for several days primarily of ongoing instructions: to walk, crawl or move in lying, to stop, to go on; together with a hands-on exercise in pairs and an invitation to move alone, in twos or small groups in front of the group. It also included sitting relaxation that I later understood to resemble Sumarah Meditation.[1] Despite the apparent simplicity of the instructions the quality of the movement work in a group, which included beginners as well as experienced movers, was exceptional. I was fascinated and could not fathom how such basic tasks and instructions could facilitate such a depth of practice.

I joined the first organised group of ten Westerners to work with Prapto in Java in 1986. This group was initiated and supported by a small group of colleagues who had travelled to Java to work with Prapto before he began offering formal courses or workshops and who also introduced his work to Europe. Three of them, Christine Stelzer, Susanne Christmann and Christian Böhringer, had previously trained in movement with Anna Halprin. So from the outset, in this generation of practitioners at least, there was an implicit inter-relationship between these two lineages of movement practice.

After years of exploring 'free movement' alone in a variety of locations in Java, Prapto developed his work initially on and with these four Europeans[2]. Through his work with them and the first group of ten he began developing his understanding of Westerners and the significant cultural difference between Western and Javanese culture that needed to be bridged in order to communicate and embody his approach to movement. Everyone involved was taking a leap of faith into uncharted waters since Prapto was barely known at the time and his work was in the early stages of its evolution. The participants were far removed from familiar surroundings, many at turning points in their lives, disrupted enough from habits and comfort zones to be available to new and life-changing experiences: willing raw material in what was effectively a creative movement and cultural laboratory.

At that point in my professional development I had stopped teaching in order to focus on my creative work. In addition to having opened to change in my professional life I found myself unexpectedly in a period of complete personal upheaval. I had a sense that my

---

1 Sumarah is a Javanese form of meditation based on surrender. It had a significant influence on the evolution of Prapto's practice and his students were encouraged to attend the regular Sumarah sessions offered in Solo by Pak Wando, a Sumarah *pamong* (guide).

2 José Mulder van de Graaf later joined the initial group of three. Prior to working with this small group, Prapto had been working in Java with Christine Rod from Switzerland.

work as a movement facilitator, while successful, had outstripped my conscious knowledge. I had an image of needing either a guardian angel or 'something' in my back. The work with Prapto filled this need.

The experience of working in Java was all the more intense because most of the teaching was not mediated by language. I experienced and understood the work, kinaesthetically, directly through my body. I could make little sense of it conceptually and would have been unable to communicate it in words. This way of learning suits me, circumventing the distancing effects of an overactive mind and connecting me to the source of my being. I need to move to understand myself and the world around me. At that point in my life I needed more than ever to ground myself in my body. Prapto's phrase *Body Body* sums up the tenor of his teaching at this time. In Indonesian, repeating a word serves to emphasise it or render it plural. The work was intensely physical, emphasising the contact of the feet on the floor and the movement of the body through space. We were invited again and again to land in the physical body, not to resist or fly away from embodiment. It was challenging and touched, at different moments, unexpected layers of both exhaustion and vitality and deep wells of emotion. Whatever was stirring we were encouraged to walk, to feel our feet on the ground, embodying a robust physicality. This offered an effective alternative when overwhelmed with emotion and contrasted with the prevalent practice of the Human Potential Movement in the 1970s which encouraged cathartic expression of emotion, fostering the belief that the only way out was through. The work with Prapto stripped back my movement patterns to repair cracks in the foundations that I had long avoided and had become adept at circumventing in my movement practice. It both brought me back to myself and moved me on. I had the image of a horse-shoe held in a red hot furnace and being re-shaped.

The only way of digesting and integrating my experiences after returning from Java was through movement. Just as my kinaesthetic being had received the teaching without the mediation of language or conceptual thought, so I digested the work kinaesthetically. Daily movement practice was less a question of self-discipline than of necessity. I *needed* to move. My kinaesthetic self was definitely running the show. I remember vividly a period when all my movement sessions were spent crawling. Each day I determined to do something different but on entering the movement space I would immediately find myself on all fours and would spend an hour crawling relentlessly. My 'animal body' knew what it needed and having been invited to come to the fore would brook no contradiction; I could not stop until it had been satisfied. I wondered subsequently if this was a process of my body filling in gaps in my movement development, returning to stages which had perhaps been passed through too rapidly, repeating particular movements just as a young child does as it learns to roll, sit, crawl, stand and eventually walk. There was certainly no question of moving on two feet during the crawling period!

When I eventually resumed teaching movement, after a further period of training in Java, ongoing intensive personal practice and working with Prapto in Europe and the UK, several conundrums presented themselves. There were challenges of both translation and of integration. Bridges needed to be built. Since I still had a primarily kinaesthetic rather than a conceptual grasp of the material I could not explain the work and needed to find a way of communicating it using language in a Western context. I was acutely aware of the chasm between myself as a Western feminist and Prapto as a Javanese man. For me there was a need for a double cultural shift in my communication and presentation of this approach to movement, not only from East to West but also from a patriarchal to a feminist approach[3]. In addition, my teaching style is consciously uncharismatic which is a reflection of both my personality and my politics. The obvious solution was to teach experientially since this is a characteristic of Prapto's work and mirrors my own approach to learning. I discovered how to apply the work in my own teaching by teaching it.

For approximately the next two years I needed to focus my attention almost exclusively on my experience of the work with Prapto. My previous work and training was temporarily unavailable as I integrated this new approach and material, and explored ways to work with it with others. One of the biggest shifts was away from the imaginative work and personal mythology which is at the core of the Halprin Life/Art process[4]. For some years, while connecting to my physical body at another, less conscious, level, I seemed to lose touch with my imagination. I no longer experienced images or narrative as I moved. I was all body. In time, images began to

---

[3] I have written in detail (1998) about the relationship between feminism and my approach to movement practice.

[4] For more information on Anna Halprin's approach, see Worth & Poynor (2004).

return but I experienced them differently; they began to flow in and through my movement without becoming primary. By continuing to follow the body rather than the image, the image does not limit the movement or become fixed, it changes as the movement evolves in a process of embodied imagination. When applied to creating performance this contributes to an experience that I can only describe as akin to 'channelling'. Language is a blunt instrument with which to capture the subtlety and immediacy of the experience I am attempting to describe in which an image or a character manifests directly in the moving body without the mediation of conscious thought. For example when preparing a solo performance for Prapto's Sharing Time Festival of Ritual Theatre and Cultural Environment (Java 1995) images of birthing and the death of a child arose directly in my movement rather than emerging first in my conscious mind or imagination. This led to the creation of a ritual performance dedicated to all women who had ever lost a child, a theme which I hadn't envisaged and which surprised me.

   The work with Prapto coupled with my training with Anna Halprin interweave to form a dual lineage which underpins the evolution of my own approach to movement teaching and practice over the past 30 years, differentiating it from other more conventional approaches to dance and theatre which I have studied. In many ways my teaching approach is different in form from how I received the work in Java. I teach by offering movement scores and tasks such as moving at different levels but only occasionally enter the space to move with people, preferring to witness and offer guidance and support, usually in words but sometimes through movement and voice, from the periphery. Although I may participate in an introductory score in a workshop to support the energy in the room, I rarely guide participants by moving with them. There are a number of reasons for this personal preference which has evolved naturally in my teaching practice. I feel one has to be very clear to be conscious enough in the moment to guide people by moving with them, which I understand as a form of teaching through transmission[5]. Personally I need the time that witnessing provides to recognise my own condition and 'check' my responses when I am

---

5 I am using the term transmission loosely to refer to spiritual practices in which experience/insight is transmitted directly from teacher to student. A related practice exists in Sumarah meditation where the *pamong* (guide) 'checks' another's condition by opening to receive/experience it in themselves thus enabling them to support the evolution of the other's meditation and life practice.

guiding others. This personal practice lies at the core of my teaching and despite the apparent difference in form directly reflects my experience of working with Prapto in Java in which, alongside the physicality of the work, there was a recurrent emphasis on 'attitude'. I understand this in the context of Prapto's Buddhism and Sumarah meditation as a practice of continual and profound self-awareness.

In individual movement therapy I choose not to enter the space, offering the mover the experience of their own space to move in (or not) in any way they choose. My intention is to support them to find their own way by offering an attentive, non-judgemental and non-intrusive presence. This approach reflects a person-centred, feminist and somatic approach to movement therapy which is deeply imbued with all I have received from Prapto.

The term non-stylised specifically indicates a desire to move away from preset movement/dance vocabularies which are taught through imitation. It also reflects the intention for each individual to discover their own way of moving. This ultimately becomes their own style which ideally remains in a state of constant evolution. When leading workshops I avoid demonstrating a movement task (unless it feels necessary or particularly helpful) in order not to encourage people to copy what they see or to create an atmosphere where 'getting it right' becomes paramount. The landscapes of different bodies shaped by different life experiences need to find their own expression in movement. Witnessing people move I perceive them coming into focus as they become more aligned with themselves, embodying their individuality and allowing others to see them more clearly. This is fundamentally different from other approaches to movement or performance that stress the need to continually generate creative material in a search for originality. Since we are all unique there is no need for this excavation of new ideas or vocabulary.

There is nevertheless a contradiction in teaching a kinaesthetic approach to movement through language and verbal scores. Language alerts our mental processes; if as we start to move we get lost in the labyrinth of our minds or seduced by our analytic understanding, we are likely to find ourselves further away from our kinaesthetic experience than ever. There is a sort of sleight of hand (or mind) that allows verbal scores to be received and mentally released, held lightly and intuitively, allowing them to filter through as our kinaesthetic self finds its way. This is at odds with educational practices that emphasise analysis and conceptual understanding. Prapto circumvents this by his maverick and poetic use of the

English language, a freedom which is perhaps easier to access as a non-native speaker.

In a synthesis of the kinaesthetic training that underpins Anna Halprin's approach and immersion in Prapto's practice of *Body Body*, the 'Walk of Life' approach uses scores based on the structure of the body, with an emphasis on the skeleton, that offer physical tasks. For example, starting from walking, working through the skeleton from the feet up gradually incorporating more of the body's structure, emphasising the interconnection and flow of movement through the whole body. The starting point is the body itself rather than a concept, theme or image. From my perspective there is a tendency for these mental functions to elicit a cerebral response that is enacted by body rather than arising directly from it. This may result in a gap, however slight, between stimulus and expression. Paradoxically this emphasis on the body as experienced in Anna Halprin's, Prapto's and my own work has the potential to liberate both personal and creative process.

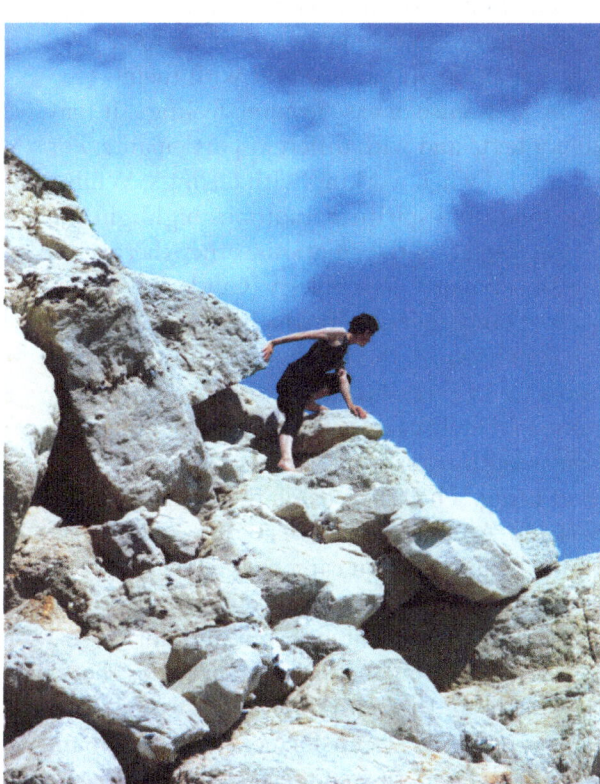

Photo: Annie Pfingst

In the context of movement in the environment, the emphasis on the body supports an embodied encounter with the land, a direct engagement of the physicality of the body with the materiality of the land in a receptive and responsive relationship. The scores offered provide a springboard and direction but the environment itself becomes the teacher with different elements eliciting different experiences and movement responses. Moving among trees may offer a clearer kinaesthetic understanding of one's verticality. Lying in tussocky grass cradled by the contours of the earth can engender a profound experience of being held and of surrender. Working in tidal environments and in different weathers offers an experience of change mirroring the changes in our interior landscape and our personal weather. Moving on the coast where I live, the constant movement of the sea combined with the clear form of the rocks supports the ability to move with clarity and fluidity – challenging us to embody both our strength and our responsiveness. The intricate microcosm of rock-pools viewed at eye level coupled with the grandeur of the cliffs offers a perspective of our place in the interconnected web of life.

Working with movement in a non-stylised and holistic way inevitably touches the emotions. To what extent and how directly a facilitator of non-stylised movement engages with emotion depends on their intention and training together with their personal perspective on, and sense of ease around, feelings. It may also vary in different contexts and with different participants. For me the body remains central when working with feelings. While some psychological methods and spiritual traditions highlight the relationship between the mind and the emotions, other therapeutic approaches, including Bio-dynamic Psychology (Gerda Boyesen's neo-Reichian approach to body therapy) in which I trained, emphasise the relationship between the emotions and the body: emotions are understood to be embedded in the body. While it is clear that changing one's attitude can result in a change of heart, from this perspective in-depth transformation also necessarily permeates our physical being. The relationship between moving and feeling is a two-way street. Anna Halprin asserts that as well as expressing your feelings by moving you can change how you feel by how you move. Moving may open the door to feelings, associations and images, the body is both the conduit and container for these. Content is elicited by the moving body which also provides the ground to process this material. By continuing to follow the body as feelings arise, they are potentially transformed, understood and integrated from a new perspective. In some respects the different Western and Eastern approaches of Anna Halprin and Prapto mirror each other in relation to the potentially transformative power of movement on our emotions.

There is a recurrent dilemma about how to understand the role of the mind in movement practice. This has been touched on briefly in relation to using verbal instructions in movement teaching and the references to the imagination. It merits a much longer discussion than can be encompassed in this chapter but I would like to offer a few further reflections here. I would suggest that the predominant function of the mind in movement practice is one of awareness rather than of description, the creation of narrative or analysis. The mind becomes an ally focusing our attention on what we are doing, on our body and where we are, rather than a distracting obstacle to be overcome. If one is fully absorbed in the physical practice of *Body Body*, there is no space to simultaneously analyse the process and thus put it at one remove. One may choose to reflect on it subsequently. There is a parallel between movement practice and the experience in meditation when the mind is empty and one simply inhabits the present moment, a sense of one's whole being (body, mind and feelings) being aligned, whether in movement or in stillness.

A more paradoxical experience of the mind in movement practice may also be echoed in meditation: through an embodied experience of moving, it is possible to calm the overactive quality of thinking which for many of us resembles a hamster on a wheel. This clears the path for inspiration or clear thought to arise and is more likely to happen if we are not focusing on a problem or dilemma in an attempt to solve it but are immersed in the movement itself. This creates the receptivity that allows something new to emerge whether we see the source of it as the inner guide of Sumarah, our subconscious mind or Life/God. The catalyst for the realisation is the moving body.

In conclusion, the practice of *Body Body* is of value to all who work with movement artistically, personally or therapeutically. The moving body is the foundation, the pathway and the means of expression. *Body Body* is an approach to movement practice which, through focusing on the physical, allows the whole being to ground itself in the walk of life.

Rahayu. [6]

~ ~ ~

---

[6] Rahayu is the expression used to mark the end of a Sumarah meditation session. It means peace, harmony, and for me it always elicits a sense of gratitude.

References

Poynor, H. (1998) *Women-Body-Movement, non-stylised movement practice as a process of personal development, empowerment and expression for women*, MA in Feminist Performance, University of Bristol

Romano, L. (2013) *Sumarah – Spiritual Wisdom from Java*, Lulu Press

Worth, L. and Poynor, H. (2004) *Anna Halprin*, Routledge

Helen Poynor runs the 'Walk of Life' Workshop and Training Programme in Non-stylised and Environmental Movement established in 1991 on the Jurassic Coast World Heritage Site in South West England.

An independent movement artist and director, Helen specialises in movement in natural environments, site-specific and autobiographical performance and interdisciplinary collaborations. Recognised by Prapto as a teacher, Helen is guest Associate Teacher for Tamalpa UK, and a Registered Dance Movement Therapist/Somatic Movement Therapist. Publications include: 'Working Like Farmer: towards an embodied spirituality' in *Dance, Somatics and Spiritualities* (Intellect, 2014) and 'Landscapes of Loss', in *Journal of Dance and Somatic Practices*, Vol. 5.2 (2013).

www.walkoflife.co.uk

24. EVER-SPEAKING BEING

Michael Dick (Germany)

What I call the 'ever-speaking being' of humanness is drawn from my investigations on elementary movements and the nature of the human instrument for performing arts. This contribution is an extract from the manuscript *Finger Exercises for Actors: An Elementary Teaching and Practice for Performing Arts.*[1]

Introducing the term 'practice' into the field of the performing arts says, first of all, that skills, knowledge and personal growth need to come from experience gained through practical activity and, secondly, that the instrument of performing arts always concerns and constitutes the whole human being. Lastly, using the term practice pays tribute to the limitlessness of our potential for humanness, both in development and attainment.

Just as fine artists use paint, canvas, and brushes for their artwork, performing artists use their own body, mind, and feeling. A pianist exercises permeability of fingering and presence of tone.[2] This chapter presents these two fundamental aspects of practice – 'permeability' and 'presence' – as they are applied to the performing arts. This is followed by a description of an introductory lesson in an acting class. The three essential elements of a performing arts instrument – body, mind/spirit/speech, and feeling/voice – are addressed with practical instructions and guidance, so the reader can 'try it out at home.' Since the explorations presented start with daily life movement, it is possible for anyone to read this chapter and relate it directly to their own experience. The chapter ends with a short

---

[1] This teaching took shape and was validated over a period of 12 years (1999 to 2011), in which I was teaching at an acting school in Cologne, Germany.

[2] For pianists, fingers are the physical part of the body that needs most practice with the instrument. So the title *Finger Exercises for Actors* highlights the main ways acting students need to apply themselves in their art-form.

description of a novel kind of blocking rehearsal that has emerged from these practices, as one example of an application for everyday professional theatrical practice.

Our Speaking Being

Human society is made up of communicative, social beings who are always inter-connected, consciously or unconsciously. Human consciousness cannot but be affected by what emanates from our bodies, feelings, and thoughts. Body, mind, and feeling are constituent elements of this 'ever-speaking-ness' of being human. In education for the performing arts, becoming more conscious of these elements is seen as most closely corresponding to becoming aware of the ever-speaking nature of humanness. Body, mind, and feeling can be seen as the agents, media, and contents of any communication happening in performing arts and in life as a whole. Students are usually quite young, coming with limited life experiences to an education for performing arts. Investigating their own character and taking on and identifying with other characters, usually expands and works on their personalities. To a certain degree, education for the performing arts can always lead to transformation for those participating. 'Practice' is an integral part of a path to enact an embodied life.

Permeable and Present

Permeability and presence are two fundamental potentials of being human. I will define what I mean by permeability and presence in the three categories of body, feeling, and mind.

Permeability

Body: For an actor, 'permeability' will express itself on the physical level as capacity for embodiment. Like changelings who can take on different forms, shapes, and physical conditions, actors need to exercise their limbs, organs, bones, joints, etc. to become permeable enough, so they can facilitate transformation.

Feeling: One could see a feeling tone being characterized and determined by its quality of vibration: amplitude and frequency. How much actors can make themselves available as a refined membrane to receive, embody, and emit these vibrations, and in this way volunteer for all possible kinds of feelings, will show the extent and limits of their permeability in this realm.

Mind: On a mind level, thinking-patterns, deeply imprinted beliefs, and unconscious orientations can become a hindrance to a more open-minded, 'translucent' attitude. To assimilate and to follow mental processes such as rationalization, reflection, analysis, and differentiation with a free mind affords accessibility and intellectual flexibility. In regard to depth of thought and the extent of understanding, actors need to apply themselves in a holistic, integrated, and organic way. It is important that the receptivity of the mind is not split off from that of the rest of the sensual apparatus. Otherwise over-intellectuality, lack of empathy, and more pathological consequences may arise. If the mind moves freely and permeably in alignment with body sensation and feeling tone, then one feels clear, open, and less fixated or controlling. The mind may even feel more tangibly knowable.

The practice of permeability refines and purifies the medium of 'ever-speaking-ness' and can lead to a sense of transparency that facilitates the embodiment of boundless possibilities. It also invokes dimensionality, in-depth feeling, and access to intelligence and freedom.

Presence

Body: In addressing 'presence', an actor would look at the relationship to him/herself first rather than in a more conventional approach to presence in terms of having an impact on others (usually an audience), or as personal magnetism or charisma. This is a crucial change of perspective. Facing myself as the bodily instrument of my art for the first time, I can see that 'I am that instrument, it is this body, my feeling, my mind'. And this is the instrument that needs to be looked at, sensed and felt, explored and exercised: I see my body as 'a forming, telling, portraying, cultivating and ever-speaking agent'. In time, this change in self-awareness will open up performers' consciousness to the presence of what could be called the *inner stage*[3]: a continuous, spatial, bodily felt, and holistic awareness of what is going on inside, while also being present in their acting on the outer theatre-stage or *stages of life* as well.

All that appears in our field of experience as human beings – inner and outer – emerges within our soul[4] or individual consciousness as an imprint, and as Martin Buber's inner *Erregungsbild* (excitement-

---

3 *Inner stage* and *stage of life* are terms taken from Prapto's vocabulary. There isn't space to define them completely in this chapter.

4 My understanding of soul comes from my studies of A.H. Almaas (2004).

picture), a "dynamic, stirring image (...) streaming through" the body.[5] These inner excitement-pictures will be noticeable to a sensitive person and can be recognized, felt, and sensed from within. It is my experience that the more an actor becomes conscious of these imprints, the more visible they will be, radiating out to an audience and by that means will become 'present.' This is a phenomenon that often amazes students, when they recognize what effect it has when they turn toward their immediate bodily experience on stage. They stop being concerned about the effect of their 'playing' and instead become increasingly able to concentrate and focus their attention on the activity, text, partner, etc.

Feeling: Presence in feeling needs involvement with heart: courage, curiosity, compassion. It feels always new and vulnerable.

Mind: Presence in mind means being awake, open, and aware of what is happening inside this mind. Simply said, what is needed is laborious exercise.

At first, practice can lead students *towards* presence. In time, they can develop a capacity to be *with* presence more often, and more continuously. Actors want to become present and be sensitive in and with their bodies all the time. They want to feel all of their emotions, and want to be able to allow the deepest, most vulnerable places within to come forth, as needed. Actors can be crisp and awake, flexible, and brilliant to grasp the depth of thoughts, to let their minds be informed and pervaded by their beauty. Further down the road, some might be ushered into a kind of embodiment that resonates with excellence and mastery. Some then might experience how to be cool and ablaze on stage at the same time, how to be fully relaxed, playful, spontaneous, and highly concentrated. *Here and now,* completely identified – and not identified – with their characters, and acting, they are then *in* presence, able to be *it*, whatever this 'it' might be.

To become permeable and present can be seen as a precondition for being able to work effectively as a performer. Its practice can become the one first ritual for one's personal studies and can be introduced as a general warm-up in any theatre company. Presence and permeability are key conditions for further application in monologue, dialogue, and ensemble work.

---

5 From Martin Buber (1999). The German term *Erregungsbild* that Buber uses, which I translate as 'excitement-picture', has not been directly translated into English, but paraphrased as quoted above. The chapter is on the evolution of language, on how before human beings speak (spoke), all outer world is (was) experienced as "inner excitement-picture".

A Practice Session

Arriving in a class of acting students learning elementary practices, I will let them know that I am more interested in their impressions than in attending to or evaluating their expression. We focus on how they feel during the exercise, and what they are experiencing. Developing a kind of neutral work-attitude becomes fundamental to this work of just perceiving and receiving impressions and learning to find a language to articulate them. Even though this usually will not make students stop judging themselves in the beginning, it can help them to enter exercises.

> "Please don't worry about your expression, rather start by shifting your attention a bit, noticing what you sense in your body. Whatever position you are in now, whether you are sitting or lying, standing or walking, start from where you are. Let yourself be informed by what you notice. You may want to touch or rub your limbs to feel your body more, to warm yourself up, or even to alleviate tension or pain you might be feeling. Explore freely what is arising from your daily life movement, where this exercise always starts. Maybe you want to relax in one part of your body and stretch another part. You can use the force of gravity as your partner in relaxing. Notice when you would like to feel your muscles more, to reach out, to expand in your movement. You can alter direction and levels. From lying, you can go to crawling and sitting, to standing up and walking. Recognize any physical or emotional impact these positions and levels might have on you. Notice mind-activity, images, memories related to the psycho-developmental stages of these postural changes. And find your way up and down. Pay attention to flow arising in your movement. At some point, please stop!"

Stopping is an essential part of this work's vocabulary. Stopping is the beginning of punctuation in movement. Just as sentences have punctuation so we can understand their grammar and direction, the movement-language of our bodies has punctuation too, starting with receiving a full stop.

> "In your stopping, receive your position and posture first and then receive your weight. Let go of any

additional tension not needed to keep the posture you are in now. Feel your organization from within, and in the space. And now, either follow the direction of weight, or choose a direction and start moving again. Now sense into possible movements of your joints throughout your body and softly explore them. Tensions often linger in joints and softly opening the joints through movement can release them. A single finger has got three joints, difficult to focus and to move singly. Each finger has its own character and feeling tone. Sense into those different characters of your fingers, recognize the extra sensitivity and the atmosphere they bring to your body when you let one of them lead the movement of your hand or your whole body.

Now check your state for a moment. This physical exercising can bring up emotions and thoughts that might distract you, let you drift and dream away at times. That's not bad; it's normal. When you recognize it, start to sense yourself again and let your body's movement be informed by those thoughts and feelings, allowing them to enter back into your physical reality, placing and anchoring their drifting quality in the here-and-nowness of body sensation."

Our next step will create a bridge to what already has been called the *inner stage*. It's always there waiting for us to enter. *Reading* is a tool for opening up, spreading, enfolding, and entering this inner stage.[6] What is it we are reading here? Every gesture, posture, inner attitude, feeling, and mind pattern is part of our gesturing. Whether we are conscious of them or not, they all are saying something.

And how do we read? Inherent to a gesture is its excitement-picture. *Reading* helps us access all inner motion, stirrings, impulses, and changing tension-patterns that we become aware of in ourselves. Later reading can expand to atmosphere, the other, our physical surroundings, and subtle realms.

"Now try it out. Make a clear gesture with your hand and stop there. Or let the fingers make little changes

---

6 *Reading* is a tool Prapto uses in his terminology, which I have explored and developed further in order to apply it in my work with actors.

> and each time try to contact the inner excitement-picture of each shape. Feel how those inner forms change alongside the outer forms. Can you feel it? This contact that you might feel now is reading. Again, don't worry too much about your expression. Just move and enjoy. See if you can let your focus open up to your whole arm, to the gesture of your arms and read. Let your awareness spread further to the whole of your body. Sense and feel the complete sculpture. Give attention to your moving sculpture and the flow of inner excitement-pictures will allow you to read in your unfolding story. Body-wisdom is willing to reveal its knowledge at any given moment, from instant to instant, and is offering its story to us. You might feel this challenging for your mind. Try to stay in contact with your felt sense even when your mind wants to figure out what it all means, where it all leads. Basically, your mind doesn't want to let go of control."

Reading implicitly fosters permeability and presence, which we are investigating here. Following movement along this line as a long-time practice can change our whole attitude and life orientation. We may start to find this immediacy of our general sense of being more important and dear to us than anything else, whichever stage we are on and whatever role we may be playing. Transparent, permeable spaciousness then may reveal the precise contours of role-play. Acting in this state feels simple, adequate, and authentic.

> "Now, before ending, follow your own guidance for a while with all the elements and suggestions that have been introduced so far. Find your object of attention, your own thread of interest, your own intention, form, and field to immerse yourself in."

So far we have been exploring our performing instrument and this newly opened inner stage from our physical presence and body awareness. The next step for our practical exploration would then be to work with our voices in three areas:

1. **Body-sound**: this means sounds that are coming from and are directed by movements of the physical body, such as sighs, groans, and moans, and sounds from rocking, shaking, hitting, kicking, etc., or simply allowing breath to become audible. This part of the practice is of great benefit in bringing together body and voice,

finding the right placement of the voice, freeing energies, and opening the joy of playfulness. This solves lots of the issues that beginners have with expression.

2. Musical sound: in the movement from sounding to singing, we recognise vibration as a support for feeling tones. Through chakra-singing, for example, we deepen our awareness of our being as a resonating cavity, and as a body made up of sound.[7] Working directly on emotions by what I call 'vowel-hiking'[8] enables us to support all possible kinds of feelings. In sounding vowels, moving slowly from one vowel to the next and pausing in between two, where the 'impure' vowels reside, we will come upon '(e)motion'.

By following profound listening practices, conducting and choosing 'right' pitch and note, we can learn how to sing emotions. By integrating movement and voice, this moving sculpture can shape and form a character, and become a character's song and feeling-dance. When finally we let text come through this conduit, feeling can colour whole passages of text into one emotion (hate, love, pride, courage, joy, whatever you like) or even more flexibly, move from one tone of emotion to another. These passages can become building blocks in developing a character through a scene or a whole play. One can learn to experience this movement as a continuous flow of a constantly transforming feeling-body, the moving and sounding sculpture of ever-speaking feeling.[9]

3. Formed sound: either pre-lingual or lingual, this is an oral-linguistic expression of sound. This is a whole field of work, especially for acting students. In practical terms, we would continue to explore words and their meanings from their constituent parts. We already have found vowels as a conduit for the vibrating body of emotion. Now we turn to the physical in consonants. To sensing into the mechanics of their pronunciation and articulation in the mouth and throat we add the experience of their quality in

---

7 **Chakra singing** is only one of several different ways of achieving this. It is a practice in which specific vowels are sung to open up certain areas and chakra-points of our body energetically. There are the three lower chakras: survival, sexual and social; the central heart chakra, and the upper three connected with expression and qualities of consciousness.

8 **Vowel-hiking** is a term I use for one of the exercises developed by English artist Guy Dartnell in his voic(e)motion practice.

9 All the steps described here have been developed on the basis of Dartnell's voic(e)motion. His exercises are highly influenced by his exposure to the Roy Hart theatre approach to voice development.

movement (squeeze, hiss and sizzle, pop, etc.), when spread onto the whole physical body. What is revealing itself then, is what we could call the words' inherent soul, a pre-lingual experience, or again Martin Buber's excitement-picture. These spirit/mind-awakening, word-birthing impressions have a palpable effect on/in us.[10] We do further research on words by investigating their experiential link to sensory roots. The word 'frog,' for example, can easily be recognized as stemming from the sensory field of sound, originating in hearing. Words are often determined through sensory linkages and their specific inner motion.

This way language will become more accessible as material for our artwork, free from incorrect accentuation, subtext, and emotional predeterminations, experienced more like an animated being with its own life and presence. Finally, a word might evolve into something more vivid than just its meaning alone. Word-bodies can attract associations, word-lineages, and word-families to play around with. We soon may feel how much more words are moving us, rather than us directing them. We recognize how much more we are in-*form*-ed by our wording and our choice of words. A word as a body in its own right; this is what needs to be imparted to a student in this part of the practice. Usually this segment of work is introduced with a lecture about the evolution and nature of language.

Eventually all the layers are included and integrated in our movement session: those of feeling, word and mind, and movement of our physical body. All move together in accord.

Reflection on experience is vital after a movement session. Emphasizing interest in discrimination, students may learn to appreciate and give meaning to their findings, rather than, as so often, wishing to be on a par with their fellow students. In this way, they may pick up the scent to find the trace *of* and *to* their own unique voice. In this context, the conversation is guided by principles like: everybody will be heard, will speak only for and of themselves, and may finish without being interrupted. Through these principles, we cultivate discourse, enjoy precise description, and invoke further inquiry.

A Blocking Rehearsal

Any drama or text used for dramatization usually gives hints such as stage directions or spoken words pointing to the nature of a character, the location of a scene, or other relevant conditions for a

---

10 I thoroughly explored this part of the teaching in a decade of research, directing, and acting in 'Healing Theatre Cologne' between 1988 and 1998.

play. Entering a blocking rehearsal with a permeable and present instrument, one can sense, feel, analyze, and understand holistically an author's intention. Hence a blocking rehearsal can become the analysis of a text's body-mind-feeling from within the location of a character and scenery, and can become a road to identification, which means feeling the character's location, situation, and position in space and time from within one's soul and body-layers. Embodying those feelings might bring about insights into a character's motives that can be adjusted to the scene and to other characters, be seen in the context of the play's topic and so on. Including all elements will show the relevance of personal experience for final artistic decisions and composition.

Where the narration comes from can be felt deeply and authentically. How it will be delivered to an audience artistically remains open. Blocking rehearsal in this way can be seen as part of a vocabulary of an elementary teaching and practice for performing arts and, with it, an aging technique can be awakened to new life.

Concluding Remark

To realize and actualize the ever-speaking nature of being through the practice of permeability and presence cleanses the mirrors that our art and life stage can become. What is said then will be plain and audible. May excellence in theatre and in the evolution of the performing arts benefit from such development and the growth of those acting in them!

~ ~ ~

References

Almaas, A.H. (2004) *The Inner Journey Home – Soul's Realization of the Unity of Reality*, Shambhala

Buber, M. (1999) *I and Thou*, transl. Smith, Ronald Gregor, T&T Clark, p.32 and p.37

Michael Dick is an Amerta Movement Practitioner who has studied continuously with Prapto since 1988. He has taught 'BeWegen' since 1995 and co-founded the 'School of/for Movement' in Cologne, Germany in 2012. He has spent 35 years as an actor, director and performance artist, co-founding 'Healing Theatre Cologne' (1988-2003), winning awards for his stagings of Kafka's *The Castle* and *A Little Woman*. Today he is a member of 'PAErsche Aktionslabor NRW' for performance art. He has been teaching drama now for almost two decades. Other practices include: Sumarah-Meditation, IOKAI-Meridian Shiatsu and Diamond Approach within the Ridhwan School Europe.

www.schule-der-bewegung.net

25. MOVING IN THE LAW

Simon Slidders (UK)

Every morning, as I come to work, I emerge from Holborn Underground Station, having raised my heart rate by walking up the two escalators ("Please stand on the right," I growl beneath my breath at the spatial awareness of hapless tourists who have not noticed the Underground rules of movement). I slip through a couple of back alleys and emerge into Lincoln's Inn Fields. I cross the park in the middle of the square diagonally. The caryatids of Sir John Soane's Museum are behind me to my left, obscured by trees, the chapel and high walls of Lincoln's Inn in front of me. I pass a catalpa (Indian bean) tree as I walk along the gravelled paths.

On summer days I cut through the tropical area where, among the ferns, a rotund man, with cigar, brightly coloured braces and mobile phone, occasionally fulfils the role of a tropical bird. I see the sky and sense the trees around me. I hear the crunch of gravel and momentarily feel I am connected to nature (listening and breathing), before I emerge, past a nineteenth-century monumental water trough, to walk down the outside of Lincoln's Inn to the back entrance to the Royal Courts of Justice. Above me, a statue of Moses (the Lawgiver), atop the central apex of the building, looks down on my approach (Jesus and Solomon are at the front with Alfred the Great).

I enter, past the security guards and metal detector, before turning sharply up a steep set of stone stairs. At the top I swipe my pass into a secure corridor which leads down and up through an Escheresque junction of stone staircases. I slip on through one exit along a wooden covered walkway. From here I can look down into the wood-panelled courts on either side below, where the ushers are slowly arranging the black-robed, bewigged barristers before the judges come in. Soon, I am out into the central office section; up along long corridors through double doors, swiping my pass and time card to reach my office on the third floor. I burst into my room as I tend to burst into any room, untangle myself from my rucksack, coat and scarf and greet my roommate. My primary movement of the day is complete. When I leave I will not be moving towards law. This is my work place. Here I spend the majority of my waking life.

The left wall is covered with shelves of law books and ends with two Zen calligraphies (one by me and one by my teacher) hanging by drawing pins from the wall, leading to my computer near the window. The window looks out over a paved courtyard to the East Wing in which judges can be seen working in their rooms late into the night, or their clerks bringing them coffee and sandwiches during the day. Judges' clerks and, occasionally, guards with prisoners cross the courtyard beneath.

I am not by nature a sedentary person, but the job involves a lot of working at a computer, phone calls, e-mails and meetings. Yet, as a manager, I take time to make myself visible to my staff in their rooms, which they also each share with one other lawyer. I am constantly in movement, delivering files, messages, consulting with colleagues, etc. I love this forward momentum of movement down straight, clearly defined corridors, the constant pushing and pulling through doors which divide them. Often I go further afield in search of judges in their rooms, finding my way through the labyrinthine passages of this metaphor of the legal system.

The Royal Courts of Justice is a huge complex of buildings, designed to express the majesty of the law, intended to bring visitors closer to an awareness of God as the lawgiver. In this building it is easy to experience law as bowing and praying. Tradition requires that lawyers bow when they enter and leave the court at all times, and all persons in court must rise when judges enter and leave the court. Still, there is also a strong sense in the courts, despite the adversarial system used in English law, that we are here for resolution: to heal, to mend, set right what has gone wrong before and to provide lines of direction for the future.

It is probably no coincidence that I chose or was chosen by a movement practice that has very few rules. I had come to movement work initially as a meditation practice, after my interaction with my own meditation practice had become so rigid that I had pulled myself to a full stop. Indeed, at first, the movement was an attempt to counterbalance my life in the law, as an escape from, or denial of it. A suit and tie seemed like a constriction I was constantly trying to evade. Suddenly, at the end of a workshop in Assisi in 1997 (four years after I had first met him), Prapto appeared to absorb for the first time the fact that I was a lawyer, and challenged me to apply movement to the idea of law and law to movement. I did not immediately find his statement that *"man is in judgement, woman is in punishment"* that helpful, but it did eventually lead me to think of my experience of law in both the active and receptive sense.

I had become used to sashaying down corridors, giving full value to my movement as I grasped door handles and moved from one area to another, crossing boundaries, contracting, then opening into each new space. I had not previously considered the law in movement terms, nor movement in terms of the law. However, I quickly saw a correlation with the development of law, at least the English legal system, with the loose framework that Prapto gave to his workshops.

For many years when he worked with groups in Europe, Prapto would split us into three groups with the intention that each group work from a different perspective. *Circle* had the theme of *Bowing and Praying*. *Oval* was about *Purification/Healing through Circulation*. *Square* has been variously described as *Creation in Reflection, Unity in Diversity, Human in Society*. What these groups actually mean in movement terms seems to be very fluid and depends on the movement teacher or applicant[1] who is leading the group. However, it is in the dialogue about, and exploration of, the meaning of these terms that we learn something about our movement. For example, I tend to think of Circle as being about my relationship with God/Soul/myself/spiritual sense; Oval as my relationship with body/nature/the other; and Square as my relationship with society and performance. Or even more simply: Circle as temple; Oval as home; and Square as stage.

When working in Avebury with Prapto as applicants (with Kristina Bourdillon and Keith Miller) we have variously described the three terms as meaning: opening to the ancestral spirit of the land – exploring ritual in the environment (Circle); opening to our body nature in circulation with the land (Oval); and opening to cultural dialogue with each other and the land (Square). These terms are always merely an entry point, a key not the door or the room. It

---

1 Prapto describes the students whom he asks to lead groups as *applicants*, because he expects them to set the content of the group by 'applying' what they do in their daily life to their movement practice and vice versa, e.g. an applicant performer might wish to explore movement in performance, and/or how our sense of performance affects our movement.

is often the quality of not knowing that enables us to start to move most freely. Nevertheless, I found myself trying to introduce these to my idea of law.

Law in society has often seemed to me to start (in patriarchal societies at least) with the idea of law being handed down from above: law as bowing and praying to a God above, whose laws we obey as an act of worship. At the same time, in the receptive sense, there are the laws of Nature like gravity, a physical phenomenon which expresses that indeed things must always come to the earth, and that from the earth there is always movement up and out. This for me is connected to movement in Circle, but also to movement in awareness of the vertical, the connection between earth and sky and the sense of oneself as a puppet of God, examining angle and proportion with our joints as we see how we connect to this line. This is taking movement back to the basic sense of the skeleton, down to the bone of things.

Then, in England there was the development of the common law. This is an amorphous human body of law that grew out of past experience and listening to the heart or conscience, feeling for what was right rather than looking to an external God. I therefore see this as law being practised in Oval. I tend to think of Oval as being an exploration of bringing the past into the present. It looks at our tendency to be behind the moment as opposed to being in the moment (and thereby in our bodies). It is often my feelings resulting from past wrongs done to me or by me and my inability to express and let go of these feelings through my body that hold me back from being in the present. My meditation teacher used to say, "Judgement comes from experience. Experience comes from bad judgements". It is only in movement that I have come to understand the importance of the 'experience' of those judgements in my body.

Eventually common law is codified or developed into legislation – statute law – whereby Government attempts to impose structure on society from the outside. This is based on thinking ahead, towards the future in clear lines, imposing boundaries, channelling society in a forward direction, and at the same time giving society a skin. It deals with the diversity of society in general rather than the individual (thankfully it is humanised by judicial interpretation in each case).

Square is about unity in diversity. As much as law tends to complexity, it is also looking for a unifying element. This leads to a desire for a distillation of the law into an ideal (an expression of the divine for the non-religious), a fundamental Bill of Rights, such as the European Charter of Human Rights. It seems that humanity is trying to create its own Ten Commandments based on a humanistic philosophy rather than theology. It is almost as if we are back in Circle again!

Did these concepts of movement applied to my idea of law affect my practice of it as a lawyer? In the everyday, it is difficult to see how they could. They did make me more conscious of the way people use the legal process to express and ultimately find their own pace of movement through pain and experience – something I had been aware of during my days as a divorce lawyer. Then I had slowly come to realise that the inbuilt delays in the system acted as a holding structure for the painful process of separation. So I am aware of the need for law to find its own pace and movement, for there to be both irrigation and clear decision-making.

In my movement practice, I try to work both with my sense of my body in relation to its own proportions and angles – e.g. the sense of the space between my horizontally bent arm and my chest, the way my hand curves in naturally towards my sternum – and with the sense of my body in relationship to other objects, living or inanimate, in the space, and the boundaries of the space itself. To this extent my movement practice is a celebration of the constantly shifting awareness of patterns of relationship that we have with our body and the environment around it. From these points of view I can also see law as offering both boundaries and channels for movement. When seen from this perspective, law becomes then not so much a restriction, but instead an access through the maze of life, always finding that ultimately the way in is the way out. In these constellations, the law does not bind but acts as a reference point for action.

When I considered what 'laws' govern the development of my personal movement, the paradigm that came to mind was the Walt Disney film adaptation of Pinocchio by Collodi. Pinocchio makes a similar journey from wood (a skeleton operated by divine strings over which he has no control, subject to wherever gravity takes him), to the acquiring of experience in muscle and flesh (including learning about his animal nature as a donkey!), before developing his own integrated conscience to give his life direction. In movement, in arriving in the space I explore the up and down, the strings, and the floor. I move into the horizontal, feeling more into the flow of my muscles, celebrating the way they wrap around my limbs, following the sense of embrace, the space that my proportion creates, not so much seen as felt and supported, inhabiting the sensual world. It is only when we have humanised ourselves by really feeling the flesh of our bodies that we can then move on to a structure that incorporates both bone and flesh, to place ourselves in society, the space to say "here I am!"

While I have already said that law can be as much about the awareness of the transcendent and experience, I have found increasingly that I am concerned with boundaries, the edges of rooms, understanding what encloses, delimits and supports spaces, the lines and senses of directions in space. I realise how comforting boundaries can be, enclosing to protect and separate us from the other.

In the office, with the very many passages and doors I go through, I find that it is at these points of transition from one space to another that I become most aware of my body. I see my hand as it pushes against a swing door or grabs the handle. At that moment I feel my attention focusing, bringing my awareness of my body to a point. Then as I come into the new space my awareness expands, my awareness both of my body and the space around me. Exits and entrances continue to interest me both internally and externally. Once, having been asked to work in Square, I tried to work with the structure of the heart, that most fluid of organs. I found myself focusing on the exits and entrances, the valves.

Prapto for a time abandoned the use of Circle, Oval and Square, and asked his applicants to just work from their own experience. This was always implicit in the way he asked applicants to work. However, I had treated the comforting structures of Circle, Oval and Square as my Body of Law, and so to start from just my own practice was both alarming and liberating.

When I first started movement, I was often anxious to get it right, to be doing what the teacher wanted, worried that I was not doing the right thing. It was only gradually that I began to realise that my greatest anxiety was when I was about to do (or doing) something that was outside my own comfort zone, that was outside *my* rulebook. It really had nothing to do with the teacher as lawmaker or judge, but about stepping into the unknown. All these references to laws are ultimately only starting points, and it is when I start to move in areas where I do not know what the rules are that I feel that I am really beginning to stretch my boundaries.

25. MOVING IN THE LAW

Laws are mutable, changing in intention and approach, as the emphasis shifts, from feeling the lines (the boundaries) to feeling the movement of the body in the substance of what is enclosed – the flesh and blood of the law.

There are always my basic reference points or rules I can rely upon if I really get lost of course: *"receive my condition"*, *"mind my own business"*, *"give value to my movement"*, and *"be awake in the space"*, but there are no laws stopping me from moving, and I aspire to law being integrated into my body.

As to man in judgement and woman in punishment, I struggled with this as some sort of law handed down from the teacher, but as I understand it, Prapto does not see his role as a lawgiver at all, only as a seed planter. I prefer to interpret that seed as: 'judgement being active and punishment being receptive'. To me, judgement is more directional, the laying down of the law, imposing, cutting through confusion (more Square). This is not to say that it is only two-dimensional. By creating lines or structures in space, there is inevitably space in and around them. Punishment can of course be active, but in this context I interpret it as more akin to suffering the consequences of judgement rather than the implementation of it. It is the containment I experience in those created spaces – in the consequences of the acts of judgement. In giving life by irrigation and ventilation to those spaces I am acting in a more Oval manner. Sometimes I confuse the two. Often I seek to impose punishment on myself, or move from an enduring sense of guilt from the past, assuming a particular quality of space, before I have checked the boundaries that have been laid down by the act of judgement in the present and what capacity they give for change. This also extends to my relationship with others in the space and my relationship with the environment. The terms judgement and punishment are intimately linked, but it is good to continually review their relationship.

Law, it seems to me, is not just about an analytical process, but also about understanding our spiritual/moral landscape and feeling our emotional landscape. In writing this chapter, I have felt constrained by a need to keep to the subject matter, to the rules, and have found myself constricted by that idea. I realise now that this is only a regression to the idea of law as being separate from myself. In fact, it is only by releasing myself from that idea of keeping to the rules that I can see how clearly they support me, that it is only my position that restricts and not the web of the law. I should not attempt to see the law as two-dimensional, but rather as living in multiple dimensions, a breathing organism, as *"moving in living measurement"*. I am walking through it as if walking through a garden, which is changing with the seasons.

Perhaps this is also an expression of my essential Englishness. England is a country of constantly changing weather, which to a city liver, like myself, who gave up geography as a subject when I was 13, appears to operate under no rules at all. I love to move in nature and feel its strength and majesty, but am often most at home in an English country garden, such as that at Michaelchurch (a country house itself situated in a border area, between England and Wales). It is there where much of the movement work I have done with Prapto has taken place. The interconnected gardens, a series of walls and hedges in terraced layers, permit varieties of movement and yet give views out into the distance and to the dark wood beyond that comfort and support me. In this environment, I can allow myself to breathe fully, feeling that nature around me is giving me both sufficient space and structure to remain in my body and yet to take it out for a cleaning and feel renewed. A sense of order brings me peace. A sense of communion with natural law rather than obedience to it. At this point service really does feel like perfect freedom.

Some of the ideas expressed here were first mentioned in a short piece for Impressions – *the Sharing Movement magazine edited by Beate Stühm.*

None of the ideas expressed here is intended to represent the opinions or views of Her Majesty's Courts and Tribunals Service or the Ministry of Justice.

~ ~ ~

Simon Slidders finished a law degree at Bristol University in 1977. He qualified as a solicitor in 1981. He then worked in private practice for a few years before taking a two-year break to consider other options. He joined the Government Legal Service in 1990. He has been a Senior Legal Manager at the Administrative Court Office since 2007. He has an MA in Text and Performance Studies completed part time at Royal Academy of Dramatic Arts (RADA) and King's College London in 2004. He also sings.

simonslidders@hotmail.com

26. THE BREATHING EYE

A Journey Towards Visual Art in an Embodied Space

Andrea Morein (Germany)

> *"The Breathing Eye" – A one-day movement workshop with Andrea Morein*
> *Date: 27 Nov. 1999*
> *How is seeing and looking related to our breathing and our movement expression?*
> *In the Hebrew alphabet the vowels are called 'movers' and the consonants 'stoppers'. When is it right to be in movement and when in stopping? When can the two mix, exchange, dialogue, dance with each other and find their own rhythm of seeing from within? These questions will be explored from a somatic, a contemplative as well as a creative point of view and will hopefully inspire the learning through our bodies."*

As I was collecting material for this essay, I came across some old workshop flyers that I had completely forgotten. I chose some sentences from one of them as the initial quote for this chapter and possibly as a motto. It can be seen as an invitation to join a 'guided tour' of how I evolved from being a movement performer and educator to becoming a visual artist through my movement practice. In this chapter, I'll attempt to draw up a map with high peaks and valleys – a somatic landscape of this process.

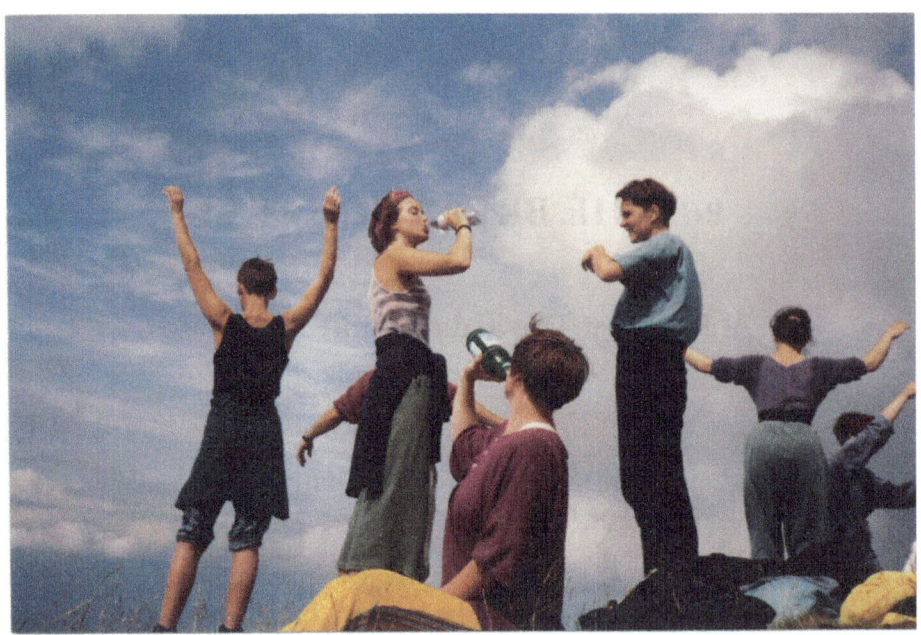

Impression from: *Meditation in Movement – Movement in Meditation*, a workshop I gave in 1991 at the Buddhist Centre Karma Ling, France. I chose this image as an example of a kind of 'incidental' composition. It feels completely natural and wonderfully alive.

Introductory Note

My focus will be on how Prapto's way of working made me look at blockages and 'black holes', eventually allowing my psychophysical and spiritual being to grow and develop, affecting my artwork to this day. The sense of breathing in my body, in my mind, and eventually in my gaze, opened up a new world for me, where movement was no longer a form of performative self-exploitation, but an opening to a more intimate dialogue with myself and my surroundings. Yet, as you can see from the workshop description above, I am equally interested in building a 'grammar' or a language for art-expression – be it in movement or in image-making.

The Space in the Gaze

Parallel to being involved in Prapto's movement practice since 1988, a shift in my nervous system occurred through the practice of Buddhist sitting meditation. During longer sitting retreats I began to relate to spaciousness, experiencing the first glimpses of a non-focused, soft gaze, 'panoramic awareness' as Chögyam Trungpa

Rinpoche called it. I discovered stillness as well as movement from within: no centre point to hold on to. A timid sort of openness was allowing inner and outer spaces to mingle more, allowing for my breathing to be felt as part of moving, seeing and feeling. My visual perception felt so very different when I was not fixating on a centre.

Prapto's way of supporting my learning process was mostly by non-verbal guiding or intuitive verbal hints – a teaching style which later on I was to discover resembles the way teachers in the Vajrayana tradition work with their students. It is called 'transmission' or 'pointing out instruction'. Somehow, Prapto was doing just that as he was guiding my movement. At the time it felt to me like the somatic translation of Vajrayana Buddhist teachings.

I realise that this way of describing Prapto's teaching style may cause misunderstandings and I never spoke with Prapto directly about it, as he was very careful not to be used as a projection for all sorts of idealisations and not to be turned into a 'guru'. But my way of 'reading' or translating his teaching experientially was definitely influenced by my meditation practice.

In 1991, during my stay in Java to study with Prapto, my learning was a sort of non-rational, non-conceptual process which had surprising consequences: one of them being that eventually my field of work shifted completely. I began to 'SEE', as I was learning to feel connected to my breathing. SEEING can be described as direct perception, with no subjective projections narrowing down the contact within and with the surroundings. It feels unhindered and vivid. Participatory.

After 1997, I started making installations, photographic artworks and mainly gestural drawings. My understanding of space as a living organism in which people and objects both co-exist and share the same essential transitoriness was my entry into the world of the visual arts. The shift was gradual and came from allowing image-making through the participatory inclusive presence which developed in the integration stage of what I had learnt with Prapto.

Who is in the Centre – or Centreless Space?

What is this notion of 'no centre' that I referred to earlier? I believe Prapto would call this *lessening the identification.*

In certain stages of meditation practice, the so-called 'watcher' is introduced as a way of focussing on one's thoughts and experience. However, for some practitioners watching their own process can become a misleading form of awareness, separating their whole-body experience from their meditation – acting like a splitting off and thus creating holdings in the mind and in the breathing. Applied in this way, the 'watcher' can cause fragmentation, affecting the breathing and movement patterns as well as the tonus of the eye-muscles.

In study periods with Prapto, I was confronted with these holdings and 'blind spots' for a long time.

Being able to make the distinction between being *in* the living moment as opposed to being *aware of* the living moment became the crux of my slowly growing ability to notice when separating off was in fact a way to maintain the 'watcher'. The new 'non-conceptual' opening arose when Being was just occurring through movement and the surrounding atmosphere. This shift from the conceptual watcher to the innate movement-intelligence is still as acute for me today as it was in 1991.

History of My Gaze

I had been expressing myself through dance and movement since the age of eight, so there was a long history of acquired patterns and psychophysical training that formed my movement expression. Dance had been an emotional release and a vehicle to develop my creative personality and kinaesthetic confidence. On the other hand, it had impaired an intuitive, receptive way of living and being in my body. What I believed had saved me at the outset from a traumatised paralysis due to my background as a second generation Holocaust survivor had later created a seemingly lively rigidity in my muscle patterns and general sense of being.

When I look back at the history/biography of my movement, several issues come to mind:

- A forward thrust in my chest area combined with tense and intense gaze during sequences of movement, to a point of seeing too sharp or blurred or both in a strange paradoxical way. Not unlike the 'dancer's stare' we have all seen on occasion.

- A tendency to express from an emotional motivation (intensification) and feeling empty afterwards. As if I had not been 'received', despite having shown myself.

- A tendency to stop breathing and feeling myself during presentations and performing situations.

- A tendency to feel separated or lost in relating to others in free movement.

As added evidence for my research into eyesight and movement, I became aware of some medical problems confirming that my 'way of seeing' was deficient. I have a 'weak' left eye which has been unable to focus since birth, and my right eye learned to compensate for this at an early age. Later on, due to other diseases, so-called 'floaters' appeared in my left eye, causing more disturbances in my gaze. My visual deficiencies have shaped my way of perceiving the world as a fuzzy or over-focussed place. And later on, I became aware of this 'special' way of seeing as a visual artist, which I shall explain later in more detail.

'Is there a split between me and my expression?'

My somatic learning or un-learning began around 1988. My postural relaxation, visual perception, eye/movement connection and the experience of myself as a moving being – rather than as a person expressing something through movement – started to highlight the blockages and limitations within my being. Where there is light, the shadows are more visible.

I discovered that if my seeing joined my movements, the sense of breathing became more present and set free the body-intelligence, allowing new movement-rhythms and vibratory sensations to emerge. A kind of 'enlivening' was unfolding. And finally, I noticed when I would split off, when I would lose contact with the surroundings, with my flow and with my breathing. In Buddhist studies of consciousness the term 'reification' is used to point to this solidified conceptualisation of an experience.[1]

Ultimately, I discovered that the moment I could sense this splitting off, the realisation would bring me right back into contact again. These realisations were slowly uncovered during the last years

---

1 "**Reification** (German: *Verdinglichung*, literally: 'making into a thing' (cf. Latin *res* meaning 'thing') or *Versachlichung*, literally 'objectification'; regarding something impersonally). Reification in thought occurs when an abstract concept describing a relationship or context is treated as a concrete 'thing', or if something is treated as if it were a separate object when this is inappropriate because it is not an object or because it does not truly exist in separation. Typically it involves separating out something from the original context in which it occurs, and placing it in another context, in which it lacks some or all of its original connections yet seems to have powers or attributes which in truth it does not have. Thus reification involves a distortion of consciousness." Wikipedia

of my movement practice, supported by somatic trauma therapy. The latter enabled me to make images that would keep me connected with myself and with the subject I was depicting. Self-regulation was slowly setting in.

Breathing in the Cross-Section...

During my first stay in Java in 1991, Prapto suggested that I work with the theme of 'Road'. I ended up exploring how to be in moving and resting *on the Road* for three months. Prapto's main instruction – *"Breathe in the cross-section, Andrea!"* – was still a challenging concept at this stage.[2] Now, looking back, I discover that already at that time I had started writing texts as visual images and had been placing banners with poems about my 'Road' exploration in the landscape. Little did I know that my future in the visual arts was actually born then. The large panels of hand-written poems on transparent paper placed in the landscape were a sort of 'marriage' between my learning to be in the present and allowing for the moment to find its own voice. Practising my movement in the landscape that held these poems was a way to be the witness of my own learning and to pinpoint and embody my experiences. My eyes could 'read' my feelings.

Eventually, the practice of 'Road' materialised many years later in creating a home-base in my life, as an answer to the questions which Prapto had often raised: *"Do you know where your place is?" "Are you coming from moving or from staying?"* Only after I had found my own sense of 'staying' could I relax my gaze and let it rest on an object, a feeling or a site, while moving – a sort of wholesomeness (homeyness).

Delight Out of Nowhere

From having found 'home-base' and soft gaze, I began trusting the open situation of a space that can hold emptiness, grace, unknowing, surprise, child's play, strange characters and sounds, forms appearing from seemingly nowhere and dissolving – the delight of sharing movement as part of a group. And all that occurs will eventually dissolve into space – full or empty, no difference, because the one feels contained in the other. This takes deep trust and a sense of

---

2 There is a more detailed description of this stage of my practice-experience in Morein (1994).

staying in the moment, rather than switching into a forward thrust which would narrow down the space, the focus and the breathing into a 'blind' survival mode.

In all areas of my life including my art-making, this has been pivotal – a profound healing, which is still ongoing. The ability to navigate between the process pacing me (which I describe above) and eventually pacing the process to build a creative language for an art-piece has given me a tool and a ground from which I felt embodied.

Knowing from Unknowing – Creating is Recognising the Moment

In the subsequent years of my movement practice, a deeply felt trust in a new way of perceiving developed: being receptive to visual input rather than hunting for it; staying in the flow of movements unfolding rather than freezing breath/posture/tonus to 'create' moments. During my study periods with Prapto, I gradually recognised that the moment need not be 'created'. It is already a creation. Instead, I found that I could merely be a witness and an ally to these moments – breathing with them. Recognising them as artistic potential or 'occurrences' rather than willing them into existence, this was something Prapto helped me to recognise and practice. Through the process I felt enabled to witness something that I was part of, to acknowledge the moment (along with my camera) and to stay in touch with my own sense of being in the space. When my gaze sharpened too much as I focused in on a visual image, forgetting my sense of being part of the whole, his warning was always: *"not for catching"*.

As recently as 2010, while participating in a group-meeting, 'Mandala for Digesting', with Prapto in France, I was moving with my camera, exploring the sense of perceiving nature directly while moving and alternating this with looking at nature through the camera while moving. The German language term I gave this exploration is: BILD UND ABBILD (image AND its representation, first-hand experience versus 'framing', elementary connection to the moment, the air, the light, the textures, the situation and the image of this experience in terms of an art-language).

The question of how an image can contain the vividness of the moment in which it is born and transmit this in art had become the key to my art-practice – and still is. Click: a warm smile of Prapto is looking at my lens!

Images from a Somatic View

Here are some examples of works of mine that exemplify this view:

- *Oneness* is one of a series of drawings made on paper or on steel plates. They are mostly 60cm x 80cm in size. The title of the work is identical with the word it depicts. The word/title also refers to a major work by Barnett Newman which he called *Onement*. Newman's writings on art and the philosophy of art have had a profound influence on my path as an artist.[3]

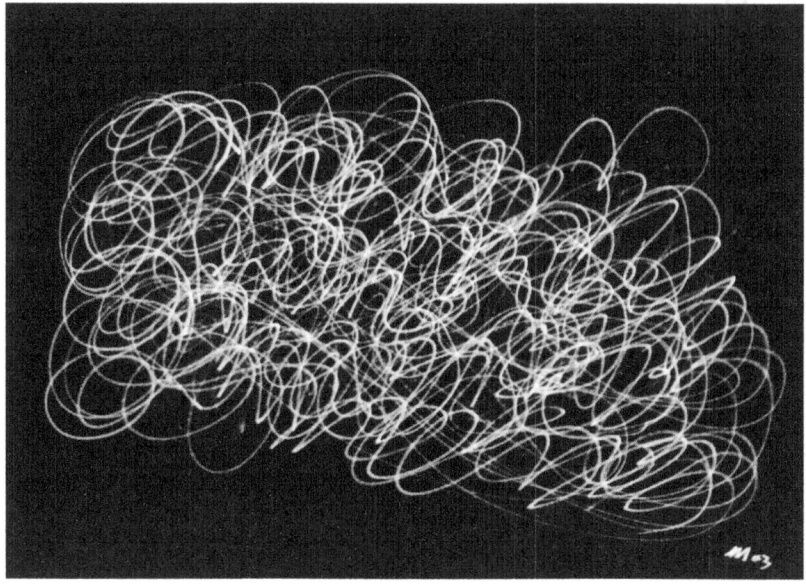

Oneness, drawing with white markers on a steel plate, 2003

Oneness was made by rhythmically re-rewriting the word over and over again on the same surface until the energy of the word became felt (and visible). The energetic quality of drawing in this way resembles moving or in moments even dancing. The interesting shift here is that I am looking at what I am doing as I am doing it. My looking and doing need to be completely joined. Again, if I separate my awareness from the flow of my hand, my line will show this. And writing the same word over and over again, as if in an incantation or recitation, I develop a kind of rhythmic trance-like 'hand-dance' which needs total concentration

---

3 Newman (1992)

and total relaxation at the same time. I oscillate between focus and spaciousness, between the process pacing me and me pacing the process.

- *Random Flow*, the second example of my gestural drawings, is a large panel made of nine separate frames making up a large scale rhythmic wave-movement. Initially, each of the nine drawings were separate complete pieces. I later joined them. Each line drawing (or movement on paper) was made with a sense of every line beginning in space, beyond the limitation of the paper, crossing the paper and allowing it to exit with the view that the line continues into infinity (invisibly). This intention of drawing was definitely affecting my breathing and hand-movement.[4]

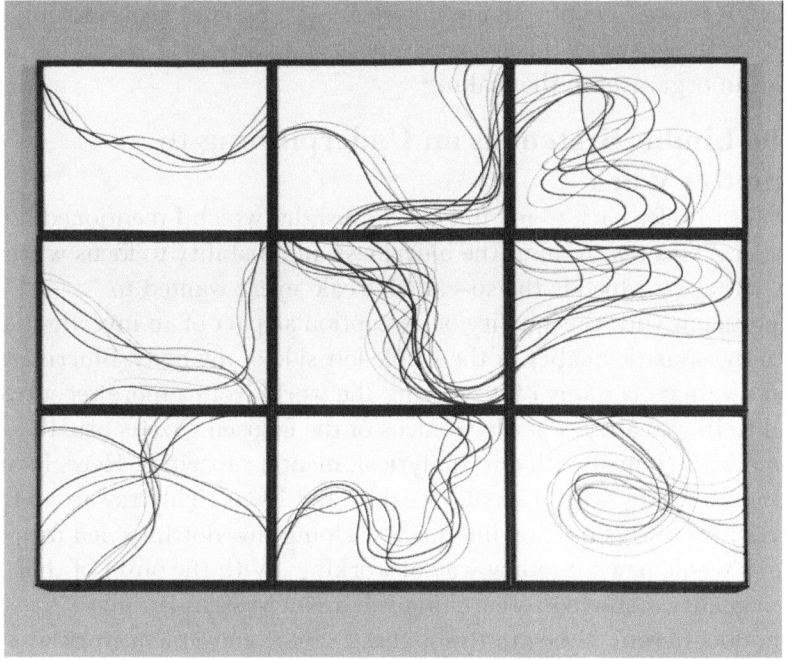

Random Flow, 2005

Eventually, I discovered that when I combined the drawings, looking to find correspondences between them, they began to interact visually and energetically, even though their lines did not always carry over from one 'frame' to the next. I could always tell whether a combination was working, because my gaze and my breath would feel congruent.

---

[4] See more of these images at http://bit.ly/ELtp20 and http://bit.ly/ELtp21

Surprisingly, we humans tend to make connections in our 'mind's eye' enabling us to see and feel 'in flow'. Our deeply rooted need to bring disparate things together as in *Random Flow* made me think of moments in movement practice when a whole group moves or stills as if they were one organism – a major characteristic of the openness of Amerta Movement, in my understanding.

In more recent drawings a shift occurred towards using tiny dots which would create fuzzy, organic kinds of shapes made of various densities and layers. This dotting activity was another form of 'hand-dance' which started totally intuitively and had some kind of obsessive quality to it. At first, I did not 'understand' at all what I was doing and what these drawings 'meant'. I just felt compelled to continue to search out the quality of this doing and let it develop by itself. It was a kind of acupuncture feeling... my hand kept wanting to pierce the paper and inject spaciousness and vibratory energy into it. Like an organism in the making.

The Limbic System as an Underpinning to Prapto's Work

I want to refer back to my impaired eyesight, which I mentioned earlier. I was researching the blurriness and inability to focus with my left eye – which is the so-called 'weak' eye. I wanted to experiment with this quality of perception as part of an investigation into the somatic quality of the whole left side of my body. Blurriness and fuzziness is a way of perceiving the world from a more receptive and feeling quality. The sharp focus of the focused gaze is usually somatically joined with our analytical, mental capacities. Here, I was delving into my way of seeing 'weakly' and I was richly rewarded in persisting in this unknowing quality. Doing my 'dottings' led me into a whole new vibratory way of working. With the onset of this new quality, I started researching the limbic system, or our 'emotional brain'[5]. I began to see that Prapto's movement work was doing nothing less than teaching us to reconnect with our limbic capacities. It would however take a whole new essay to write more about the convergence of the two, although it is most relevant for somatic studies. Shown below are some works related to my 'Weak Eye' – research and a limbic form of seeing. They are marker drawings on transparent paper-layers[6].

---

5 On the limbic system, see Lewis et al.(2000)

6 See more of these images at http://bit.ly/ELtp22

26. THE BREATHING EYE

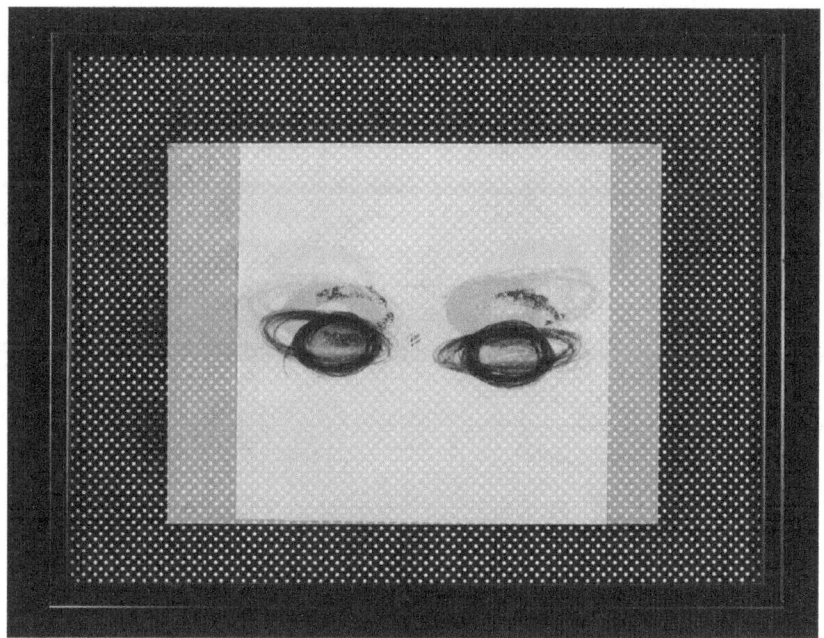

Eye (I), 2011

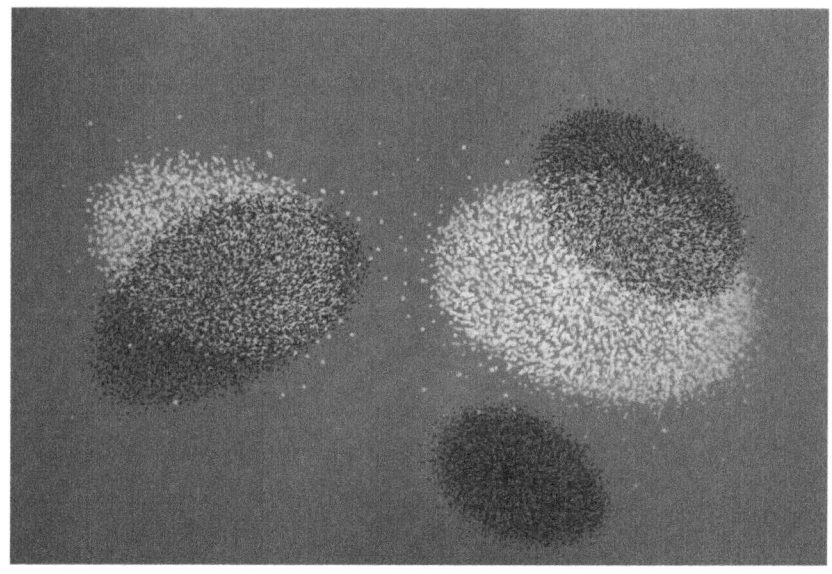

Limbic Landscape, 2010

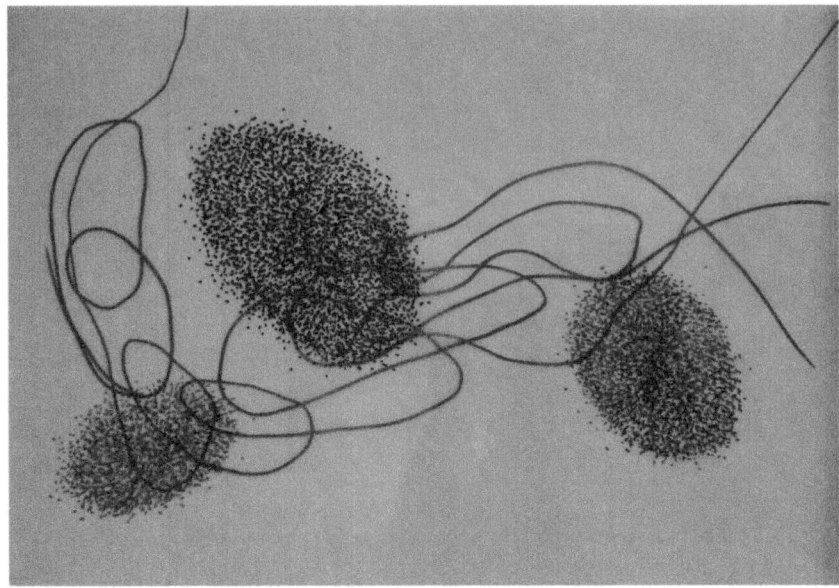

Limbo Three, drawing on transparent papers, 2011

Photographing Movement – Vividness and Resonance with the Space

As a conclusion, I want to say a few words about my current research and process. The first image at the beginning of this essay was a photo of a group of movers randomly standing on a hillside which I included for its vividness and uncontrived quality. My last two images are recent photographs. They are part of an ongoing project about joining photography of movement/spaces and writing as drawing... Maybe I've come full circle?

- *Work-Dance(r)* – has been collaged from more than 20 images. The man's movements as he painted the gallery walls were so dynamic and swift that I felt an electric spark in the space and joined in with my camera. I simply wanted to follow his 'work-dance' with the camera as if we were dancing a duet in space. Collaging three of these moments as I did, I feel that the space dances with him.

26. THE BREATHING EYE

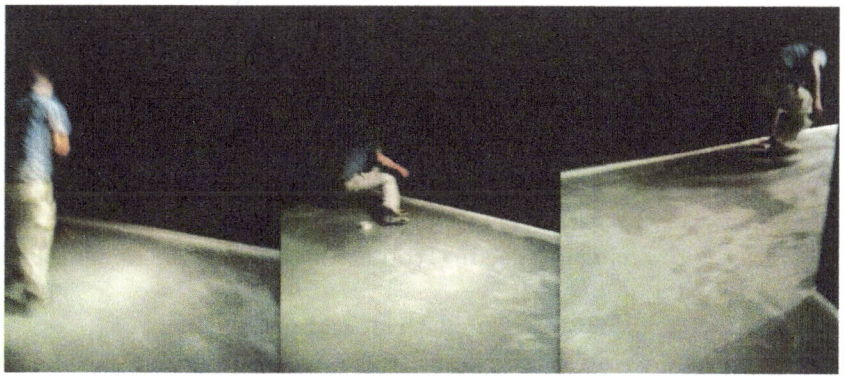

Work Dance(r) Triptych, 2012

- *Dancing On Space* was shot during a performance at the opening of a Group Show called *On Space*. Here, the dancers' movements and the architectural references of a video-work behind them creates a synchronicity and aliveness of the exhibited works in the space through the dancers' positions linking them. My breath is held for a split second while making contact with the dancers through the camera. This quality I found later was present in the photo.

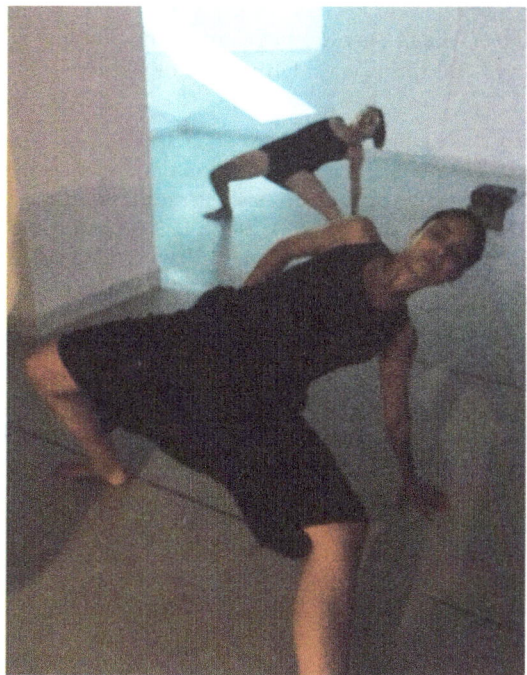

Dancing on Space, 2010

Both works were shot in the same location – a gallery in Tel Aviv, which in the last couple of years showed my work. *Work-dance(r)* was in preparation for my Solo Show *Night My Light* in which I created a darkened space with a combination of the 'dotted' works and photographs in a spatial setting transforming the gallery-space into a 'limbic environment', affecting the audience not only visually, but holistically. I wanted visitors to relate from their limbic brain, engaging with seeing and feeling, contacting a spaciousness within as well as without.

I want to conclude this essay with an acknowledgement of gratitude and love for Prapto without whom this journey would not have happened.

~ ~ ~

References

Lewis, T., Amini, F. and Lannon, R. (2000) *A General Theory of Love*, Random Books

Morein, A. (1994) "A Practice called 'Road' – Studying 'movement in meditation' with Suprapto Suryodarmo in Central Java, Indonesia", *Contact Quarterly* Winter/Spring 1994. Vol.19 #1

Newman, B. (1992), 'The Plasmic Image' and 'The Sublime is Now', Selected Writings and Interviews, University of California Press

Andrea Morein was born in Vienna, Austria and lives in Cologne, Germany. Her early studies included German dance, movement and theatre studies in Germany and Israel. In 1973 she graduated from the Director's Course at the Drama Centre, London. Since 1985 she has undertaken numerous Performance Art and Movement Projects. Between 1989 and 2000 she studied with Prapto in Indonesia and Europe. Since 1988 she has given Somatic and Creative Movement Trainings in institutions, universities and her own 'Re-source Institute'. From 1998, her work shifted to the visual arts – mainly dealing with perception, spatial relations, architecture and poetics. Andrea's performances, media works, drawings and photographs have been widely shown in museums and galleries in Germany, Italy, France, Netherlands, Portugal, Israel and Indonesia.

www.andreamorein.com

27. JOY

The Stony Way

Anita Lüdke (Germany/Bolivia)

A deep love and passion for space inspired me to study architecture. Years later I discovered within movement the same laws of creativity and inspiration that I knew from my process of creating a design for space. In this relived discovery I could reflect on these laws with renewed attention and could widen the area of their validity for my growth as a human being.

From then on, a general exploration and understanding about the growth of human beings began to develop.

I started learning from Prapto 27 years ago, because of my contemplations about how to teach architecture students. Working as a university tutor, I experienced from the very beginning that most of the students were drawing decorative patterns out of lines without apparently feeling the line as a wall or feeling that a meeting of lines makes a corner, or how light enters and affects the atmosphere of the space created between the lines. I knew that they needed to experience existing architectural spaces by moving through them with their senses open and then to reflect on their experience. So I improvised learning situations for them but I always felt that I was missing something. Amerta Movement work, as I got to know it from Prapto, inspired me to integrate this way of practice into my teaching. It helped to open up consciousness and the recognition of the density of space and of the play of light. Besides this, the movement work gave students the experience of how it feels when their creative source is flowing.

Right now I am about to finish a book with the cover title *Seemingly Nothing Special* and the inside subtitle *and yet it has changed my life....* It contains a retrospective account of how all this process came about. Parts I and II below are excerpts from this text. The poetic word-installations in Part I stand alone, independent from their original context, which includes accompanying paintings.[1]

This transcript is also an homage to Prapto the teacher as thanks for his in-devotion-offered, wonderful gift to the world in the form of Amerta Movement.

Part I: The Fulfilment

Here I express, what this kind of movement without a given form means to me, which to me is the essence. The words were allowed to move all over the sheet and in different ways they found their distance and location or their connection.

'Space of Being' (used below) is translated from the German '*Raum des Seins*'. The German language allows a more complete expression. In '*Ra aum des Seins*', Ra is the goddess of the sun and aum understood as the basic sound of infinity and unity leading into stillness.

---

[1] See: http://bit.ly/ELtp24

27. JOY

In the essence
reduced to one sentence
this kind of movement practice means to me
to experience myself in being
                            in the **Space of Being**

                                          which exists independent of time
                                                    and independent
                               of functionally and emotionally oriented thinking

on the following pages I tell about the most fundamental
discoveries, experiences and recognitions

in this **Space of Being**

                                                on the way to this **Space of Being**

                          . . .

Embodied Lives

                      this discovery

which

       when I was first allowed to feel it
                 exploded chains
   triggered astonishment and euphoria in me
         I felt light as a butterfly and
             free like a bird

that through me

                                              can happen

what is appropriate
        for this moment

     in this context

                                             for me
                       for the whole and
         for any element of being within it

                   . . .

27. JOY

recognition

that

this adventure

is even richer

the less I intervene

the less inhibited I allow
my thinking as well as my bodily and psychical capability
always with a fuller consciousness

to be

as living tool
of something much superior

. . .

....
....

. . .

Embodied Lives

this **Space of Being**

                                          is the place

                                                                where

                                      life feeds from the source

where
   creativity arises

                 as its purest and most original impulse

                        to find

through us   *its expression*

be it in word, in matter, in dance, in gesture, in songs, in music, in healing .....

or

      in everyday life

                    . . .

....

....

                  . . .

27. JOY

and

        once I am opened
        to be guided through life
        then

             I feel my being
as

    rhythmically flowing
            rhythmically dancing
with always new surprises
             as adventure
        as joy
    as deep touch
as gratitude
    as melting towards
  the enchantment

          life
          . . .

this freedom for risk

                        being shared with others

                                              fulfils a dream

                  which started
when I many years ago – suddenly –
the first time being in movement
was allowed to enter

    this **Space of Being**

                        beyond my thinking
              and beyond my emotional 'I'

to experience

            the guidance of

                                    something superior

        which since then
I call the jazz of movement

                                        and to this
                            belongs a wide swinging

                red dress

                   . . .

Part II: Fruit Along the Way

In this section I give an overview of the structure of my own teaching in this practice, as I offered it to students of architecture and of graphic and product design.

Everybody has seen dance or martial arts. Recalling those skills immediately shapes and develops our internal criteria of how movement should be and what it should look like. These ideas may initially prevent us from getting involved with our own impulse towards movement and with following that as it really is. But that very impulse, when it is realized with honesty and with an acceptance of the limits of its own potential, creates beauty, which deeply touches the heart of whoever is there. This is a beauty beyond form, which nevertheless needs embodied expression to manifest itself. If someone in their movement sequence reaches this quality of being for just one moment, the entire room is changed. It is like a miracle, like something magical; all those present are suddenly very awake, alert and involved.

This law of the effect of truth and presence applies not only in the context of movement practice; it is visible in every form of human expression: architecture, graphic and product design and, of course, in daily life.

Suggestions and commands in movement practice will help us to experience what prevents us from being in this state of simplicity, as well as to explore the creative aspect of this state. Over time and by practicing movement in a variety of situations, so that we can experience this state again and again, our being learns to find the way by itself towards this quality of being. And through teaching others I myself have learnt more about the practice of movement.

For example, given the enormous power that lies within intention, I start every course and every day with the intention that whatever I put into the room should be good and should encourage the personal growth of participants. Without much thought, that intention has always helped me swiftly to find myself in the 'Space of Being' (described above) from where I could follow my impulses in guiding others. I speak of 'guiding' because of perceiving within myself an absence of thinking (although I am also not necessarily in a condition of intuition or inspiration). Thinking becomes important in retrospect, in the reflection and classification.

I can call this condition 'the condition of the open heart and dedication,' the condition of love for all lives, love beyond all need, love for the being in my body, for the being in the body of others, for the being in the plants, animals, mountains, wind, water, fire, earth, clouds, rain, sun, the air, the being that permeates everything and unifies us with everything.

Those words can easily be understood as being romantic and kitsch. To avoid this I shall describe the above-mentioned condition once more but now from a different point of view. I can also call it the inner place of neutrality, in which there is no emotion at all, just receiving and acting; in which there is a bright light (immaterial white with a bit of coloured grey in it) floating through the whole of my body and what's more flowing through all forms and beings in my surroundings. It is not at all comparable with any artificial light and is not even like the light of the sun or the moon, it is something peculiar to itself with its own characteristics.

The sensation of depth, purity, truth and clarity in this quality of being has given me the confidence to express it or to act, simply to do what in my spontaneous perception needed to be done, without doubting, without questioning. It has not always been enjoyable, and even to me not always immediately understandable or comprehensible. But I learned to stay in that condition, even if it was clear to me that it would probably cause an unpleasant reaction, I learned to accept, to respect and to do it anyway without falling into an emotional pattern of self-protection or self-assertion. I started to recognize and distinguish whether my impulse came from this 'Space of Being' or came from an emotional condition – at least for the space-time of a workshop in this practice. The latter is very important! It makes a big difference whether I am with a wholesome intention in a guiding role in the space-time practice, or if I am in the challenge of daily life. This experience and recognition I have felt to be essential and valuable as at least during the time of my courses I was spared the condition of persistent arrogance.

While being in the 'Space of Being', and accompanying others I was also aware that all the beneficial things that happened – and which participants expressed gratitude for – were due to the guidance that we were given together, and not to my personal skills and knowledge.

This recognition has changed my attitude again and again into one of necessary humility and tolerance. The guidance does work through my personal skills and knowledge and by this becomes visible and gets body, but its basic existence is not attributable to me – nevertheless I accept the responsibility that is attached to the role of teacher.

Through and especially in the movement practice, I find my way into the freedom of being able to look with wonder and compassionate respect at another human being in their own way of living. Daily life with myself and others does, however, as already mentioned, still have abundant emotional difficulties and re-entering the 'Space of Being' in daily life is a permanent practice.

Part III: The Art of Daily Life

In 2007 my life changed as the result of an illness. Since then and because of this I got the chance to concentrate on my daily-life practice while living mainly in Bolivia.

In my movement practice as I had got to know it, my inner awareness was trained to be very detailed and accurate, which fitted well with my own mentality. This was a big help in 'guiding' the students who were discovering the unique creativity present in each one of them.

And now this quality is supporting my intention to be fulfilled by finding my way into the 'Space of Being' in daily life. Whatever action gives me the impulse to move, with the luck of grace more or less immediately after having started it I find myself sensitive to not just the function of the action itself, but to being in the objects, the forms, the colours, and the textures.

So, for example, I feel my hand going deep down into the dry white rice, the little long grains, one beside the other slipping through my hands, as if they were made of silk, sinking into a measuring cup; from there like raindrops falling into the pot and then changing their whole consistency just by me adding some water. All at once they are heavily stacked one on top of the other...

Thus I find a little pleasure here, another little pleasure there; my inner chemise is changing and in this my 'looking at' is changing into seeing, my hearing is changing into listening and my touching is changing into feeling.

Granted the gift of awareness my daily walking along the snail footpath (which leads through trees and flora and connects our different rooms) results in an experience of rhythm itself, giving me a massage through my body from toe to top.[2] My hands pulling up weeds destroy those so-called bad plants but in this same act I also feel the joy of the surviving plants and the suffering of other plants that are unhealthy. Slowly, slowly, through all this, something very fundamental is changing in me; a shift which is supported by hearing, morning and evening, the symphonies of birds, insects, crickets, frogs and wind, which at this moment in my life can't be topped by any symphony in a concert hall.

Equally I can experience that same path through the same nature-temple with the same light falling through the leaves as dry and grey only because of my heart not being open and, as a consequence, my eyes and ears which are physically open, being closed. It is the touch of my own (personal) sense of beauty that lets me jump into the 'Space of Being.' It is not even jumping – it is an instant change of all that I am.

I used to be utterly convinced in my mind and in my feeling that living in town was the very best thing for me – the bigger the urban jungle and chaos the better. Nothing else was worthwhile. That was my home, the place I identified with. Now I live in the jungle of nature. It is not that I jumped from there to here in one step. There was quite a long path in between, where I had not really let go of the one and had not really landed in the other. But now after just a few years, especially during the jungle concerts mentioned above, I can feel nature entering my cells and my cells changing into tentacles that are moving deep into the green surroundings and my body dissolving and widening into the infinite space. This is like my most precious jewel. If ever I felt something holy from the deepest part of my heart then it is this feeling of unity. I also could say my whole situation at the moment, this opportunity of being in every sense free for this extraordinary experience, is holy. And of course there are a lot of obstacles, both internal and external, that can easily throw me out of this smooth condition, so this is how I am in my day-to-day movement practice.

These obstacles are the stones, which are mentioned above in my subtitle. In my writing here I describe just the joy. The joy, even in its details, appears to be more of a shared, similar experience for one person or for the other. The stones are much more individual; they are the result of the bunch of gifts we bring with us from wherever in being born and, as we all know, we complete this bunch mainly

---

2 See: http://bit.ly/ELtp24

with the experiences we have during our first years in this world. I like the word Gift because it has in my German-English a double meaning, which fits well in this context: in German the word *Gift* means poison. What happens in life is that one or another of the Gifts, in the English meaning, turns out to be a Gift in the German meaning. It is these stones that provoke unpleasant and emotionally complicated situations within ourselves and in our contact with others, which have to be revealed for what they are, respected and accepted and, in this way, hopefully transformed.

Often at the beginning of a practice session there is a lot of movement because of all the impressions and emotions that have been gathered during the day and need attention. Then suddenly every impulse in the body stops and there is only going down to the earth and staying there in silence. For me, this is always an astonishing moment. I don't know how long it will last but it is the point zero from where at its exact time a new movement will arise like the famous phoenix out of the ashes. Sometimes it takes quite a long time. To end it by choice is hard, nearly impossible if you are no longer a beginner in movement work, because that would mean cutting or breaking and then whatever comes next will be, for sure, a frustration. So one has to wait for the right moment. It is also always astonishing to me that sometimes I even fall into something like sleep, but in a second I am again totally awake in a new movement with a much deeper quality and sometimes entering directly in the so-called 'Space of Being'. This moment in my life I am living just now here on our land in Bolivia feels a bit like this point zero.

There are some periods of great activity with a lot of movement beside the daily necessities, but most of this is happening in my inner world. Meanwhile the outside world is shrinking more and more and my inner space is expanding enormously; I need all my strength, all my force and all my creativity for this internal journey.

None of the professional activities I undertook in my former life continue, except for my love and creative fire for architectural space. Until now this creative fire has remained without manifestation in the outer world: but I can smell the possibility. I do not know how long the outer stillness of my moment will stay and toward what it will, if ever, lead me. This is the dance of adventure one can experience in movement practice surrendering to the inner guidance by listening and seeing, by just being, and now it is my life.

~ ~ ~

Anita Lüdke is an architect and freelance artist. She has 20 years experience of teaching in the field of space and form (Raum and Gestalt), including 12 years as a professor at the University of Düsseldorf in Applied Sciences. In 1985 she began the practice of Amerta Movement; in 1995 Prapto invited her to be on his list of teachers; currently she lives in Germany and Bolivia.

anita_luedke@gmx.de

28. "RE-MEMBERING" BUTTERFLY BEACH

Melinda Buckwalter (USA)

Memory

Butterfly Beach – I happened on it while riding my bicycle around Santa Barbara, California, during a vacation. I was visiting my best friend who had just moved there; this was back in the 1980s. I remembered it for years as the perfect beach. I had come upon it at the end of my stay so I didn't have time to go back, but I marked it in my memory. Shady, there was a wall, a descent, not much beach. Was it high tide? Heavenly swim. That sip had potency. Meanwhile, my friend moved to the mountains, and Butterfly Beach entered my dreamscape, enhancing its status. Then began the long slide, from consciousness to sunken treasure. And there it lay.

Words

I am a dance writer with a curiosity for making dances out of improvised movement, a practice sometimes referred to in the US as compositional improvisation. I noticed that several artists had developed unique ways of going about it. I decided to study with them; maybe I would learn something about making my own dances! In this process, it seemed natural to keep a journal. Then, a friend asked me if I would write a book on the topic. I was fascinated by what I had read about Indonesian dance maker Prapto and his Amerta Movement, and I wanted to include his work in my book. So, in 2005, I sent a passage of my dance writing, a chapter on Amerta Movement, to him for review. I had some trepidation about what he might think of it, since I hadn't actually experienced his work. Were my hunches on target? Prapto and Diane Butler, a dance scholar and native English speaker, looked at my writing. They sent brochures, context pieces, and explanatory emails.

In our editorial process, there were issues regarding tenses. Prapto preferred possibility and ongoing present – "*if feeling flying, be embodied;*" I translated into time-based, dependent clauses – "while having the feeling of flying, remain embodied." I would try to make some sense of their wording and then I would send back a reworked section. Sometimes my suggestions were accepted, but in a few persistent places Prapto and Diane would not shift. I was afraid the writing wouldn't make it by my editor. What to do? I decided to quote Prapto's material as is. The quotes had enough context to give a gist of what was meant to an English speaker, and more importantly, to give the particular flavor of the way Prapto uses language. Our exchanges intrigued me and piqued my curiosity for study in person with Prapto.

Practice

My first opportunity to study with Prapto was at *The Prayer of the Butterfly*, a workshop in the woods of Western Massachusetts. From my notes on the workshop:

> Adapt to language of wind, finding place where wind doesn't blow you, like butterfly, how may find the land of wind?

I remember Prapto pointing to two butterflies in the orchard – playing, dancing with one another, sparring as they do mid-flight, flickering like shadows and light make dapples under a tree when the wind blows. *"Like that – find the land of the wind."*

In the workshop there was a lot of angst among the ten or so of us from around the globe about finding our right place in the world, our home, where to live, how to live. We were all vagabond dancers, either mid-vagabond, wondering 'what next?' or post-vagabond, wondering how to deal with the stationary world in which we found ourselves. Kerplunk. With Prapto dancing, singing, or drumming along with us, we practiced anchoring, coming and going, and staying in relationship. He adapted his work to our situation and context. It made perfect sense.

Toward the end of this workshop, Prapto told us about a nun he had encountered while teaching and how, in her spiritual practice, she was very seriously striving for connection with God. From Prapto's perspective, her striving for was an obstacle and kept her from *being with*. An attitude of striving positioned one's God out of reach. This need for a switch of perspective, of tense if you will, in order to be with made sense to me. It was along the same lines of perspective-switching that we practiced in our dancing. For example, in one exercise we used our arms and legs as frames to look through, as if looking through various windows of a house. Prapto explained that in doing so we cleaned the windows of our perception; we became more fluid in shifting between sensory modes and from internal to external impulses. In the case of the nun, Prapto spoke of a shift from vertical – living in a time-sequenced progression, to horizontal – an expansive, continuous present kind of place. Sometimes I felt this place when we danced under Prapto's direction. How to find it on my own?

I asked Prapto how we might continue to practice once the workshop was over. He gave me two suggestions. One was to *re-member* how we worked. I understood this to mean that I should not copy exercises by rote or recreate the experience of them as they had happened, but rather that I should reconstruct them from my present circumstance. The second was a pointing exercise. He asked me to *"Please try."* When Prapto asked for a physical reply in response to a question, I found it unusually difficult to focus. However, I did my best. In this case, I was to point with my finger and name what I pointed to – simple enough. I squirmed a bit under the microscope, but demonstrated to Prapto's satisfaction. I was happy to have something to work on.

Semaphore

In Steve Paxton's workshop, *Material for the Spine*, we learned to point with other parts of our body – our sitz bone could point to our heel. Internal pointing led to external shaping of the body and this work gave volume to my pointing practice. Steve had recently read that pointing had been identified as an evolutionary step toward language. Evidently, being able to point at snakes, to warn and be warned not to step on them, was a survival tactic that led to more advanced modes of communication. If dance is a universal language, then pointing is its Morse code.

In Daniel Lepkoff's workshop, *Making and Seeing Dance*, we worked with bamboo poles. The long sticks served as extended pointers. Their heft helped inform me about the physical and multisensory effort involved in pointing. While the forces at play in wielding a fingertip are minimal and so familiar as to go unnoticed, the unwieldy poles magnified the act of pointing – the time, energy, and muscularity of it – and brought it into conscious awareness. Daniel asked us to notice the objects of our environment. As we pointed and measured with our poles, we inserted ourselves through movement into the composition of the room. Our poles, pointing from one object to another, became magicians' wands with which we conjured space and time into being. Through this expanded pointing, I experienced how my body actively interprets my surrounding environment and brings life to it by adding dimension.

I made an outdoor performance called *West Halifax Study No. 5* to work on my pointing practice. I enjoyed pointing to obvious things in the immediate vicinity and naming them, then I mixed them with things that were minute like ants, or inside me like my liver, or very far away, whose locations I had to guess at. I enjoyed how it played with the imagination of the audience, sending them on an instantaneous field trip of macrocosmic or microcosmic proportion. I finally had an 'ah ha' moment – I realized that in pointing I was actually locating myself. I used not only vision but also proprioceptive senses to point; there was a felt component in the act. I was locating, remembering myself in space through the external. How else to know where I am?

Blossoming

In October 2011, I flew once again to Santa Barbara after twenty-odd years, this time to study with Prapto. We met daily in a Unitarian Church and a public park across the street. We practiced *stopping in not moving, stopping in no moving*, and *stopping in moving*. Ducks were our mentors. We practiced with them on a little island in their pond at the park. Stopping in not moving was when they slept, beak tucked under wing, oblivious. Stopping in no moving was their habitual paddle – lazing about, nibbling at the water, and throwing in a preen. Stopping in moving was when they took off after something, a rival duck or proffered breadcrumbs, darting with single-mindedness. This one-pointed focus during the duck's dart created the stopping effect. Even though they were moving at top speed, they kept an unwavering attention on the object of their dart that translated into a kind of stillness. We observed, then practiced. I often got it backwards. Nevertheless, I practiced something, blindly, somehow finding my faith in the process.

Later, we moved on to *not leaving*. In not leaving, we worked indoors with chairs. We sat in and moved in and around our chairs, but never left them. Even if we stood up to shift position, our attention was to stay focused on the chair. The chair was our anchor. This is a difficult practice for busy Americans, always on the run. Prapto mimicked, to hilarious effect, how we move from one thing to another with our minds already on the next spot – where we are going to be rather than in the transit.

In a development of the exercise, one person sat in the chair, not leaving, and another person moved around them, not leaving. Prapto explained that the person in the chair was more of the flora variety and the person moving was more of the fauna variety. This exercise makes excellent couples therapy! Prapto and Diane did a fabulous duet-lecture-demonstration, including dialogue from their personal relationship. Prapto tiptoeing, strayed a bit far from the chair and Diane, perfectly timed, harrumphed that she would rather stay home and take care of herself, thank you very much. We explored our own comfort zones, just how far could we push the envelope before it felt like we had left our companion-in-chair? Were we more flora, a rooted homebody? Or more fauna, enjoying a bit of independence now and then?

Before we knew it, we were *Being Blossoming*, the name of the workshop and pun on the name of the organizer, Katya Bloom. Prapto brought us into the courtyard and explained the lotus sutra (a lesson on immortality which many consider to be the Buddha's final teaching) to us as we gathered around the orange daylilies in various stages of bloom. In order to be blossoming, we used the practice of not leaving in order to stay inside the lily bud where we would *show our face*, rather than buzz around outside the flower – bizzy, busy, buzzy, buggy mind. In *The Prayer of the Butterfly* workshop, there had been many sitting sessions. In this workshop there was just this one, adapted from the lotus sutra for present-day Santa Barbara Unitarian Church purposes. Simple ingredients: we re-membered and relocated the sutra from our multi-voiced perspectives, a gathering of ducks. The result: we did blossom!

Our blooming was somehow accomplished through all of our moving practices – our moving had secretly been informing us. When it came time to sit, we just knew what to do. We were outwardly sitting, but inwardly (is it really inward?) we were showing our face, basking in our blossoming, finding our stopping.

I wish I could explain the movement that we do so that it could be pictured. That is how I have been taught to write about dance, 'Please paint me a picture.' All I can remember is that when Prapto asked, *"Please come,"* I just moved, and if I didn't start just moving, I wouldn't be able to find it. It is the exact opposite of many improvisation classes I have taken. In these I am told, "Don't noodle around! Make a phrase! Learn to be still! Learn when to exit!"

Come to think of it now, in Prapto's work we do have our stoppings, so it's not like we are noodling. Our stoppings help us. Prapto says composing while dancing is recognizing ourselves in the dancing. *"Find your stoppings,"* he reminds us, *"then you can recognize your composition."*

At first, it is hard for me to trust the moving that Prapto asks of us. *"Please come,"* he says, which means come here and start moving. I don't mean that it's hard to begin just moving around. It's not! It's just that I've been trained to want something more, to look for something. Prapto asks me to stop looking for something else, to stop leaving the dance. As I drift from words to workshops – alighting, flitting, and re-membering – I am slowly learning to trust those invisible currents that the butterfly calls home, the land of the wind.

I could say something about the way the movement feels. On watching it, it feels silvery, like a thread, like the weaving of a web, a quicksilver web. In dancing, it feels like entering a slipstream of movement that is always almost right here, being woven just beyond normal, if I could only catch it. Then I do. I find myself moving and I forget that I ever needed something more.

Seraphim

My last day of *Being Blossoming* was beach day. Prapto often works on the beach at his home in Java and in Bali. How lucky to have the opportunity to do that work with him here in the US! We carpooled and arrived at the beach in the afternoon, squeezed into the last few parking spots we could find, and clambered down the stairs onto the beach. It's Butterfly Beach! My memory returns – the perfect beach, and here with Prapto to do his amazing yet ordinary work.

We immediately ran to the water's edge, dipping our toes, making overtures to the waves to let us in, like little kids on holiday. Prapto admonished us not to lose ourselves. He then showed us how to find the horizon and to find ourselves *in relation*. Our dances that day were a way to find our *human measurement* amid this infinite backdrop. We danced in duos and trios, in and out of the water, on and in the sand. *"Please come,"* Prapto said, over and over. I struggled and flagged in the hot sun, grit, and beach gnats. What was I doing? I would find some strand of a dance to hang onto, only to have it drift away. The tide shifted around us. I felt a familiar sense of being lost, at sea in my improvisations.

Finally, as the sun set, I made my goodbyes to the group; I was too tired to register sadness at my departure. The next morning, as I sat in a brief predawn meditation before a full day of flying, I felt, quite unexpectedly, the ocean moving. It was a physical echo, like a sailor experiencing land sickness. Slurping, slapping, rocking, laughing, washing. I was feeling myself in relation to the ocean, and for a moment, in my stopping, it made perfect sense: the endless movement, the ducks and butterflies, the coming and going, the not leaving. In measuring myself against the ocean, in pointing to that vastness, I had been reflected back. In that moment, I recognized my self – ever changing yet always right here. And then, an ocean of activity swallowed me as it does every day. But for that moment of stopping, I could feel its gentle caress: I am here, I am here, I am still here. What a treasure!

~ ~ ~

Melinda Buckwalter is a writer and researcher, the author of *Composing While Dancing: An Improviser's Companion* and has been co-editor of *Contact Quarterly*, the dance and improvisation journal, since 2005.

She studied dance at Bennington College where she received her MFA and teaches anatomy and kinesiology at Wesleyan University. Currently she works for the Five College Center for East Asian Studies at Smith College in Northampton, MA, and continues to develop a constellation of interests in Asia, including practice in Qigong, Jin Shin Jyutsu, and yoga.

melindabuckwalter.com

29. I WILL TRACE THE CONSTELLATION OF MY STARS WITH MY FINGERS

Ellin Krinsly (USA/Australia/Mexico/Ethiopia)

Preface

My metaphor is not complete
My constellation is on the path of becoming

If you gaze up at the turquoise blue ceiling of Grand Central Station in the heart of New York City, stars glisten and the constellations are connected into their images by golden threads: Pegasus the winged horse, Pisces the fish, Leo the lion. The ceiling is a memory from my earliest years, powerful and exalting. It is a grand urban and architectural wonder, revealing both day and night, an honoring of nature.

The metaphor for my life's journey is stars in the sky. Someday my stars will become a constellation, a revealed pattern, but for now the stars are within the ever-present flux of life: new ones are added, some flash brighter, some move farther away.

The stars of my metaphor are both symbols of the places I live with my partner Arie van Duijn, the collaborative intercultural performances we have performed around the world and the performance rituals I have done to mark the anniversary of my father's and mother's deaths.

Golden threads connect the stars in my metaphor. The golden threads are my training and apprenticeship with Prapto in Amerta Movement.

Introduction

I was born in New York and have lived half my life in Sydney, Australia. We rent a small casita in a mountain village in Mexico and we volunteer each year at a community in Ethiopia. Each of these places is home when we are there. In each country, a different aspect of my creativity is evoked.

In New York the urban intensity brings energy and a connection to my heritage. When we live in Sydney, the walks in the sand and swims in the ocean bring a transformative calm. Mexico feeds my soul through the ancient beliefs that are still alive in the Mexican culture today. My heart expands with the generosity of the Mexican people. Ethiopia is a new home, a small community in Aleto Wondo where we volunteer: a community where a hundred local women come each day to learn to read and write and where I collect local stories to make books for the school children. Ethiopia is a land where people still walk long distances.

For fifteen years, Arie and I have been participating in intercultural collaborations in physical theatre and movement with artists from Sulawesi (in Indonesia), Mexico, and Mongolia. We perform in nature, in sacred sites and in theatres in those countries. Our Glass Studio and the performing garden attached to our tiny Sydney home is where we recreate our intercultural performances for community evenings, to share our lives artistically and culturally. The performances in Sydney are the bridges.

My life, lived as a metaphor of stars in the day and night sky, is in flux. My life is open to life.

Metaphor

The strands of Amerta Movement have emerged at different times and in different ways in my life, not as a set pattern.

Prapto seeks to discover and offer metaphors for his students as they study and practice Amerta Movement as a way for them to understand themselves and to guide their practice. Sitting in the soft moist air of Solo, Prapto would answer questions after a practice session. Often he would say, understanding what your practice means may not be revealed for a long time, years.

The notion of metaphor always eluded me. I first entered the practice with Prapto in Amerta Movement in Solo in 1992. In 2008 Prapto came to New York City to give a workshop. It had been some years since I had last practiced with him in Java and my life had changed dramatically.

During the workshop I was seeking to understand how Amerta Movement resonated with my heritage in the city where I was born and to find a metaphor for where my life had taken me. Prapto asked me if Sydney, Australia was still my home from where I radiated out to collaborate and perform interculturally.

No, Sydney wasn't any longer my one home.

Suprapto then suggested that Sydney might be a terminus for me. But that did not resonate with my feelings either. I didn't have roots in Sydney or New York or any one place. My metaphor still hadn't emerged. Prapto then opened a question for me, one that deep in my unconscious was seeking an answer through metaphor.

Where was my home?

Now years later my metaphor of stars in the sky has emerged and reveals to me how Amerta Movement and Prapto's wisdom and brilliance continue to guide my life.

I Will Trace the Constellation of my Stars with my Fingers

...as I trace the influence of the golden thread of Amerta Movement and *kejawaan* in my life.

Kejawaan is an Indonesian term meaning 'Javaneseness' and 'Javanism' and harks back to a time when animism was the mystic belief of the Javanese people. *Kejawaan* derives from the Hindu Buddhist period of Javanese history. It shapes the cultural values, the conduct in daily life, and the ethical and spiritual values of the Javanese people. Prapto's cultural and spiritual heritage in *kejawaan* was passed down through his parents.

In *kejawaan* the creator and created are not separated. Humans are part of the whole, of the universe; and the universe lies within each human. Each of us has the possibility to find unity with nature and spirit.

The strand of Amerta Movement touched by *kejawaan* that has been a trajectory in my life is the view that life can be experienced as a continuum and is interconnected: the notion of non-duality expressed in the belief that nature/spirit/human have equal value, not separated but connected into one unifying existence.

Alice Pitty studied with Prapto over an intense year and lived in other communities in Indonesia. In her writing she maintains that

Prapto is teaching his own culture or *kejawaan* but in unique ways:

> "I believe Prapto is indeed teaching Javanese culture, but he is not teaching Javanese culture from the perspective of Java. He is teaching Javanese culture within this broader framework of placing Javanese values, philosophy and psychology within a global mapping of cultural exchange that is stimulated by the broad range of nationalities represented on his courses." (1997, 5)

This "global mapping of cultural exchange" in Amerta Movement has guided me to discover my own relationship with intercultural performance and collaboration.

Framework of Practice

Prapto's framework for Amerta Movement may be seen as a system illuminating multiple ways for making connections. In the 1990s Padepokan Lemah Putih had four physical areas for practice: the *Pendopo*, with a tiled roof and strong wooden pillars representing home; Square, an open grass area that alluded to marketplace; a red concrete octagonal shape called Mandala, for circulation; and Road, a place of intersecting paths for journeying.

At a cultural level, *Pendopo* as home could also be seen/experienced to represent the traditional Eastern village culture where people stayed and lived at home within the collective *We*. In contrast, Road could be seen/experienced to represent Western culture, where people travel and leave their homes for work and for new opportunities. This is more the culture of the individual *I*.

One of the reasons I left New York was that it was such a driven culture and city. Individualism is a characteristic of the city, and often isolates people, which was my experience.

Prapto invited us to move in each area and to choose one for our practice. I chose the Mandala set into a bowl of hills. Mandala embodied the theme of 'purification in circulation.' Circulation is a quality that connects people in a collective feeling, unifying not separating. I was seeking the flowing connection I had felt between the Javanese friends on our workshop. Mandala was a firm and safe base to explore my fear of my awkward movements and my insecurity in entering into communication with others. The shape of the red Mandala, the energy of the hills, the flowing movements of other practitioners moving in Mandala encouraged my movements to flow.

I learned a more sensitive way of connecting through the exercise of moving in 'The Passive in the Active'. The flow of movement allowed me to begin to feel when another practitioner was open to me joining in movement, rather than my habitual New York 'drive' to just enter, whatever. I learned to wait, which in my New York culture would be passive, but in Amerta Movement was actively being attentive to another.

The interconnectedness of 'circulation' in movement offered me ways of exploring how to find a dialogue with those people I didn't have much in common with, as well as discovering the areas that we did share, thus discovering a vastly richer personal and intercultural world. Here were the roots that became my life in intercultural performance.

Amerta Movement Beyond the World of Mojosongo

Through Amerta Movement, Prapto enables his students to understand that life is in constant change, flux. How do we find balance, calm when everything is always changing? Changing our sites of practice supported our ability to be in flux.

Parangtritis, a place of dunes and ocean on the Southern coast of Java where everything is constantly changing, is the home of the mythological Queen of the South Seas. It provided the ideal environment to confront the reality of flux and constant change. I gained the courage to balance in not having balance, to not know what would happen when I entered into circulation with the shifting sands, with another person, or with the group. I began to seek flux.

Seeking flux has become my life, discovering new 'homes,' new stars to form my constellation. My home is where I am.

Studying with Prapto was like emerging from a two-dimensional life into a three-dimensional being-in-my-life. I had found the nourishment that I was seeking. It was out of this aspect of Amerta Movement, this system illuminating multiple ways for making connections, that my desire to perform interculturally was born.

Intercultural Performance

When I muse about the ceiling of Grand Central Station, stars that are connected by golden threads into constellations, I feel that practicing within the "global mapping of cultural exchange" has been the inspiration for Arie and me to create our lives with 'homes' in different cultures, our *pendopo* on the road. We have created our own continuum of belonging and individuality.

In 1999 Prapto was invited by the founder and director of *Teater Kita Makassar*, Asia Ramli, to give a workshop to artists from Ujang Pandang (now Makassar) in Sulawesi. Arie and I were apprentices with Prapto in that workshop.

Pak Ram, as he was affectionately known, had with a group of young artists moved to live in Sombu Opu, a cultural and nature site on the edge of the city. They lived there for two years, practicing trance, delving into animistic rituals, exploring alternative improvised movement, as a way of creating contemporary theatre emerging from their own cultural heritage rather than from a modern Western aesthetic.

The Sulawesian artists were professional performers and Arie and I were drawn to collaborate with them. Like a comet streaking across the sky we didn't know then where we would land, but the energy unleashed towards collaborative intercultural performance was born out of that workshop. We began an intercultural performance collaboration that spanned twelve years. Arie's and my performing name became 'Between' – translated from the Indonesian word *antara*. 'Between' because we wanted to find ways of creating performance that connects cultures. My Masters of Theatre in Intercultural Performance at Wollongong University, Australia was based on our collaborations and performances.

An Intercultural Performance that Traveled from Spain to Mexico and then on to Australia and Sulawesi

A friend who I met while studying for my Masters was exploring the work of Nicolás Núñez, a director of alternative theatre from Mexico City. Núñez had studied with Grotowski and lived for a year with a Tibetan community in India. His theatre, performed at Aztec and Mayan pyramids, was often based on traditional Shakespearian and Mexican drama. Núñez was going to walk the famous Pilgrim Road in Spain, with a group of his performers, to develop a performance.

Most people know the *Camino de Santiago de Compostela* as the famous Catholic Camino. Núñez wanted to walk the *Camino del Dragon* (walk of the dragon, as the camino was known before it became the Catholic Camino). We walked in the spirit and meaning of the Mexican God Quetzalcoatl, the feathered Serpent. Quetzalcoatl was related to the gods of the wind, of the dawn, and of arts, crafts and knowledge, and the patron god of the Aztec priesthood.

The Camino along the north of Spain travels through three

distinct regions. Núñez connected each region with one of three creative states: facing our condition, finding our creative meaning, and spiritual transformation. Arie and I were invited to join. Forty days and forty nights we walked across Spain.

Each evening, I would practice movement in windswept trees, in fields, on ancient stonewalls. I would practice to arrive anew, to feel within my body and being the journey and my connection to the spirit of the *Camino del Dragon*, to nature, and to the others on the road. I would practice to have the resources in my body and being for creative work.

> "From the *kejawaan* perspective, real knowledge, is both mysterious and subjective, it is personal insight into the true nature of things that cannot be formulated objectively." (Muldar 2005)

Six months later we went to live for half a year in Mexico City to be part of the performance based on our individual and group journey on the Camino. Each member created his or her own story mainly within the tradition of psychodrama.

Arie and I created three separate performances based on the three geographical and creative directions of our journey: facing our condition, finding our creative meaning, and spiritual transformation. For us the synthesis and meaning of nature and the spiritual entwined with our experience inspired our performance.

These three individual performances were a continuum representing the whole journey. *Caseria des Estrellas* (Home of the Stars) was performed Friday, Saturday and Sunday nights in a small theatre in Coyoacán for two months.

Upon returning to Sydney we recreated the three performances into a performance called *Eye of the Dragon*, which we performed in our Glass Studio and garden. Life offered us a gift. Hamrin and Pak Ram from *Teater Kita Makassa* happened to be in Sydney collaborating with Aboriginal artists for a performance at the Sydney Opera House. Hamrin was able to play music for our three performances sitting on top of the large rock shelf, hewn from an old quarry site, bordering our garden. He offered us the feathers we moved with when, in the essence of Quetzalcoatl, we transformed into the Plumed Serpent in the third section of *Eye of the Dragon*. The continuum, the golden thread of the Camino's journey had now traveled in our performances from Spain to Mexico to Australia.

Pak Ram felt that the mythological story, the connection to nature, the completeness of our journey in performance would speak to audiences in Sulawesi and invited us to perform *Eye of the Dragon* in Sulawesi at a festival in Barru and also at the Art House in Makassar. The performance spoke to the audience in ways we could have, but didn't, predict.

The festival in Barru was in a small *pendopo* and almost 500 people were surrounding the *pendopo* on three sides. In the middle section of the performance I faced my struggle with human relationships using a ragged piece of bark, howling. Instead of the intense feeling of pain that many in the audience felt in Mexico and Australia there was surprised laughter. One of the features of *kejawaan* and Indonesian culture is finding equilibrium in emotions and not directly expressing anger, fear or any overt emotion. The laughter expressed their discomfort at these raw emotions. When I flew into Arie's arms expressing the transformation of the Dragon to a Plumed Serpent the audience cheered.

And so the journey on the *Camino del Dragon* in Spain, which became an intercultural performance in three parts in Mexico, was a performance in our Glass Studio and garden for our community in Sydney, Australia, wove its way back to Sulawesi where we had first begun our collaborations in intercultural performance.

The deep satisfaction of this artistic pilgrimage was that the "global mapping of intercultural exchange" had become a constellation in itself, the Plumed Serpent, which was shining brightly in my metaphor.

Ritual Performances

Outside the Hall of Golden Buddhas in Candi Mendut, the Buddhist monastery connected to Borobudur, is a long stone corridor. One dark night, illuminated by the brilliant reflections of lights shining from the Golden Buddhas inside the hall, we practiced movement with Prapto.

We practiced in the rain, frogs hopping everywhere. It was a time of purification through rain, frogs, and Golden Buddhas. The intense atmosphere and energy of practicing monks filled the space. My inner feeling of life through the improvised movement practice was joy, freedom and connection beyond anything I had ever known: my life was being purified.

Years later we visited Koyoasan, the Buddhist Monastic Centre established twelve centuries ago on the top of Mt. Koya in Japan. Walking beneath the looming pine trees in the ancient cemetery,

29. I WILL TRACE THE CONSTELLATION OF MY STARS WITH MY FINGERS

the wish to create a ritual performance to honor the recent death of my father came to me. I had no personal tradition or rituals in my life to guide this. Even with all the feelings and experiences of ritual through Amerta Movement and through many intercultural collaborations encompassing rituals on Sulawesi, Bali and Java, ritual was still not a daily part of my life.

Inspired by the walk in Koyoasan, on the first anniversary of my father's death in New York I gathered fifteen of my close friends at 7.30 in the morning in Sydney. On that sunny morning far away from New York and Japan, I shared my love and sadness in a ritual performance for my father.

Starting in a small park above our home I had hung ties in trees, my father's ties, ties worn over 60 years of his working life. My friends gathered and drank fresh orange juice, and I waited in a park below. Picking the ties from the trees as I had requested, they walked down the public stairs where I had chalked sentences, short sentences about my father: my father wasn't an easy guy, but he loved us dearly. They walked down the stairs to the park with an open vista to the valley below, where I sat. My friends hung my father's ties in the large spreading trees. I moved in and with the trees, and air and valley, I moved with the ties, I read a quirky, funny letter my father had once sent to me and when I was done, we all went back to my house for breakfast. I had created my own ritual performance for my father.

Many years later, my beloved mother died, also in New York. As she was dying she would take my hand and press it to her cheek. I knew immediately that I wanted to have a lunch with friends in Australia who had met my mother, sharing my mother's favorite food. That was arranged. After the funeral in New York and before returning to Sydney I had a dream. In the dream my sadness and grieving was like deep blue dye seeping into me.

The dream inspired me to create a ritual to honor my love of my mother. Returning from New York to Sydney, I had two weeks before the lunch. Ana, my dear friend Ana, who has helped us create many costumes for our performances in Sydney, helped me sew an indigo blue top and pants, and a simple, white, Japanese-style, sleeveless, wraparound coat. I ordered dark blue indigo dye and a BBQ for the fire to heat the dye. I practiced in a small flat grassy spot in our garden surrounded by a stone wall where my friends would sit.

In the performance ritual my hand touched my cheek, just as my mother had taken my hand to touch her cheek. The coat, as I took it off, became a symbol of my wish that my mother's soul would leave her body and find peace.

I plunged my hands into the dye heated in the fire and stroked my face and arms, covering myself with the dye, my grief. I moved my love.

The sun was full and warm that day, and as I shed the white coat, a gentle rain began to fall while the sun still shone. And the rain fell, like loving tears from heaven until the moment the ritual ended.

My life of intercultural performances, homes on the road, rituals for my parents, are stars that have emerged and are connected through the golden thread of Amerta Movement. I will trace the constellation of my stars with my fingers. The stars that shine in the never ending possibilities of life.

Rahayu.

Thanks to life and thanks to Prapto.

~ ~ ~

References

Lavelle, L. (2009) 'Embodying the present moment: Basic features of an Asian movement improvisation.' In Dance, Movement, Mobility, Proceedings, 9th International NOFOD Conference, October 23-26, 2008. Leena Rouhiainen (ed.), University of Tampere, pp.106-113.

Muldar, N. (2005) *Mysticism in Java – Ideology in Indonesia*, Kanisius

Pitty, A. (1997) *Questions in My Hand Luggage: Exploring The Cultural Context of Amerta Movement* (unpublished)

Stange, P (1994) 'Silences in Solonese Dance', *Southeast Asian Journal of Social Sciences*, vol.22

Ellin Krinsly entered the world of Amerta Movement with Prapto in Java in 1992. Amerta training has led to intercultural collaborations and performances in Java, Bali, Sulawesi, Mexico, Mongolia and Australia. Volunteering at a small community in southern Ethiopia with her partner, Arie van Duijn, has inspired performances in Australia and Mexico. Their most recent performance, performed in the Night Garden of the Glass Studio in Sydney, 2014, was stimulated by travels in Iran and based on a poem by Hafiz.

ellin.krinsly@gmail.com

30. AWAKENING ART AND DHARMA NATURE TIME

Participatory Approaches to Interculture in Cultural Environments

Diane Butler (USA/Indonesia)

There is such a rich ground for creative dialogue when, as Prapto has suggested, all societies can gather, share and *"interact concretely inter-culturally by various disciplines"*. In this chapter, I hope to convey some of the ways that my involvement with Sharing Movement, since its initiation in 1997, and subsequent practice of Amerta Movement with Prapto has informed my approach to interculture in cultural environments. To give a sense of why and how, I decided to begin by 're-membering' some seeds in earlier stages of my life and then describe practices that I have been developing in my 'Awakening Art' workshops and share examples of public programs of International Foundation for Dharma Nature Time.

Re-Membering my Movement, Creative and Awareness Practice Heritage

I am deeply grateful to have shared and collaborated with artists from diverse cultures and faiths in the Americas, Europe and Asia through my work as a movement artist, teacher and program director for the past 25 years.

Interestingly, in my birthplace of Ohio, when I was five years old my first class was in Dalcroze Eurhythmics, a non-stylized improvisational movement practice to awaken one's kinesthetic awareness and expressive experience of music. Then I studied classical ballet and at the age of 13 began to study classical modern dance. At 17, I moved to New York City where I trained amidst dancers and companies from various traditions and countries. I first engaged in site-specific dance events with American, Asian and European artists and local communities from 1984 to 1989 while assisting and performing with Sino-Japanese American choreographer Ruby Shang in the USA, France, Japan and UK. During that same period of time, I also began to engage in daily *shamatha-vipassana* (mindfulness-awareness) meditation, solitary and group retreats, and dharma studies and in 1986 took vows in the Mahayana Buddhist tradition.

Yet I longed to integrate my everyday life, meditation practice and prayer life, and my dance and creative life. I was also interested in how the language of art fosters a common field for people of varied cultures even when their art forms and spoken mother tongues differ. I wondered how to support creative dialogue and a sense of community among artists and with the larger society.

The Basic Orientation and some Movement-Based Practices in my Early Work

As I was teaching movement and creative process workshops at colleges and studios in the USA and Europe and leading a new InterArts Studies program in the field of contemplative education at Naropa Institute (now Naropa University) in Colorado, movement-based awareness practices and improvisation were the main vehicle.

Though I had only heard about Prapto's work in 1993 from my friend Nancy Stark Smith (after she attended the 1st Sharing Time in Köln) – in retrospect I sense that the basic orientation in my teaching and cultural exchange work from the early to mid-1990s had an affinity with Amerta Movement, such as

- fostering an experiential, contemplative, self-directed, noncompetitive learning environment

- practicing the arts by engaging the five senses (sight, hearing, smell, taste, touch), thought, and kinesthetic awareness as a process whereby body-mind synchronization can occur

- experiencing pedestrian postures, movement, and gestures as a bridge between daily life and dance/movement studies to develop presence in awareness

- utilizing improvisational structures to deepen and expand one's movement vocabulary and to cultivate sensitivity toward others and the surrounding environment in the present moment

- recognizing the interdependent relationship between varied art forms and developing an ability to be creatively responsive to, and collaborate with, others

- encouraging a sense of community.

Two societal activities also sowed seeds in my early work. One was speaking *and* moving with colleagues as we developed The Mariposa Collective, a community of artists to support the creative process and performance. The other was, at the age of 35, being invited to join a weekly multi-faith Spiritual Eldering group with religious leaders and practitioner-teachers who shared prayers, meditations, readings, and discussion *and* were also willing to try a movement improvisation practice that I shared as a means for dialogue.

My hope was that students and practitioners could experience the art of life, appreciate the diverse views and ways of others, and be willing to open to the possibilities of creativity while staying awake.

Nurturing Seeds with Prapto and Sharing Movement Colleagues

Though full-time teaching ripened me in many ways, I felt a need to dialogue with peers in other countries, to experience their approaches, and to know *if* and *how* my work resonated in other cultural environments.

So it was quite timely that my involvement with Sharing Movement began in April 1997 (its initiation year), when Prapto sent me an invitation to join the month-long international Movement Arts Teachers Society Meeting (MATS). Held at Padepokan Lemah Putih and Central Java heritage sites such as Candi Boko, Kalasan, Borobudur, the Parangtritis seacoast, Candi Ceto and Sukuh; and the Surakarta Cultural Park – some 40 practitioners of a variety of disciplines from many cultures gathered daily to, as Prapto wrote, *"dialogue in movement; finding colleague, impression–expression at the pendopo, in nature, in temples"*.

Particularly meaningful to me was the diversity of ways that people engaged in movement, creativity *and* prayer in the arts while in dialogue with others *and* the environment.

How did intercultural exchanges with Sharing Movement colleagues during the MATS in Java and other gatherings such as the 3rd Sharing Time in Dartmoor, UK and the 2nd annual Movement Arts Meeting in Amsterdam, as well as practicing Amerta Movement with Prapto in the USA, Europe, Java, and Bali, inform my practice? It 'slowly-slowly' stimulated three interrelated aspects:

- **Living prayer**: Practicing the arts as a way to bring to life an attitude of bowing, offering, and praying in a context of humans, nature, and God/the Source of Life. This is from the view that an individual or community's manner of daily life and creativity can be the living out of prayer itself.

- **The practice of dialogue**: Beginning by a dialogue with oneself in movement to explore and develop an embodied awareness of one's own cultural roots. Then, when the meeting of one's cultural background and that of a person from another culture stems from a need for understanding, there can be respect for each other in dialogue. In this way, the practice of dialogue can be a gateway opening toward interculture in cultural environments.

- **Interculture in cultural environments**: An ongoing dynamic process within a cultural group and between people of different cultures – each with their respective world views and practices – based on equality, mutual respect, sharing and cooperation that is also in connection with living nature and the unique tangible cultural elements and socio-cultural and spiritual dimensions of the environment in which it occurs.

Just as significant, I experienced the garden as an environment where *both* traditional and modern cultures can share art rooted in their traditions *and* also engage in creative dialogue. This was very vivid in 2000 when I witnessed Prapto with Hindu, Buddhist, Muslim, and Christian dancers and musicians perform a ritual forging of a gong for Pura Samuan Tiga in Bedulu, Bali and when I joined 100 rural and urban artists from Indonesian provinces, Asia, and Europe creating ritual art and installations for the Collaboration Asia-Europe in Art and Environment RONG at the Tejakula, North Bali seacoast.

I began to deeply consider how living prayer and the practice of dialogue are sources for creativity in the arts and could, as Prapto proposed, be *"placed in a garden concept"* to foster unity in diversity.

All these previous experiences then inspired me in 2001, at the age of 40, to develop my 'Awakening Art' workshops and also inspired me to co-found with Prapto an international cooperative foundation, Dharma Nature Time. Since then, I have resided in the villages of Bedulu and Tejakula, Bali and joined in the initiation of several Sharing Art programs with Prapto and colleagues from many cultures.

In other words, my experience of interculture in cultural environments while practicing Amerta Movement with Prapto and during exchanges with Sharing Movement colleagues nurtured seeds in the development of my approach in the field of movement arts and also with society.

'Awakening Art' Workshop Themes and Practice Environments

'Awakening Art' is a workshop series that I currently lead based on my prior work in Eastern and Western Europe, Northern America and Indonesia; and deepened by my practice as a Dialoguer in Amerta Movement. The name refers to awakening the creative process of art and also to art that awakens the people who offer or witness it and the surroundings. Actually, after naming it, I learned that 'art' stems from the Latin root *ars* meaning 'a way of being' and *ar*, to 'fit together or join elements' into an aesthetic form.

Movement-based awareness practices and improvisation are still my main vehicle. I can say that, from studying Amerta Movement with Prapto, my practice has more relaxing and settling, natural vitality, pausing and recognizing, surrendering, and tuning in a contextual sense. I feel at home in prayerful movement and more *"in communication with a quality of dialogue"* with my cultural roots, with others and nature.

I have initially developed four 'Awakening Art' workshop themes, which I hope can provide a participatory environment for people of all ages and backgrounds to engage in intercultural creative dialogue through the arts.

To allow the body to relax, settle and change in its place and time, I invite people to begin in a daily life posture, to rest like a living tree or in a silent atmosphere yet also be alive in the context of the environment. Then, stay or move to a new posture in accord with the place, time, and conditions. In this way, we practice being awake in every moment of movement and dwelling in *Twenty-One Moments of Stillness*.

The theme of *Tri Hita Karana in Environmental Art* is inspired by the Balinese principle of *Tri Hita Karana* (three causes of goodness and prosperity), which are a harmonious relationship between human beings and with nature and with God/the Source of Life. By placing and moving three small stones and two bamboo sticks, each person can practice an architectural sense of how their posture and movement forms space as well as how the shape of a place affects their posture and movement. After that, in small groups, we create environmental art compositions in dialogue with nature and the social and spiritual dimensions.

Embodied Movement Relief begins with daily life walking to become aware of place and space. I like to say from the 'soul' of the foot gesture can arise like the centuries-old engravings on a *candi* (temple). As our bodies transform in movement relief, gradually the presence of our gestures comes to life. In composing attuned with the surrounding environment, our physical narratives unfold as an offering, expressing awakening.

Awakening Art & Religiosity is an opportunity to practice how one's feeling of religiosity can be present in art and how art can communicate a feeling of religiosity. We explore dance, chant, prayer, music, poetic recitation, and ritual offerings as art that reflects the diversity of humankind's manner of bowing or reverence for God/the Source of Life.

Since January 2012, I have been offering three-hour 'Sharing Awakening Art' sessions on Sunday mornings at the Goa Gajah Temple garden in Bedulu Village. For me this site is enlightening, as it is associated with the seminal eleventh-century meeting of interreligious creative reconciliation between Bali Aga, Çiwaist, and Buddhist faith groups at Samuan Tiga. Some Sundays, I share 'Awakening Art' in the garden of the home where I reside in a family atmosphere. Usually, two to five people participate. These sessions are not a formal workshop; just really sharing.

People engage in living prayer and the practice of dialogue in such diverse ways. Some bow their head with hands clasped or palms open, others join the palms at the heart-center or forehead or raise the hands up or hold hands with others. Some prostrate on the ground, others sit or kneel or stand. Some walk, others dance, whirl or sway. Some recite prayer from memory, others read from a book or spontaneously compose a prayer. Some play music as a form of living prayer. Some speak, others chant or sing with or without music. Some face in a specific direction. Some light incense or candles or place a cloth or arrange flowers or food or stones or sprinkle water. Some are outwardly silent and offer inner prayer.

Sharing 'Awakening Art' as a guest teacher has raised my confidence that living prayer and creative dialogue is not only fitting in so-called recognized natural or built heritage sites; but can also be practiced in a wide range of settings. For instance, people of varied cultures dwelled in *Twenty-One Moments of Stillness* in a museum garden at Candi Borobudur; while people of varied faiths practiced it in a convention center corridor during the 2009 Parliament of the World's Religions in Melbourne; and Body-Mind Centering practitioners engaged in the same practice in a forest studio in North Carolina. Architecture students explored *Tri Hita Karana in Environmental Art* in a university foyer in Jakarta, while students in Yogyakarta improvised in an assembly room. I am glad that, like my experiences in an Amerta Movement workshop, even when the practice environments and the cultural backgrounds of the participants differ, an ambiance of kinesthetic awareness and creative dialogue still emerges.

Yet, Amerta Movement has not only informed my approach to interculture in cultural environments in 'Awakening Art' and my everyday life. Since 1997, I have also been inspired by public intercultural events offered by Padepokan Lemah Putih and Sharing Movement that provide space and time for sharing among people from *and* in different cultural environments. In truth, since 2000 my dialogue with Prapto has been more thinking about giving birth in the form of events, rather than thinking about, feeling, and cooking Amerta Movement in my movement presence and work. So, I would also like to mention a societal approach in the programs of Dharma Nature Time.

Participatory Public Programs of Dharma Nature Time

One of the most pivotal questions that Prapto posed to me was what is the contribution of sharing in the arts, religiosity, and nature for the world today and in the future? And, how can that be reconnected to education? On my fortieth birthday I knew that I wanted to create an organization to work with these ideas in practice.

Dharma Nature Time is a non-profit public charity and international cooperative foundation that Prapto and I co-founded in 2001. Its programs and the activities of cooperative members (currently 14 in South-Eastern and Eastern Asia; Europe, and Northern and Central America) aim to foster creative dialogue among people from diverse cultures and faiths and among non-formal and formal educational approaches through sharing in the arts, religiosity, and nature to support interculture in cultural environments.

Given the multicultural reality of more and more places in the world, one approach has been to develop public, participatory, practice-based art programs conceived and implemented with local communities to foster creativity, reflection and sharing among cultures. 'Sharing Art' (*Srawung* or *Pasamuan Seni*) is an intercultural space that:

- takes shape and evolves in relation to the particular places it occurs and is, in that sense, site-specific

- offers an open forum for participation that can last from a few hours to several days

- is a unique context in which local and visiting participants from varied cultures, faiths, fields, age groups, and socioeconomic spheres work together to establish themes and formats of artistic collaboration; and share perspectives and creative activities through dialogues, workshops, prayers or meditations, artworks, and ritual arts.

The cooperative efforts of Dharma Nature Time with Padepokan Lemah Putih and Sharing Movement colleagues as well as other organizations and the participation of hundreds of artists, teachers, scholars, and interreligious leaders (both tradition-bearers and contemporary practitioners) have contributed significantly to the actualization of inter-village, inter-province, international intercultural Sharing Art events in Indonesia and other countries. This has opened my 'under-standing' of a way that all societies can gather, share and *"interact concretely inter-culturally by various disciplines"*.

From an outside perspective, it is an honor that Dharma Nature Time was granted roster consultative status in 2009 by the Economic and Social Council of the United Nations, accrediting it to attend UN meetings and conferences and contribute to the work programs and goals of the UN.

What Does 'Sharing Art' as an Approach to Interculture in Cultural Environments Reveal?

There are many profound moments that I could recount. As a dancer, I can tell you about one that was particularly illuminating for me.

I remember when I attended the decennial celebration of the Museum of World Religions in Taipei with 50 interreligious leaders and scholars from around the world in 2011. I asked a European professor of religious studies if he could address the contribution by the arts to the dialogue among the world's religions. During a symposium discussion, he shared a story about two traditional drummers from adversary tribes who were invited to improvise together at a music festival. Each began with solo drumming but gradually the improvisation transformed into a lively musical duet. Hence, they engaged in more than just speaking and listening to one another. Rather, each musician was engaged in expression through sound and rhythm yet simultaneously capable of listening to *and* dialoguing with the other person's expression in sound and rhythm.

After the panel, I took a walk in a garden and remembered dancing in *Tari Sesaji Tri Yoni Saraswati* with Prapto from Solo; Gusti Koes Murtiyah and Eko Kadarsih from the Karaton Surakarta palace; Bali Hindu high priest Ida Pedanda Arimbawa and Ni Ketut Arini from Bali; Nurlia Ruddin from Makassar, South Sulawesi; and the World Peace Barong for the International Plenary of the 2009 Parliament of the World's Religions in Melbourne attended by over 6,000 participants from 80 countries. I truly experienced that movement arts involve more dimensions in terms of creative dialogue. Each of us began with solo prayer and movement, yet were simultaneously capable of perceiving and dialoguing with the other artists' expression in movement and rhythm *and* spatial sensibilities as well as the surrounding environment.

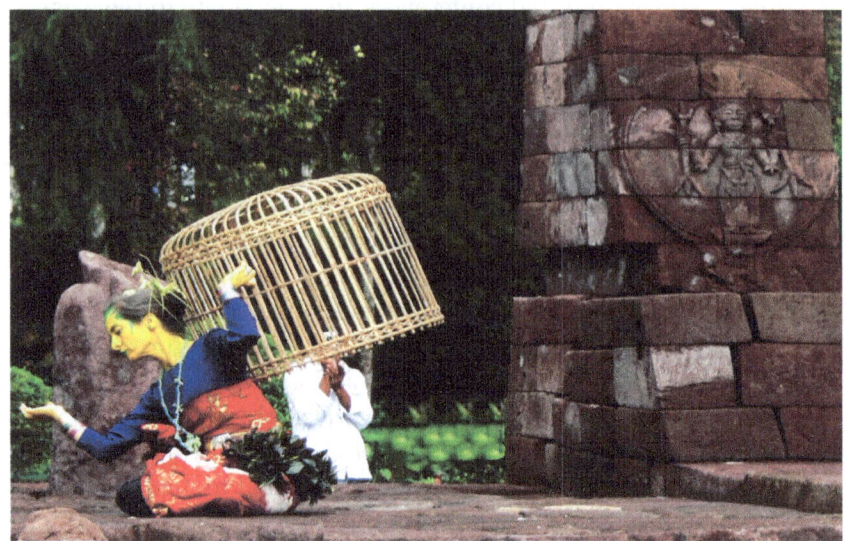

Dewi Ruci by Diane Butler, Rusini Sidi, Nurlina Syahrir, Waluyo S. Sukarno for 5th Sharing Temple Art at Candi Sukuh, Central Java. 11th January 2009. Photo: R.S. Lawu. Usually the way of inner enlightenment is Dewa Ruci (male). What is the way of Dewi Ruci (female)?

This capacity to engage in intercultural creative dialogue is something that I have witnessed in many rural and urban settings over the years such as during 'Sharing Art & Religiosity' at Samuan Tiga and 'Sharing Art Ocean-Mountain' in Tejakula, Bali; 'Sharing Art & Religiosity' in Assisi, Italy; 'Celebration Ethnic Art in Time' at Xochicalco, Mexico; 'Art Human Nature' in the Redwood Forest of California; 'Infinite Humanity: World Religions & Art for Peace and Respect of Life' opening 21 December 2001 at 12 noon in the United Nations Meditation Room, the 'World Meditation Gathering' in Solo, Java; 'Sharing Art & Religiosity: 1,000 Years Wisdom of Samuan Tiga' in Bedulu, Bali; and 'Sharing Art Garden Ocean Mountain' at Candi Borobudur. Intercultural exchanges through sharing art reveal that people can and do create both traditional and modern art offerings stemming from their cultural roots, sense of community, connection to nature, and ways of living prayer in a variety of contexts together with people of other cultures and faiths. I find even the names Prapto has given to these events stimulates sharing and speaks to the creative potential of each environment.

I believe that sharing art in these ways is a model for how to mutually foster interculture in cultural environments.

A Vision for an Institute to Support Interculture in Cultural Environments through the Arts and Culture

These are only a few of the seeds that have blossomed on a small and larger scale over the years, of which even more moved me to include reflective essays by several Sharing Movement colleagues in my doctoral dissertation on religiosity in art.

I would like to close this chapter by sharing with you a vision that Prapto put forth in 1997, which has been in my heart and thoughts since then. Truly sharing in the arts, religiosity, and nature fosters a common field such that traditional rural and modern urban cultures can study and engage in creative dialogue together. With blessings, future activities combining non-formal and formal education can serve as the basis for an ongoing curriculum to form a cooperative institute dedicated to supporting interculture in cultural environments through the arts and culture to foster unity in diversity for the benefit of infinite humanity and the Earth.

~ ~ ~

References

Butler, D. (1996) The Mariposa Collective: Pilot Project Year, MALS thesis, Wesleyan University: Connecticut.

Butler, D. & Suryodarmo, S. (2001) Articles of Incorporation of International Foundation for Dharma Nature Time, drafted May/June in Solo, Java.

Butler, D.C. (2011) *Religiosity in Art inspired by Samuan Tiga and Tejakula, Bali: Unity in Diversity*, PhD thesis, Universitas Udayana: Bali, summary online at: http://bit.ly/ELtp14

United Nations (2009) Resolutions and Decisions of the Economic and Social Council, UN Publications. Available from: http://bit.ly/ELtp15

Diane Butler is a movement artist/teacher/program director who has collaborated with artists from diverse cultures and faiths in the Americas, Europe, and Asia for 25 years and resided in Bali since 2001. She and Prapto co-founded International Foundation for Dharma Nature Time. Previously, Diane served as an Associate Professor, Founding Chair of InterArts Studies and Director of Dance/Movement Studies at Naropa University. She holds a BFA in Dance (The Juilliard School), MALS in Dance & Culture (Wesleyan University), PhD in Cultural Studies (Universitas Udayana) and is an alumna of the 2011 UNITAR Series on the Management and Conservation of World Heritage Sites.

dianecarolbutler@gmail.com

http://awakeningartworkshops.wordpress.com

AFTERWORD: A PRAPTO COMPANION

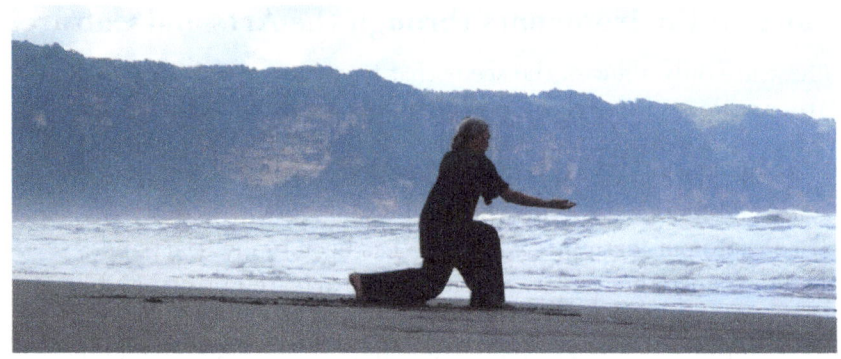

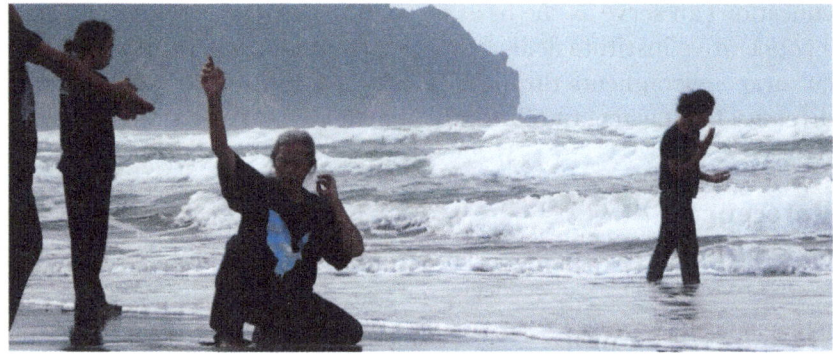

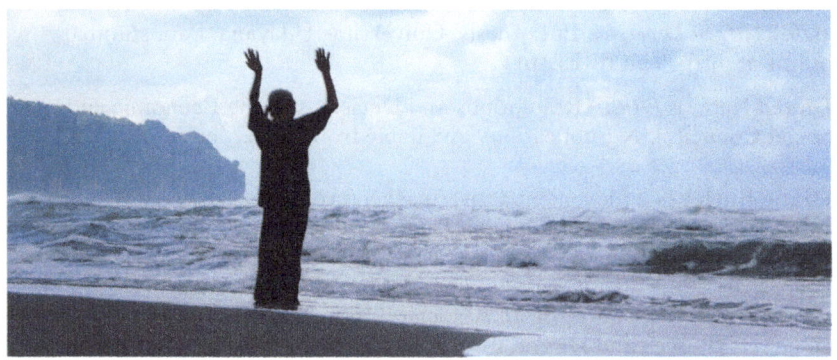

Parangtritis, Java, 2014. Photos: Karolina Nieduza

"I am in the atmosphere of story. But, at the same time, I have an awareness of the ability to create my own story. I am not just in the story of others, or of society, of my family or of the ancestors. But I am also not nullifying them. They still exist in my life story. And to hold both is not so easy."

SUPRAPTO SURYODARMO: AN INTRODUCTION

Joged Amerta is a practice developed by Suprapto Suryodarmo (Prapto), a Javanese movement artist and teacher. The following material describes some of the background to his teaching and movement workshops.[1]

The practice was developed at Padepokan Lemah Putih[2] (Prapto's interdisciplinary arts institution, located near Solo, Central Java) and also throughout the world where he has travelled and taught, in conversation with participants from many different countries.

In 1970, Prapto started *"to practise movement with the approach of exploring like a child..."* He practised *"in many conditions of time and space, in nature, temples exploring the qualities of freedom and limitation"* (Suryodarmo, 2010). He perceived the world through movement rather than from stasis, or, as he initially described it, *"from the Buddha walking, rather than from the Buddha sitting"*. Alongside Buddhist practice and observing the movement of children, his practice was influenced by studying the elements and movement in nature, the practice of Sumarah (a traditional Javanese meditation practice of 'letting go' or surrender) and, through his parents' influence, Javanese mysticism.

In his seminal performance *Wayang Buddha* (Buddha's Shadow Puppet), first performed in 1975, Prapto demonstrated his innovative combining of traditional and contemporary forms by moving as a self-articulating shadow puppet, as puppet and puppeteer in one. He embodied the central Buddhist precept that the only constant in life is change, as exemplified through movement: he was moving, the sound was moving, the light was moving, the screen was moving and the members of the audience were moving. This performance could be seen as one of the early examples of developing contemporary performance without losing the roots of Javanese traditional culture.

In 1982 Prapto travelled to Europe for the first time with the

---

[1] For a full picture of Prapto's artistic work please visit http://bit.ly/ELtp11

[2] Padepokan Lemah Putih offers a vision of contemporary art in which the natural landscape and social environment, including their historical backgrounds, are determinants in the creation of the works. It provides opportunities for local, national and international participants to exchange and share experiences through the process of creating artworks, conceptual projects and joining in workshops, performances, gatherings, festivals and other activities.

Sardono Dance Company for the Milan Siladek International Pantomime Festival in Cologne, Germany. As a result of contacts made during that trip and during a subsequent trip to Switzerland in 1983, three Westerners travelled out to Solo to work with him for two months in March 1984. They included Christina Stelzer[3] who has written a chapter in this book.

Thus began an avid exchange of movement practices, of attitudes and approaches to life, an in-depth process of meeting between East and West that lasted for over three years. Some of Prapto's Western colleagues practised Tai chi and/or had studied with Anna Halprin, amongst other somatic movement traditions. Among a variety of cultural backgrounds, the main language, passion and tool for research was movement itself. Over time each person, including Prapto, developed their own particular approach to movement in dialogue with their own traditions and by "cooking" their own particular approach as they shared experiences with their colleagues. Prapto called the emerging work Amerta Movement, meaning the 'nectar of life' movement.

More formal movement workshops in Java began in the Spring of 1986 and gradually Prapto established the course programme at the Padepokan Lemah Putih. His stated intention is *"lessening the sense of identification through the practice of movement arts"*[4] (Suryodarmo, 2010), which explicitly informs the cycle of his movement workshop programme to this day, as well as the design of his garden school and his performance work. After 28 years his practice-as-research methodology, although constantly evolving and becoming more refined through movement, is basically complete.

In 2010 the name of Prapto's work evolved and became Joged Amerta. This change was due to his feeling that his moving being had also become a dancing being *"moving dancing, dancing moving"* and he wanted the name of his work to reflect that development. *Joged* is a common word for dance in Indonesia and also carries a sense of social culture, ranging from children who dance for fun right

---

[3] They were Christian Böhringer, Susanka Christmann, and Christina Stelzer. In 1985, during a further year of intensive practice in Java, this pioneer group was joined for some months by Christine Rod and by José Mulder van de Graaf. For full details of the timeline please visit the book's webpage: **www.triarchypress.net/ embodiedlives**

[4] This is an approach coherent with a Buddhist view of no fixed sense of self, a view based in the constancy of change.

through to the dances in high society. For example, *joged* exists in the palace culture in Yogyakarta up until this day.

Today Prapto uses the term Joged Amerta for his own work. This has released the term Amerta Movement as a more generic term for the garden of work inspired and influenced by his practice.

Unlike most similar practices, Amerta was never meant to be passed down to students in the more formal, teacher-student style of pedagogical training, which he refers to as a 'pyramid approach'. Although there is a series of courses that comprises the framework of Joged Amerta, and a logical progression from one course to another, there is no formal training to become a teacher.

Instead of teachers, Prapto has created over time a list of around 90 'dialoguers' who have his permission to share practice within the tradition of Amerta Movement. Prapto encourages these dialoguers to offer practice from the attitude of 'gardener' rather than from the attitude of 'teacher'. A gardener is creative and tends to the needs of the soil and habitat as well as to each particular organism. Each plant has different requirements to grow and blossom. A gardener/teacher is trained to *"open the atmosphere first in space and time"* and then *"to see the condition, the habit of body, the character of person, like nutrition of growing"* (Suryodarmo, 2010) with the intention of supporting the growth and 'blossoming' of the mover.

So the gardener is invited to see from the mover's potential (*"like nutrition of growing"*) rather than from the mover's problems or difficulties. This is coherent with a view of no fixed sense of self, a view based in the constancy of change. In practice it demands a dynamic, creative, responsive approach and cultivates an atmosphere and an attitude of loving-kindness.

~ ~ ~

References
Suryodarmo, S. (1999) 'Web Art Garden Statement', http://bit.ly/ELtp23

Suryodarmo, S. (2010) 'Joged Amerta: Art in Joged Amerta Programme 2010-2011' http://bit.ly/ELtp11

INTERVIEWS WITH PRAPTO: SOLO, AUGUST 2013

These are extracts from public interviews with Prapto which have been transcribed and minimally edited. All the words are spoken by Prapto.

The Art of Joged Amerta

"Joged Amerta is a practice that arises from the view of art.

Creation is never-ending and has the quality of blossoming in the garden. I put myself in creation itself as evolution, rather than creativity being one part of evolution.

How can I be an involved witness, how can I bring together the qualities of actor and audience within my breathing Being-in-Creation?

In fact, through being born we are already connected with the creation of the life, we are already in the pool of life, but we find it difficult to recognise what we have, to recognise our own unique potential.

In our need 'to get', we forget ourselves. How can we understand and create from what we have already, how can we find our point of growing from what we have already? How can we grow our sense of embodied but not remain 'flat' even when we are embodied?

As a way of approaching being embodied, I like the idea of our movement itself as a 'costume' or as our clothing. Clothing includes the sense of beauty, design, choice, filtering and an individual's signature in the signs of nature. We are all just part of an environment.

Many ideas in writing, in painting, or even in the movies give us the sense of flat. Sometimes I see everything from the awareness of flat, be it in the Reality world or the Dream world. Even the Tree of Life can be flat – in the perception of our understanding, it is flat. We cannot really feel it as alive.

Sometimes movement is flat – it has no nuance, no sensing, no impulse and our receiving of the world and of the other remains flat. How can we wake up our recognition in the pool of life, wake up our understanding, our awareness and our sensorimotor life so that we can feel 'not flat'?

Awareness itself is not flat. It can be likened to a piece of fabric that is not taut. If it is taut, it cannot breathe. It loses its 'living' nature. It loses sensitivity, and that is 'flat'.

How can we find a position or a place where we can have safety but where we are still able to feel present within the moment-to-moment creation? How can we be alive in the changing and still riding the changing without losing ourselves?

My whole approach in Joged Amerta is one of relax, of the Being Breathing, and of giving time and space for blossoming.

I am only one part of the circulation. I see it as my duty in Joged Amerta, as a gardener, to wake up the potential of each person – all that they have – so that they can find their own Being-in-Creation. But maybe, in fact, Time or the Garden or the Ancestors will speak to them – not only me. I can learn from what they all speak.

Through resonance we can wake up the potential of each person. The resonance is different for each person and for each culture and comes from what we each already have as an offering for humanity. We need to practice tuning with each other and with the situation, like instruments in an orchestra; same tuning but also different.

The unknown is shared but each person's description of the unknown is different and each person's way/stay/process to finding the unknown is different – it depends on their particular sensibility.

This really needs to be understood by all, otherwise the reaction is 'I've got it! – what Prapto says is like this' and the practice becomes a monolith.

In fact, Joged Amerta is not like that, it is not for that. It is for the freedom of how to grow but can still have sharing. Sharing for me is the holy itself. Communication is the holy itself because it is like the growing for freedom. If we can have more diverse expressions or languages to speak with and to listen from, that is beautiful.

Joged Amerta exists for each person to find through movement their own Being-in-Creation in the pool of life and sharing what they have, like sharing garden movement.

Oh ah hum rahayu."

(Transcribed and adapted from two public interviews with Prapto by Sandra Reeve, Solo 2013.)

AFTERWORD: A PRAPTO COMPANION

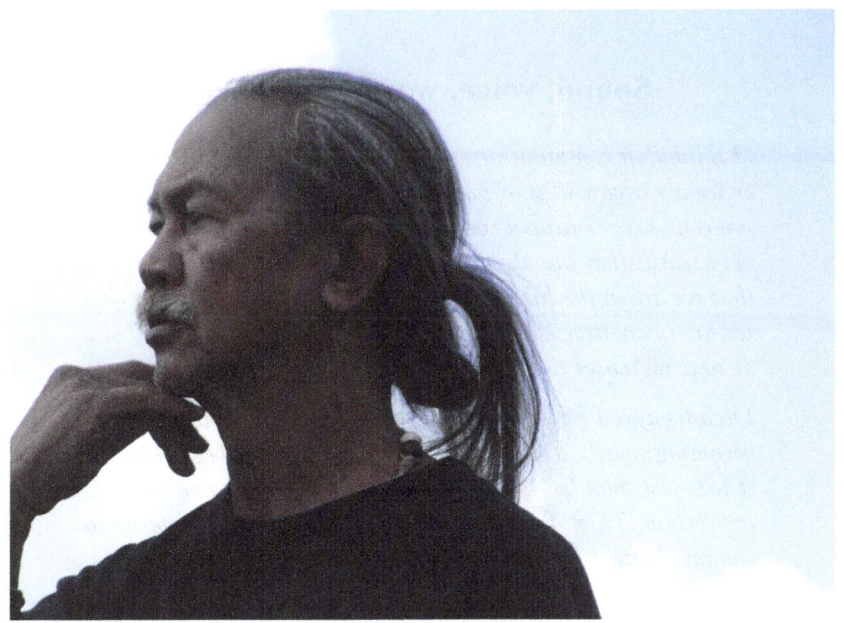

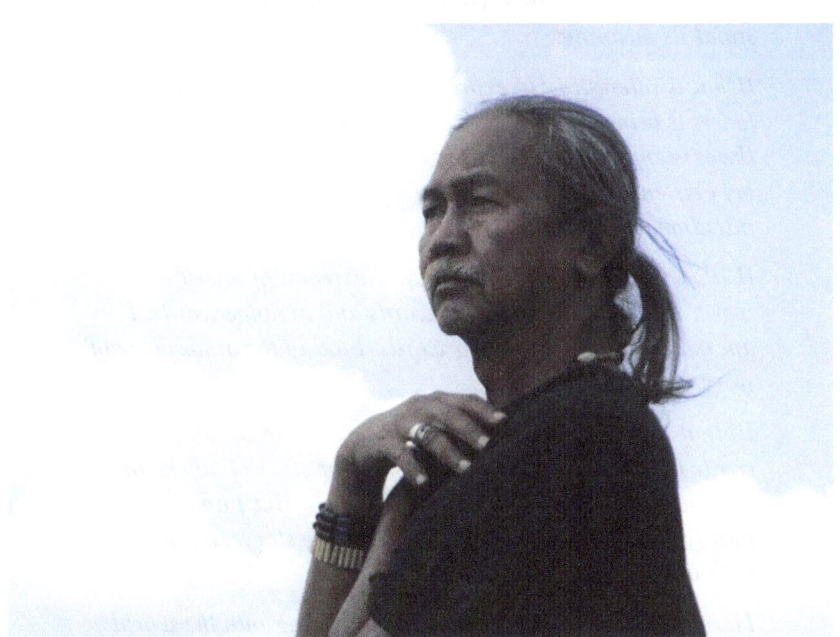

Avebury, UK, 2009. Photos: Keith Miller

"A world without words is still in communication, but there are no words."

INTERVIEW WITH PRAPTO

Sound, voice, words, sentences

"I think that communication already exists in this life, whether we are aware of it or not. Actually, it is a bit strange when someone says, 'I cannot communicate' even though by those very words they are already communicating. I prefer to feel that we are in the life of the world of communication and that we are in creative evolution to create new ways, new symbols, or new sentences within that world of communication.

Decades ago, I tried to explore sound becoming voice, becoming words, and becoming sentences. In the beginning, it was just sounds. As time passed, the sounds became an expression. Then, from that expression, I really felt a desire to communicate, to convey something, to create words.

From there, a word was born though I could not understand its meaning. But also a word was born that I could understand its meaning.

What is interesting in expressing sound, voice, words, sentences is being able to bring a word into presence as a fact of the existence of the word. This word feels as if it is a form in my existence, in the existence of my body, mind, heart, intention, and seed.

Within that process there was an awareness of myself as a word; my presence can create words and arrange words. I am in an evolution creating words. I am in the atmosphere of story.

But, at the same time, I have an awareness of the ability to create my own story. I am not just in the story of others, or of society, of my family or of the ancestors. But I am also not nullifying them. They still exist in my life story. And to hold both is not so easy.

Here lies the existence of a polemic: entering into the world without words and into the world with words. A world without words is still in communication, but there are no words.

An example of the world without words is the main stupa at the temple of Borobudur which has neither bas-relief sculptures, nor a statue of the Buddha. It is empty. But, we can see that the stupa has given birth to many books from the world with words – from storybooks to holy books.

I really like the story about Siddhartha in the Lotus Sutra, when he pointed to a lotus with the movement of his hand and in that same moment the lotus blossomed. Simultaneously a monk understood and recognised Nirvana.

I interpret that happening as the Unity of the World of Nature Reality and the World of Symbol (or words), which is able to communicate embodied understanding.

The blossoming of a lotus also gives meaning to beauty in life – enlightenment. Both the blossoming of a flower and the awareness of being in the bud free up the illusion of a boundary between the inner world and the outer world, between space inside and space outside.

I put this as a symbol of the idea of my awareness being in relaxed, empty axis, in empty space within the life story that comes into existence by designing signature in sign nature.

This is the basis of Joged Amerta, combining the World of Nature Reality and the World of Symbol, the Reality world and the Dream world in human movement, nature movement, space and time.

Oh ah hum rahayu."

(Interview material recorded and translated by Diane Butler, Bali 2014)

Embodied Lives

PRAPTO'S ARRANGEMENT OF THE JAVANESE ALPHABET

Being able to bring a word to presence as a fact of the existence of the word

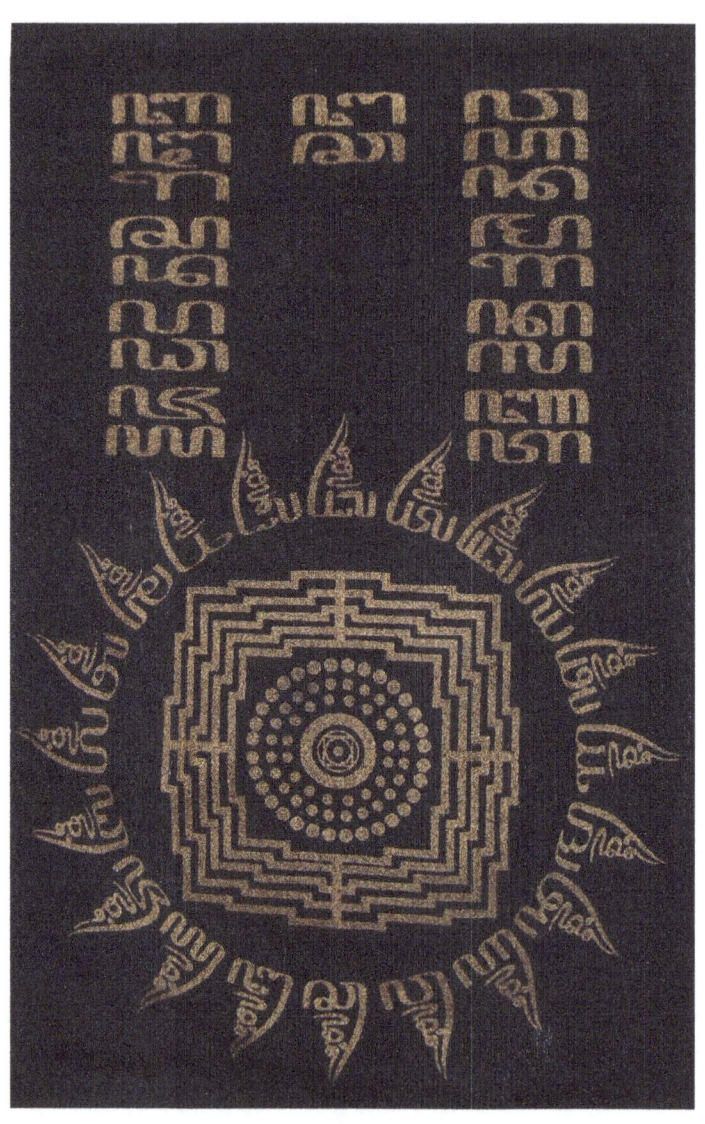

AFTERWORD: A PRAPTO COMPANION

In 1991, at the Taman Budaya Jawa Tengah (Central Java Cultural Park) in Solo, Prapto made a new arrangement of the aksara Jawa (Javanese alphabet). The old arrangement of the alphabet had been as follows:

> Ha Na Ca Ra Ka Da Ta Sa Wa La
> Pa Dha Ja Ya Nya Ma Ga Ba Tha Nga

These carakan consonants, when run together in a certain way, create the following saying:

> **Hana Caraka, Data Sawala, Pada Jayanya, Maga Baṭanga**

This means:

> **There were two messengers in conflict due to each one's faith in the word of their leader.**
> **Both messengers were equally *sakti* (powerful) and that conflict became their death way together.**

Prapto's new arrangement was:

> Ba Tha Ra Sa Da Pa Dha Ja Ya
> Nga Ca Wa Ha Na Ma Ga Ka La Nya Ta

This in turn created the following saying:

> **Bathara Sada Padha Jaya**
> **Ngaca Wahana Maga Kala Nyata**

This means:

> **Humankind by bowing and meditating towards the God that is the Great Unity has an attitude of life *sama-sama jaya* (win-win) by mirroring the space, way, time reality.**

Thus, by bringing these new words into presence as an alternative fact of the existence of the alphabet, Prapto was able to bring into being a harmonious poem reflecting the current Javanese cultural values of Unity in Diversity.

INDEX

A

Archaeology 19–28, 58
Authentic Movement 214–220
Autism 201–210

B

Blossoming 2, 3, 17, 53–54, 76, 81, 129, 175–184, 203, 280–282
  Blossoming in Europe 168, 174
Body-Mind Centering 218, 220, 301
Borobudur 39, 67–74, 212, 292, 297, 301, 304
Buddhism 24, 37–44, 57, 72, 167, 213, 226, 250, 251, 253, 287, 292, 296, 300

C

Candi Sukuh 37–44, 304
Chi kung (Qigong) 110, 130, 136, 283
Children 76, 97, 154, 175–184, 195–200, 201–210
Choreography 106, 124, 128, 183, 187, 296
Circle, Oval, Square 26–27, 94, 109, 170, 243–244, 246
Constellation 68, 69, 70, 103, 107, 108, 112, 283, 285–294
Costume 113–126
Crystallization 27, 41, 83, 127–136, 168, 174

D

Dreaming 19
  Dreamworld/Realityworld 113, 119, 121–123, 167
  Social Dreaming 165–174

E

Empty Axis 46–47, 51
Environment 3, 10, 12–13, 20–28, 30–31, 69–74, 90, 92, 104, 114, 116, 120–126, 131–136, 145–146, 150, 158, 165, 166, 168, 181, 195, 205–210, 213–216, 217, 221, 227–230, 245, 247–248, 280, 297, 298

F

Family 70, 97, 175–184, 204, 209
Feldenkrais Method 1, 106, 107, 112, 146, 183, 195, 199
Filmmaking 45–56
Free Association 8, 139

G

Guiding 17, 35, 62, 72–74, 87, 90–96, 134, 195, 197, 198, 215, 222, 225, 229, 237, 251, 271, 272, 273

H

Halprin, Anna 16, 17, 35, 146, 221–230

I

Improvisation 10, 68, 69, 105, 113, 122, 128–136, 160, 161, 173, 212, 213, 263, 277, 282, 283, 290–294, 295–306
Infants 143, 185–194, 205
Intercultural 199, 285–294, 295–306
Inter-independence 109, 110, 159

INDEX

K

Ki 88
Kung fu (Gong fu) 130, 136

L

Law 241–248, 271
Limbic system 16, 98, 258–260, 262
Living measurement 23–24, 25, 189, 248

M

Mantra 147–156
Meditation 1, 2, 12, 15, 24, 38, 42, 43, 45–46, 49–50, 63, 69, 91, 100, 153, 170, 229, 242, 244, 250–252, 283, 297
   Mindfulness 10, 24, 28, 54, 70, 87–88, 88–90, 98, 100, 132
   Vipassana 2, 91, 92, 100, 213, 296
Memory 20–23, 90, 93–94, 158–159, 190, 277, 285
Metaphor 3, 113, 118–122, 242, 285–287, 292
Movement therapy 137–146, 185, 192–193, 226
Mudra 67–74, 188
Music 42, 53, 74, 157–164, 173, 208–209, 215, 238–240, 300, 303

O

Organism, Organisation 13, 71, 137–146, 186, 189–191, 205–207, 251, 258

P

Parangtritis 14, 289, 297
Pendopo 33, 34, 39, 119–120, 288, 289, 292, 297
Performance 14, 28, 31, 52, 75, 103, 106, 109, 111, 113–126, 127–136, 149, 155, 160, 225, 226, 243, 261, 280, 285–294
Permeability 107–108, 159, 231–240
Photography 46–49, 260
Presence 9–18, 34, 73, 89, 103–112, 159, 160, 161, 168, 211–215, 226, 231–240, 251, 271, 317

R

Reading 4, 20, 23, 57, 58, 68–73, 152, 236–239, 251
Receiving 2, 10, 14, 24, 30, 34, 39, 41, 60, 63, 68–72, 82, 130, 160, 176–178, 181, 185, 191, 193, 225, 232, 235, 247, 252
Ritual 3, 26, 28, 58, 70, 119, 134, 153, 155, 193, 197, 211, 225, 234, 243, 285, 290, 292–294, 298

S

Samadhi/Semadi 98–102
Seiki 87–96
Sharing Movement 3, 17, 248, 295–306
Sharing Time 154, 225, 296, 298
Shiatsu 44, 74, 87–96, 165, 174, 210, 240
Singing 39, 43, 74, 157–164, 190–191, 208, 238–240
Somatic Experiencing 15–18, 85
Song circle 159–160
Sound 10, 32, 42–44, 52, 83, 89, 94, 149–156, 157–164, 165–174, 176, 187–191, 206, 208–209, 237–240, 303

INDEX

Sumarah 2, 12, 17, 35, 92, 127, 134, 136, 199, 222, 225, 226, 229, 240

T

Tai chi (Taiji) 1, 35, 57, 130, 136
Theatre/Theater 70, 77, 125, 129, 134, 183, 221, 225, 231–240, 286, 290–291

ABOUT THE PUBLISHER

Triarchy Press is an independent publisher of new alternative thinking (altThink) about organisations and society – and practical ways to apply that thinking.

Of course, thinking isn't the most obvious place to start talking about Prapto's work and its influence in the world. And alternative movement isn't helpful. It suggests there's a conventional way of moving that Prapto somehow defies – which is not the case. Perhaps we could best draw from his work the idea of altGardening – the sense that we, as publishers, are trying to prick out, pot on, thin, mulch and stake the best ideas that come our way: giving authors a chance to breathe freely and make a tendrilous stretch. In which case, here are some other titles in the Triarchy Press garden:

A forthcoming book from Lise Lavelle (one of the contributors to this collection) describes Prapto's programme in the 1980s and 1990s – and the ideas and approaches that underpinned it. *Attending to Movement: Somatic Perspectives on Living in this World* (also due out in 2014) explores a number of the movement themes raised here in *Embodied Lives*. Sandra Reeve (co-editor and contributor here) has also written *Nine Ways of Seeing a Body* – which tracks different conceptions of the body within western thinking, right up to the latest notions of the 'ecological body'. She is also the editor of a revealing collection of essays on *Body and Performance*.

In nearby garden beds, Phil Smith's books *Mythogeography* and *On Walking* take on the psychogeographers and W.G. (Max) Sebald and offer some exhilarating alternatives. His two books on Counter-Tourism will also make it hard for you to visit a tourist attraction in the same way ever again.

Restoring practical hope and inspiring wise initiative are two of the intentions of International Futures Forum – one of Triarchy's Publishing Partners. IFF's books on designing resilience, transformative innovation in education, Three Horizons thinking and *Ten Things to Do in a Conceptual Emergency* have all been published by Triarchy Press.

In a similar vein, Jean Russell talks about the deadening effect of 'breakdown thinking' and the world of possibility opened up by 'breakthrough thinking' in her captivating book on *Thrivability*.

Details of all these titles (as well as Thought Papers and Idioticon entries) can be found at:

Triarchy Press
www.triarchypress.net

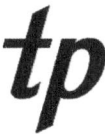

Lightning Source UK Ltd.
Milton Keynes UK
UKOW06f0341270515

252292UK00012BB/135/P

9 781909 470323